Radical Prostatectomy

James A. Eastham • Edward M. Schaeffer

Editors

Radical Prostatectomy

Surgical Perspectives

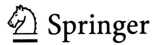 Springer

Editors
James A. Eastham, M.D.
Sidney Kimmel Center for Prostate
    and Urologic Cancers
Memorial Sloan-Kettering
    Cancer Center
New York, NY, USA

Edward M. Schaeffer, M.D., Ph.D.
Brady Urological Institute
Johns Hopkins Medical Institution
Baltimore, MD, USA

ISBN 978-1-4614-8692-3   ISBN 978-1-4614-8693-0 (eBook)
DOI 10.1007/978-1-4614-8693-0
Springer New York Heidelberg Dordrecht London

Library of Congress Control Number: 2013953259

Printed on acid-free paper

Springer is part of Springer Science+Business Media (www.springer.com)

Preface

Radical prostatectomy is among the most complex operations performed by urologists and optimal results are sensitive to fine details in surgical technique. Outcomes research has repeatedly documented how markedly the results and complications of this operation vary among surgeons. The elusive goals of radical prostatectomy are to remove the cancer completely with negative surgical margins, minimal blood loss, no serious perioperative complications and complete recovery of continence and potency. No surgeon achieves such results uniformly.

The purpose of this textbook is to provide surgeons with a comprehensive overview about an anatomical approach to radical prostatectomy, whether done through an open (retropubic) or robotic-assisted laparoscopic approach. The focus is on the procedure itself, not a summary of outcomes or a comparison between various techniques. The book is structured to provide a step-by-step approach to the appropriate performance of what many consider to be the most technically demanding surgery performed by urologists. We are optimistic that this text will serve as the definitive surgical reference for what is the most common oncologic procedure in urology.

Contents

Contributors

Mohamad E. Allaf, M.D. Urology and Oncology, Minimally Invasive and Robotic Surgery, Brady Urological Institute, Johns Hopkins Hospital, Baltimore, MD, USA

Trinity J. Bivalacqua, M.D., Ph.D. Urology Department, Johns Hopkins Hospital, Baltimore, MD, USA

Arthur L. Burnett, M.D., M.B.A. Urology Department, Johns Hopkins Hospital, Baltimore, MD, USA

Stacey C. Carter, M.D. Urology Department, UCLA Medical Center, Los Angeles, CA, USA

Michael S. Cookson, M.D., M.M.H.C. Department of Urologic Surgery, Vanderbilt University Medical Center, Nashville, TN, USA

Anthony Costello, M.D., F.R.A.C.S., F.R.C.S.I. (hon), M.B.B.S. Department of Urology, The Royal Melbourne Hospital, Richmond, Victoria, Australia

Anahita Dabo-Trubelja, M.D. Anesthesiology and Critical Care, Memorial Sloan Kettering Cancer Center, Weil Cornell Medical College, New York, NY, USA

James A. Eastham, M.D. Sidney Kimmel Center for Prostate and Urologic Cancers, Memorial Sloan-Ketttering Cancer Center, New York, NY, USA

Jim C. Hu, M.D., M.P.H. Director and Henry E. Singleton Chair of Robotic and Minimally Invasive Surgery, Associate Professor Department of Urology, David Geffen School of Medicine at UCLA, Los Angeles, CA, USA

Elias S. Hyams, M.D. Section of Urology, Dartmouth-Hitchcock Medical Center, Lebanon, NH, USA

Gautam Jayram, M.D. Brady Urological Institute, Johns Hopkins Medical Institution, Baltimore, MD, USA

Samuel D. Kaffenberger, M.D. Department of Urologic Surgery, Vanderbilt University Medical Center, Nashville, TN, USA

Eric R. Kelhoffer, M.D. Anesthesiology and Critical Care, Memorial Sloan Kettering Cancer Center, Weil Cornell Medical College, New York, NY, USA

Vincent P. Laudone, M.D. Sidney Kimmel Center for Prostate and Urologic Cancers, Memorial Sloan-Kettering Cancer Center, New York, NY, USA

Aaron A. Laviana Director and Henry E. Singleton Chair of Robotic and Minimally Invasive Surgery, Associate Professor Department of Urology, David Geffen School of Medicine at UCLA, Los Angeles, CA, USA

Christian P. Pavlovich, M.D. Brady Urological Institute, Johns Hopkins Bayview Medical Center, Johns Hopkins University School of Medicine, Baltimore, MD, USA

Stephen A. Poon, M.D. Southern California Permanente Medical Group, Fontana, CA, USA

Adam C. Reese, M.D. Brady Urological Institute, Johns Hopkins University School of Medicine, Baltimore, MD, USA

Jaspreet S. Sandhu, M.D. Department of Surgery, Urology Service, Memorial Sloan-Kettering Cancer Center, New York, NY, USA

Peter T. Scardino, M.D. Department of Surgery, Urology Service, Memorial Sloan-Kettering Cancer Center, New York, NY, USA

Edward M. Schaeffer, M.D., Ph.D. Brady Urological Institute, Johns Hopkins Medical Institution, Baltimore, MD, USA

Robert L. Segal, M.D., F.R.C.S. (C) Urology Department, Johns Hopkins Hospital, Baltimore, MD, USA

Jonathan L. Silberstein, M.D. Urology Service, Department of Surgery, Memorial Sloan-Kettering Cancer Center, New York, NY, USA

Joseph A. Smith, M.D. Department of Urologic Surgery, Vanderbilt University Medical Center, Nashville, TN, USA

Lincoln Tan, M.B.B.S., M.R.C.S. (Edin), M.med (Surgery), F.R.C.S. (Urol) (RCPSG), F.A.M.S. (Urol) Urology Unit, Royal Melbourne Hospital, Melbourne, Victoria, Australia

Lincoln Tan and Anthony Costello

Abbreviations

IHP	Inferior hypogastric plexus
NVB	Neurovascular bundle
H & E	Haematoxylin and eosin
nNOS	Neuronal nitric oxide synthase
CN	Cavernosal nerves
RP	Radical prostatectomy
EPF	Endopelvic fascia
ATFP	Arcus tendineus fascia pelvis
PPF	Periprostatic fascia
PF	Prostatic fascia
LAF	Levator ani fascia
DF	Denonvilliers' fascia
pPF	Posterior prostatic fascia
SVF	Seminal vesicles fascia
APA	Accessory pudendal arteries
DVC	Dorsal vascular complex
BPH	Benign prostatic hyperplasia
EUS	External urethral sphincter
IUS	Inner urethral sphincter

L. Tan, M.B.B.S., M.R.C.S. (Edin), M.med.
(Surgery), F.R.C.S. (Urol) (RCPSG), F.A.M.S. (Urol)
Urology Unit, Royal Melbourne Hospital,
Melbourne, VIC, Australia

A. Costello, M.D., F.R.A.C.S., F.R.C.S.I. (hon),
M.B.B.S. (✉)
Department of Urology, Level 3 Centre,
The Royal Melbourne Hospital, Infill Building,
City Campus, Grattan Street, Parkville, Richmond,
VIC 3050, Australia
e-mail: cosurol@bigpond.net.au

Surgical Neuroanatomy of the Male Pelvis

Sympathetic

The sympathetic innervation is responsible for the secretory functions of the prostate and seminal vesicles as well as ejaculation (contraction of the vas deferens and synchronous activation of the internal smooth muscle urethral sphincter). Sympathetic innervation of the lower urogenital tract arises from thoracolumbar segments T10–12 and L1–2 [1].

Sympathetic preganglionic nerve fibres leave the spinal column, and instead of synapsing in the sympathetic chain ganglia, they pass through the ganglia and travel medially to form the aortic plexus. The nerves continue downward as the superior hypogastric plexus (sometimes called the presacral nerve) which divides into right and left inferior hypogastric nerves (also known as presacral plexus). These fibres then mingle with pelvic splanchnic nerves (parasympathetics and accompanying sensory nerves) to form the inferior hypogastric plexus (IHP), also known as the pelvic plexus, after which postganglionic fibres terminate at blood vessel, prostate, seminal vesicles and the urethra [2].

J.A. Eastham and E.M. Schaeffer (eds.), *Radical Prostatectomy: Surgical Perspectives*,
DOI 10.1007/978-1-4614-8693-0_1, © Springer Science+Business Media New York 2014

Parasympathetic

The sacral parasympathetic system originates from spinal segments S2–4. Sacral fibres emerge shortly after exit from the sacral foramina as pelvic splanchnic nerves, which follows the rectum and the dorsolateral boundaries of the prostate [3].

The pelvic plexus acts as a relay station for sympathetic and parasympathetic fibres. The detailed anatomy of the pelvic plexus and the neurovascular bundle (NVB) that leaves it will be discussed in greater detail in a subsequent section.

This mesh of parasympathetic and sympathetic fibres caudally amongst other nerves forms the cavernosal nerves (CN) of the penis, which innervate the cavernosal tissue. Together with the deep artery and vein of the penis, the cavernosal nerves of the penis enter the crura after exiting from the muscular pelvis. Penile erection arises from parasympathetic dilatation of the smooth muscles lining the cavernosal sinuses with resultant influx of blood.

Somatic

Pudendal Nerve

The pudendal nerve is composed of ventral rami of spinal segments S2–4, which together with accompanying parasympathetic and sympathetic fibres form the pudendal plexus.

After leaving the pudendal plexus, it passes around the ischial spine and reenters the pelvic cavity through the lesser sciatic foramen. It then courses under the levator ani muscle on top of the obturator internus muscle. Along its course in the ischiorectal fossa, the nerve gives off small inferior rectal branches and one or two perineal branches [4]. After leaving Alcock's canal, the nerve divides into its terminal branches—the perineal nerves and dorsal nerve of the penis [5] (Fig. 1.1).

Superficial branches supply the skin of the perineum and posterior scrotum. The rectal nerves innervate the external anal sphincter. The dorsal nerve of the penis penetrates the suspensory ligament of the penis and supplies the penile shaft skin and glans penis and striated urethral sphincter [6, 7].

The deep branches of the perineal nerves give motor supply to the striated urethral sphincter, ischiocavernosal muscles and bulbospongiosus muscle [8, 9]. Contraction of the ischiocavernosus muscles produces the rigid–erection phase. Rhythmic contraction of the bulbocavernosus muscle is necessary for ejaculation.

Takenaka found that the distance from the lowest point of the endopelvic fascia to the point where the sphincteric branch of the pudendal nerve entered the urethral rhabosphincter was a mean of 5.5 mm (range 3–8 mm) [10]. Narayan similarly found branches from the dorsal penile nerve innervating the rhabdosphincter were in close proximity (3–13 mm) to the prostatic apex. Thus these branches can potentially be injured during the apical dissection of the prostate [7]. Direct injury to the branch of the pudendal nerve as it extends into the dorsal penile nerve has been reported with the perineal approach [11] (Fig. 1.2).

It is generally accepted that the pudendal nerve has purely somatic function and that the cavernous nerve only regulates autonomic function. Consistent with their functions, the pudendal nerve is located inferior to the pelvic diaphragm in the ischio-anal fossa and the pelvic plexus lies superior to the pelvic diaphragm. Cadaveric studies and more recently computer-assisted dissections of foetal cadavers have shown that the pelvic structures responsible for sphincter continence and sexual function receive dual innervation from the autonomic supralevator (cavernous nerve) and the somatic infralevator pathways (dorsal penile nerve) with communicating branches between them [3, 12–14]. This suggests possible plasticity in the supply of nerves for penile erection.

The Pelvic Plexus and Neurovascular Bundle (NVB)

Sympathetic fibres of the superior hypogastric plexus, the sacral sympathetic chain ganglia and parasympathetic fibres of the pelvic splanchnic nerves, as well as somatic afferents, feed into the pelvic plexus. This is the main coordinating centre for pelvic autonomic innervation.

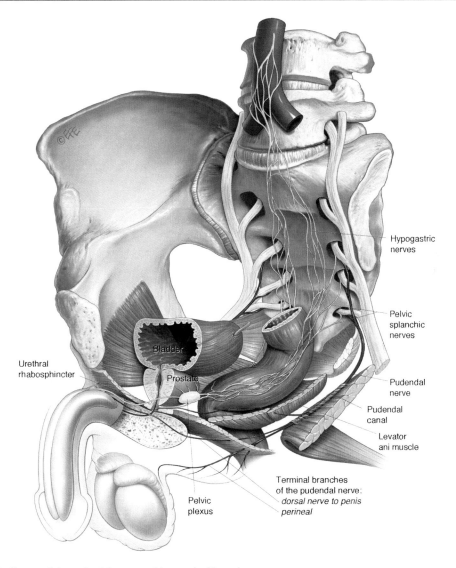

Fig. 1.1 Course of the pudendal nerve and its terminal branches

In 2004, our team at the Royal Melbourne Hospital performed a series of detailed anatomical studies on 12 adult cadavers [15]. Four of the 12 cadaver specimens were hemisected. The fascial sheaths overlying the sacral nerve trunks were excised. The parasympathetic pelvic splanchnic nerves were identified branching from the anterior sacral nerve trunks S2–S4 and dissected as they descended anteriorly to pass beneath the lateral border of the rectum. The rectum was transected at the level of S1–S2 and its anterior surface reflected from the posterior aspect of the prostate.

Extreme care was taken when freeing the anterior surface of the rectum from the prostate, as dispersed throughout the separating fascial layers (collectively known as Denonvilliers' fascia) and adipose tissue laid the neurovascular tissue under investigation. Both layers of Denonvilliers' fascia (prostatic and rectal) were left on the posterior surface of prostate to ensure an adequate safety margin for preserving neurovascular tissue. The mobilized rectum was displaced posteriorly, revealing the underlying pelvic splanchnic nerves entering the pelvic plexus.

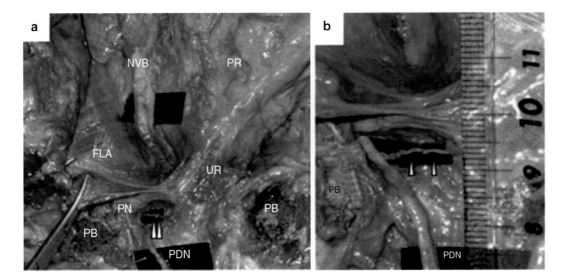

Fig. 1.2 Relationship between the fascia levator ani (FLA) and the sphincteric branch from the pudendal nerve (in the *right* pelvis). (**a**) Dissection around the membranous urethra in the fresh cadaver. A small branch from the pudendal nerve entered the rhabdosphincter, representing the sphincteric branch; (**b**) Close-up photograph of the sphincter branch in panel (**a**). The distance from the lowest point of the fascia levator ani (FLA) to the entry point into rhabdosphincter was 7 mm. *PDN* penile dorsal nerve, *PN* pudendal nerve, *PB* pubic bone, *UR* urethra, *PR* prostate, *NVB* neurovascular bundle; arrowhead, sphincteric branch from the pudendal nerve. Reprinted from Takenaka A et al. A novel technique for approaching the endopelvic fascia in retropubic radical prostatectomy, based on an anatomical study of fixed and fresh cadavers. BJUI (2005); 95(6):766–71, with permission from John Wiley and Sons

In the remaining eight cadaver specimens, the dissection sequence was altered with an en bloc pelvic resection adopted. Pelvic blocks were excised from the remaining eight cadaveric specimens. Both lower limbs were amputated at the upper extremity of the thigh and the abdomen transected 1 cm above the iliac crest (with previous removal of lower abdominal viscera). The lateral and posterior aspects were sectioned exposing the levator ani musculature and the posterior wall of the rectum. Remnants of the bony pelvis and perirectal adipose tissue were removed, clearly exposing the lateral surface of the levator ani musculature and the posterior and lateral walls of the rectum, respectively. The rectum was reflected and displaced posteriorly, exposing Denonvilliers' fascia with an investing layer of perirectal fat. When reflecting the rectum, care was taken to preserve its neurovascular supply. The perirectal fat was excised and Denonvilliers' fascia carefully dissected, with the anatomy of Denonvilliers' fascia and its relationship to the interposed and underlying neurovascular tissue

noted. Loose connective tissue and adipose tissue surrounding the prostate, seminal vesicles and bladder was removed, rendering them clearly visible. This dissection sequence enables the pelvic plexus to be dissected in full, and exposed the additional branches innervating the bladder, seminal vesicles, anterolateral prostate and levator ani musculature. Although innervation to these structures was noted, the focus was directed on documenting the nerve branches descending within the NVB. The levator ani musculature was excised to varying extents, and the lateral pelvic fascia resected to gain greater exposure of the NVB and anterolateral surface of the prostate. The prostatic apex, external urethral sphincter, perineal membrane and membranous urethra were exposed. The cavernosal nerves were traced to the corpora cavernosa.

With both methods of dissection, the pelvic plexus and NVB were meticulously dissected under magnification (×6) with the interposed adipose tissue and fascial layers carefully removed. The relationship of the NVB to surrounding

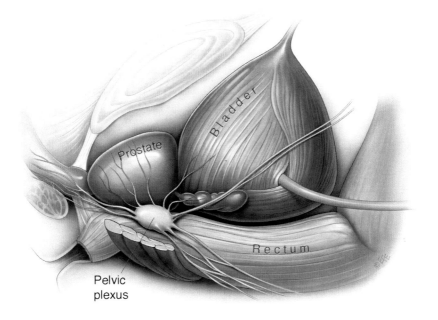

Fig. 1.3 Illustration of the *left* pelvic plexus and its relations

structures and the target organs of its constituents was documented.

The fenestrated pelvic plexus is a retroperitoneal, rhomboid shaped collection of ganglia with a longitudinal diameter of 3–5.5 cm. It is situated on the lateral surface of the rectum—separated by the pararectal fascia and 1–2 cm of perirectal adipose tissue. It extends as far as 1.5 cm posterior to the dorsal edge of the rectum and 1 cm superior to the rectovesical pouch (Fig. 1.3).

We found that there is a quantitative relationship between the size and mass of neural tissue within the pelvic plexus and the number of nerve branches within its projections. The branches of the pelvic plexus form three major projections: (1) anterior, extending across the lateral surface of the seminal vesicle and the inferolateral surface of the bladder; (2) antero-inferior, extending to the prostatovesical junction and obliquely along the lateral surface of the prostate; and (3) inferior, running between the rectum and the posterolateral surface of the prostate, forming the neural constituents of the NVB (Fig. 1.4).

The pelvic plexus is closely associated with branches of the inferior vesical vein and artery. These large vessels are predominantly in a sagittal plane that is superimposed on the lateral surface of the pelvic plexus. On removing investing adipose and connective tissues, these vascular and neural (pelvic plexus) structures generally lay in distinct separable layers posteriorly, only to converge at the level of the pelvic plexus projections.

Course of the NVB (Fig. 1.5)

The inferior projection of the pelvic plexus unites with several vessels to form a prominent NVB, where it descends between the rectum and posterolateral border of the prostate.

In all 24 dissections, the plexus of nerves running within the NVB branch from the postero-inferior aspect of the pelvic plexus are 0.5–2 cm inferior to the level of the tip of the seminal vesicle.

The number of macroscopic nerves present varies, with 6–16 noted. On branching from the pelvic plexus these nerves are spread significantly, with up to 3 cm separating the anterior- and posterior-most nerves.

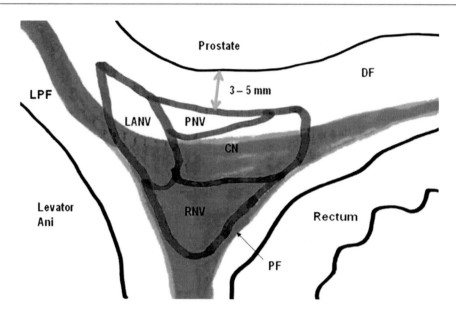

Fig. 1.4 The fascial compartments of the NVB. *RNV* neurovascular supply to the rectum, *DF* denonvilliers' fascia, *PF* pararectal fascia, *LPF* lateral pelvic fascia, *LANV* neurovascular supply to levator ani, *PNV* neuro-vascular supply to the prostate, *CN* cavernosal nerves. Adapted from images courtesy of Department of Anatomy, The University of Melbourne

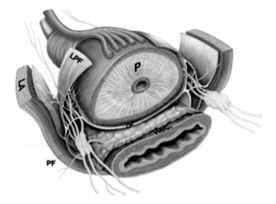

Fig. 1.5 Illustrative representation of periprostatic autonomic innervations. Denonvillers' Fascia (DF), Levator ani (LA), lateral prostatic fascia (LPF), pararectal fat (PF), rectum and prostate (P), rectum (Rec). Reprinted from Costello et al. Immunohistochemical study of the cavernous nerves in the periprostatic region. BJUI 2010;107:1210–15, with permission from John Wiley and Sons

The nerves located most anteriorly are intimately associated with the seminal vesicle, coursing along the posterolateral surface, while the nerves located posteriorly run dorsal to the posterolateral verge of the seminal vesicle.

Generally, most of the NVB descends posteriorly to the seminal vesicle. The nerves converge en route to the mid-prostatic level, forming a more condensed NVB, only to diverge once again when approaching the prostatic apex.

The nerves of the NVB are intimately associated with vessels branching from the inferior vesical vein and artery. As these vessels course distally toward the prostatic apex numerous terminal branches are given off which, in most cases, mimic the course of the nerves.

The nerves running in the NVB innervate the corpora cavernosa, rectum, prostate and levator ani musculature. Nerves running in the NVB pass through slit-like openings in the lateral pelvic fascia to innervate the superior and middle sections of the levator ani musculature. Many nerve and vascular branches pierce the lateral pelvic fascia distally to supply the inferior portion. The nerves innervating the posterior aspect of the prostate are intimately associated with capsular arteries and veins of the prostate. These structures penetrate the prostatic capsule along its base, mid-portion and apex.

The cavernosal nerves and several small vessels pierce the urogenital diaphragm posterolateral to the prostatic apex. At this level the clearly visible cavernosal nerves divide into numerous small branches that descend along the posterolateral aspect of the membranous urethra, before penetrating the posterior aspect of corpora cavernosa.

These findings confirmed the course of the cavernosal nerves in the posterolateral groove between the prostate and rectum as described in the seminal work on foetal cadaveric dissections of Walsh and Donker [16].

Functional Compartmentalization of the NVB

The constituents of the NVB are organized into three functional compartments (Fig. 1.4). The neurovascular supply to the rectum is generally in the posterior and posterolateral sections of the NVB, running within the leaves of Denonvilliers' and pararectal fasciae. The levator ani neurovascular supply is in the lateral section of the NVB, descending along and within the lateral pelvic fascia. The cavernosal nerves and the prostatic neurovascular supply descend along the posterolateral surface of the prostate, with the prostatic neurovascular supply most anterior. Part of this anterior compartment runs ventral to Denonvilliers' fascia. The functional organization of the NVB is not absolute and is less pronounced proximally at the levels of the seminal vesicles and the prostatic base. In addition to the nerves descending within the NVB, a scattering of nerves extends from the medial margin of the NVB to the prostatic midline. The deepest nerves (from an anterior aspect) innervate the anterior surface of the rectum at the level of the prostatic apex. The more superficial nerves descend posterior to the prostatic apex and merge laterally with the NVB.

This significant discovery of distinct fascial compartments within the NVB showed that the synonymous use of the terms NVB and cavernosal nerves in previous publications was not appropriate.

Sural nerve grafts to treat post radical prostatectomy erectile dysfunction were in vogue at the time of this study. The finding of additional innervation beyond that of the carvenosus nerves within the NVB meant that one could no longer just anastomose the sural nerve graft to any intraoperatively identified nerve fibre in the NVB.

Are There Parasympathetic Nerves Outside of the NVB?

The concept of the well-defined NVB posterolateral to the prostate was challenged subsequently by several investigators. Kiyoshima found a recognizable NVB in the posterolateral region of the prostate in only 48 % of radical prostatectomy specimens, while the rest of the specimens showed vessels and nerve trunks sparsely spread from the lateral aspect of the prostate to the anterior, without a definite bundle formation [17]. Eichenburg found in his study of radical prostatectomy specimens that a quarter to one-fifth of nerves are found on the ventral surface of the prostate [18]. In his study of foetal and adult cadavers, Lunacek found that the growth of the prostate influences the topographic anatomy of the cavernous nerves, with the nerves displaced more anteriorly and dispersed along the convex surface of the prostatic capsule [19]. These findings supported the cadaveric studies by Takenaka, who found that parasympathetic nerve components joined the NVB in a spray-like distribution at multiple levels [20].

These authors speculate that these anteriorly placed nerves contribute to the pro-erectile cavernous nerves. However, no study ever showed the actual function of these nerves. Despite this lack of evidence, some institutions developed nerve-sparing techniques aimed at preserving these structures. This new nerve-sparing approach, dubbed the "Veil of Aphrodite" technique by Menon's group in Detroit or curtain dissection by Lunacek, releases the lateral prostatic fascia high on the anterolateral margins of the prostate above the midpoint of the prostate [19, 21].

Immunohistochemical Study of the Cavernous Nerves in the Periprostatic Region

Our team felt there was little anatomical evidence to justify this approach, given that based on our previous work, the higher placed nerves were most likely destined to innervate the prostatic stroma and not the cavernosal tissue of the penis.

To provide more evidence for the different nerve-sparing approaches, we embarked on our study focused on characterizing the position and nature of the autonomic nerves surrounding the prostate using specific immunohistochemical stains to clarify the likely functionality of the more anteriorly located nerves [22].

Four blocks of pelvic tissue from the hemisectioned pelves of two embalmed and two fresh cadavers were serially histologically sectioned, from the prostatic base proximally to the apex distally. The hemisected pelvic blocks were then divided into 4-mm sections and embedded into paraffin for histological analysis. All of these initial slides were stained with haematoxylin and eosin (H&E) and, based on a primary analysis, 50 representative blocks from only the fresh cadavers were selected. From these 50 blocks, a further two slides were cut at 3 μm and mounted from each block to undergo immunohistochemical staining using both tyrosine hydroxylase (sympathetics) and neuronal nitric oxide synthase (nNOS) (parasympathetics).

To localize the parasympathetics an antibody directed against nNOS was used. nNOS is a 150-k Da protein that is found in peripheral parasympathetic nerves and catalyzes the formation of nitric oxide. Nitric oxide is released by parasympathetics and is a potent vasodilator, implicated in the physiology of the male erection.

To localize the sympathetic nerves, we used a primary antibody directed against tyrosine hydroxylase. Tyrosine hydroxylase is the rate-limiting enzyme in the synthetic pathway of norepinephrine, which is a neurotransmitter found in peripheral sympathetic nerves and their associated ganglia.

Each slide was analyzed according to nerve fibre number, type (somatic, parasympathetic

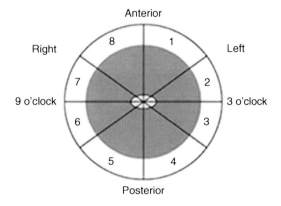

Fig. 1.6 Method of sector analysis. Reprinted from Costello et al. Immunohistochemical study of the cavernous nerves in the periprostatic region. BJUI 2010;107:1210–15, with permission from John Wiley and Sons

or sympathetic) and position relative to the prostate. The analysis allocated nerves as they were observed to a particular sector as shown (Fig. 1.6).

Results

Parasympathetic nerves accounted for 43.3 % of all nerve fibres present at the prostatic base, increasing to 45.5 % at the apex. Parasympathetic nerves found ventrally above the 3–9 o'clock level accounted for only 4 %, 5 % and 6.8 % of the total number of nerves at the base, midprostate and apical regions, respectively.

The proportion of sympathetic nerves was relatively constant from base to apex: 38.7–39.1 %. Sympathetic nerves found above the 3–9 o'clock level represented ≈15 % of the total number of nerves at any given prostatic level.

Somatic nerves corresponded to 18 %, 16.5 % and 15.5 % of the total nerve fibres at the base, mid-prostate and apex, respectively. Somatic nerves found above 3–9 o'clock level represented 7.5 % of the total nerves at each level of the prostate.

About a quarter (27.4 % base, 26.5 % mid-prostate and 29.6 % apical) of all the nerve fibres identified were found on the anterior half of the prostate, above the 3–9 o'clock level.

Table 1.1 Distribution of parasympathetic nerve fibres as a percentage of total parasympathetic nerves fibres at that level

Position	In NVB[a]	Above 3–9 o'clock[b]
Prostate base	69.4	9
Mid-prostate	65.3	11.1
Prostate apex	57	15

[a]Within sectors 4 and 5
[b]Within sectors 1, 2, 7, and 8
NVB—neurovascular bundle
Reproduced from Costello et al. Immunohistochemical study of the cavernous nerves in the periprostatic region. BJUI 2010;107:1210–15, with permission from John Wiley and Sons

Parasympathetic Nerve Fibre Distribution (Table 1.1)

At the prostatic base, parasympathetic nerves accounted for only 14.3 % of the nerves located on the anterior aspect of the prostate. However, these nerves correspond to only 9 % of the total number of parasympathetic nerves found at the base. A significant proportion of the parasympathetic nerves at the base were localized to the region of the NVB (sectors 4 and 5). At this level, 69.4 % of the parasympathetic nerves were found within the anatomically defined NVB.

Similarly, at the mid-prostate, 65.3 % of the parasympathetic nerves were found inside the NVB. Only 11.1 % of parasympathetics at this level were found above the 3–9 o'clock junction, which, as a proportion of the total nerves at this level, represents 18.8 % of those nerves found on the anterior aspects of the prostate.

At the apex, 57 % of all parasympathetic fibres were found within the region of the NVB, with 15 % found above the 3–9 o'clock level. Importantly, the proportion of parasympathetic nerves found within the NVB dropped slightly from the base to the apex.

The fascial architecture of the posterolaterally located NVB was also analyzed and in 18 of the 32 slides examined the NVB exhibited a fascial architecture with three separate compartments as previously described. Figure 1.7 illustrates the compartmental architecture found within the NVB on a slide. Three compartments containing nerves and blood vessels can be clearly seen, the most medial of which conveyed a significant proportion of the parasympathetic nerve fibres.

Do the Anterior Parasympathetic Nerves Innervate the Corpora Cavernosa?

Our immunohistochemical staining study suggests that the anteriorly placed parasympathetic nerve fibres are likely destined for innervation of the prostatic stroma rather than the penile corpora cavernosum. This observation is supported by two pieces of evidence.

First, the total number of visible nerve fibre was smaller at the prostatic apex as compared to the base. This decrease in the number of fibre has been reported by some authors and may be related to a significant proportion of nerves penetrating the prostate to innervate the gland itself [17, 18, 23]. In the fresh cadavers in this study, 134 nerve fibres were located at the base as opposed to 115 at the apex. Of these, the absolute number of parasympathetic nerves found on the anterior half of the prostate at the apex was only eight—further supporting this hypothesis of nerves entering the prostate as they course along it.

Second, the fascial architecture of the NVB itself supports the view that prostatic innervation is the role of these anterior nerve fibres.

This study has confirmed the compartmental structure of the NVB shown in our earlier work with 12 micro-dissected cadavers [15].

Apically the absolute number of the parasympathetic fibre above the 3–9 o'clock junction increased slightly. This is consistent with studies that show the cavernous nerves ascending to assume a higher position distal to the apex. Takenaka et al. claimed the cavernous nerves assume a higher 2–10 o'clock position at the apex [24]. This study did not confirm his findings. However, careful dissection and ligation of the dorsal venous complex is recommended to preserve the neural anatomy.

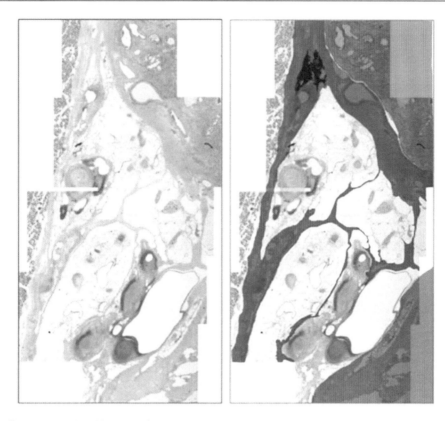

Fig. 1.7 Compartmental architecture of the neurovascular bundle (mid-prostate). *Left*: haematoxylin and eosin slide showing compartmental neurovascular bundle architecture. *Right* (overlay): prostate (*green*), fascial bands (*blue*), nerves (*yellow*), pararectal tissue (*grey*), levator ani musculature (*spotted pink*). Reprinted from Costello et al. Immunohistochemical study of the cavernous nerves in the periprostatic region. BJUI 2010;107:1210–15, with permission from John Wiley and Sons

Nerve Quantification: Numerical vs. Surface Area

Cross-sectional area may be a more appropriate measure of the periprostatic nerve distribution since nerve bundle quantification does not account for bundle size. To further elucidate the topography and function of the periprostatic nerves, we investigated the precise periprostatic nerve distribution in cadaveric specimens by calculating the cross-sectional area of nerve bundles [25].

Hemipelves from five fresh and two embalmed male cadavers were serially sectioned, and 4 μm serial sections representing the prostate base, mid and apical regions were prepared into slides. Mounted slides were stained with haematoxylin and eosin and digitized with a high resolution Mirax Scanner (Zeiss®) with a 20× objective.

Digital sections were covered with an overlay dividing the hemiprostates into six equal sectors at a 30° angle and numbered 1–6 clockwise and counterclockwise (Fig. 1.8). Sector 5 corresponded to the posterolateral region, where Walsh identified the prominent NVB. The 13 hemiprostates were treated as independent units.

Upon analysis the periprostatic nerve bundles between the lateral prostatic fascia and Denonvilliers' fascia posterior, and the prostatic capsule were identified and counted for all six tissue sectors. All sections were viewed using Mirax Viewer (Zeiss) software at ×5 magnification. Nerve bundles were classified as periprostatic (between the lateral pelvic fascia and capsule) or capsular (within the fibromuscular capsule). When identified, nerve cell bodies noted within sections were considered

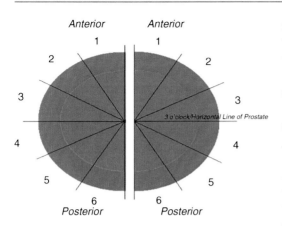

Fig. 1.8 Sector analysis used to describe nerve bundle distribution around prostate. Each sector is 30° apart from central point. From Clarebrough EE, Challacombe BJ, Briggs C, Namdarian B, Weston R, Murphy DG, Costello AJ. Cadaveric analysis of periprostatic nerve distribution: an anatomical basis for high anterior release during radical prostatectomy? J Urol. 2011 Apr;185(4):1519–25. Reprinted with permission from Elsevier

the same as nerve bundles. Cross-sectional area was calculated for periprostatic and capsular nerve bundles in each sector.

In all specimens analyzed a total of 1,199, 1,065 and 1,017 periprostatic nerve bundles were counted at the prostate base, mid part and apical regions, respectively. Total neural cross-sectional area in the base, mid part and apical periprostatic regions was 24.7, 19.7 and 13.7 mm², respectively.

Significantly more nerve bundles were counted in the periprostatic region than in the capsule of all regions. A total of 465, 478 and 426 capsular nerve bundles were recorded in the base, mid and apical regions with a periprostatic-to-capsular ratio of 4.1, 2.4 and 3.4, respectively. The cross-sectional area of all periprostatic nerve bundles was calculated for each of the 6 sectors to determine the topographical distribution of neural tissue with respect to the prostate. The maximum neural cross-sectional area of any single sector across all specimens was 19.1 mm² in sector 5 in the base of the prostate and the minimum was 0.2 mm² at the sector 1 base and the sector 6 mid zone.

Sector 5, the classic location of the NVB, had a significantly higher proportion of neural cross-sectional area than all other sectors at the base,

mid and apical prostate. Sectors 1 and 2 had low total neural cross-sectional areas but this increased from the base toward the apex (Table 1.2).

The highest median percent of neural tissue cross-sectional area was in sector 5 with 77.4 %, 82.2 % and 75.5 % of total periprostatic neural cross-sectional area at the prostate base, mid gland and apex, respectively (Fig. 1.9).

The percent of neural tissue surrounding the anterior part of the prostate was far lower than that around the posterior part. However, this varied and increased from base through to apex with 6.0 % at the base, 7.6 % at the mid part and 11.2 % at the apical anterior prostate.

Ganzer et al. similarly investigated the distribution of nerve bundles of prostatectomy specimens using the cross-sectional area of nerve bundles or planimetry rather than simple nerve quantification [26]. They reported that only 7.2 %, 19.4 % and 14.2 % of neural tissue surrounded the anterior part of the prostate at the base, mid zone and apex, respectively. Also, there was a significant decrease in total nerve surface area from the base over the middle toward the apex of the prostate as the periprostatic nerves penetrated the capsule to directly innervate the prostate.

The limitations of these studies were that, while the distribution of the neural tissue could be quantified, the contribution to erectile physiology was unknown because of the use of nonspecific staining. Ganzer et al. addressed this problem with their recent detailed characterization of the topographic distribution of periprostatic nerves, including immunohistochemical differentiation of pro-erectile parasympathetic from sympathetic nerves of 49 radical prostatectomy specimens [27].

They confirmed our previous findings that more than 75 % of neural tissue is distributed in the dorsolateral position, with less than 15 % of parasympathetic neural tissue found ventrally. In addition, they found that the proportion of parasympathetic tissue ventrally did not increase towards the base. They concluded that high incision might help preserve more parasympathetic nerves at the base and the middle but is of little help at the apex.

Table 1.2 Periprostatic nerve bundle and neural cross-sectional area per sector

Cross-sectional area							
–	Section 1	Section 2	Section 3	Section 4	Section 5	Section 6	Totals
Periprostatic nerve bundles							
Base (mm^2)	–						
Total	0.2	0.4	0.8	3.2	19.1	1.0	–
Median (range)	0.0 (0.0–0.1)	0.0 (0.0–0.1)	0.0 (0.0–0.2)	0.1 (0.0–1.2)	0.8 (0.4–4.5)	0.0 (0.0–0.8)	24.7
Midzone (mm^2)	–						
Total	0.4	0.5	0.7	1.1	16.7	0.2	–
Median (range)	0.0 (0.0–0.1)	0.0 (0.00–0.02)	0.0 (0.0–0.2)	0.1(0.0–0.4)	0.8 (0.4–4.8)	0.0 (0.0–0.1)	19.7
Apex (mm^2)	–						
Total	0.4	1.0	0.8	1.7	9.5	0.3	–
Median (range)	0.0 (0.0–0.1)	0.0 (0.0–0.2)	0.1 (0.0–0.2)	0.1 (0.0–0.7)	0.7 (0.3–1.5)	0.0 (0.0–0.1)	13.7
p value	0.35	0.14	0.84	0.19	0.21	0.45	–
Neural tissue							
Median % (range)	–						
Base	0.2 (0.0–4.7)	1.2 (0.0–11.4)	4.6 (0.9–9.6)	10.3 (3.5–26.7)	77.4 (62.4–94.2)	1.0 (0.0–12.3)	–
Mid part	1.9 (0.0–10.1)	2.7 (0.0–8.6)	3.0 (0.0–19.4)	5.3 (0.0–18.8)	82.2 (63.7–99.3)	0.1 (0.0–5.5)	–
Apex	1.8 (0.0–13.3)	4.8 (0.2–27.2)	4.6 (0.0–28.8)	6.7 (0.0–43.6)	75.5 (37.8–89.7)	0.0 (0.0–8.6)	–

From Clarebrough EE, Challacombe BJ, Briggs C, Namdarian B, Weston R, Murphy DG, Costello AJ. Cadaveric analysis of periprostatic nerve distribution: an anatomical basis for high anterior release during radical prostatectomy? J Urol. 2011 Apr;185(4):1519–25. Reprinted with permission from Elsevier

The drawback of all these anatomical studies is that none are able to confirm if these anteriorly placed parasympathetic nerves contribute to erectile function. Kaiho et al. measured the increase in intracavernosal pressure after intraoperative electrical neurostimulation of the lateral periprostatic nerves by a small bipolar electrode [28]. This small study demonstrated that every electrostimulation of the nerves found between the 1 and 5 o'clock positions on the lateral surface of the prostate resulted in an increase in cavernosal pressure. Of note the mean pressure response was most powerful for 5 o'clock stimulation and decreased with stimulated points further from the 5 o'clock position. While this is suggestive that the anterior periprostatic nerves contribute to erectile function, artificial electrical stimulation may be too crude a technique to provide anatomical proof of function.

As long as the physiology of these nerves is not clearly verified by functional studies, one should undertake every effort in nerve-sparing prostatectomy procedures to preserve as many of these nerves as possible. With this in mind, we suggest that a slightly modified incision technique be used to dissect the NVBs off the prostate, making a sweeping incision that climbs anterior up to the 1 o'clock position at the apex but not in the more proximal regions of the gland.

Relationship of Pelvic Fascial Layers to Nerve-Sparing Prostatectomy

Having described the location of the CN in relation to the NVB and periprostatic area, understanding the location and distribution of the fascias around the prostate and their relation to the NVB becomes key to achieve the desired degree of nerve sparing during the radical prostatectomy (RP). There are four main fascial layers surrounding the prostate and NVB, which serve

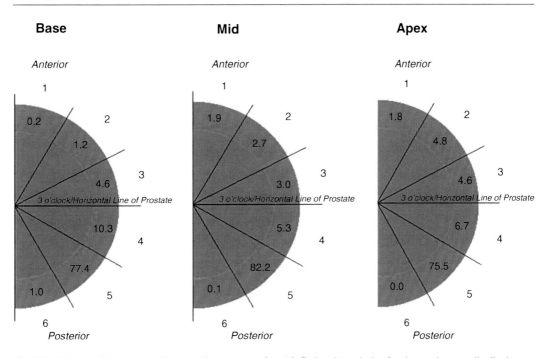

Fig. 1.9 Values in *blue areas* indicate median percent of periprostatic neural cross-sectional area per sector at prostate base, mid part and apex. From Clarebrough EE, Challacombe BJ, Briggs C, Namdarian B, Weston R, Murphy DG, Costello AJ. Cadaveric analysis of periprostatic nerve distribution: an anatomical basis for high anterior release during radical prostatectomy? J Urol. 2011 Apr;185(4):1519–25. Reprinted with permission from Elsevier

as surgical landmarks that will help determine the layers that should be incised in order to remove or preserve different amounts of cavernous nerve tissue during RP.

Endopelvic Fascia (EPF)

The endopelvic fascia has two components: parietal and visceral. The parietal EPF covers the levator ani lateral to the fascial tendinous arch of the pelvis. The visceral EPF covers the detrusor apron and anterior surface of the underlying prostate. The parietal and visceral EPF are fused at the lateral side of the prostate and bladder. This fusion site is sometimes recognized as a whitish line and is called the "arcus tendineus fascia pelvis" (ATFP) [29]. The ATFP runs from the puboprostatic ligament to the ischial spine.

Conventional wisdom is that the EPF should be incised lateral to the ATFP to avoid unnecessary haemorrhage from prostatovesical veins [30]. Takenaka and colleagues showed in cadaveric studies that preserving the fascia of the levator ani helps to protect the levator ani muscle, rhabdosphincter and pudendal nerve branches to the rhabdosphincter [10]. This concurs with what other pioneering prostatectomy surgeons advocate—that the correct location to incise the fascia is medial to the fascial tendinous arch—thus leaving the levator ani muscle covered by its fascia [31].

Occasionally, part of the endopelvic fascia over the prostate coalesces with that lying over the levator ani fascia at its deepest point of reflection. This fusion of layers needs to be detached for an adequate incision of the endopelvic fascia. Applying countertraction on the prostate facilitates identification and dissection of the contour of fascial reflection where the endopelvic fascia forms a cul-de-sac between the levator ani fascia laterally and the prostatic fascia medially. It is easier to identify and correctly incise this cul-de-sac when this dissection is initiated close to the base of the prostate (as opposed to close to the apex) where the endopelvic fascia seems to be thinner and the space between levator ani and the prostatic fascia is wider.

Periprostatic Fascia

The fascia on the outer surface of the prostate has been given several different names by different authors. It has been referred to as periprostatic fascia by Myers and Villers [32], Stolzenburg et al. [33] and Tewari et al. [34]; as lateral pelvic fascia by Costello et al. [15], Takenaka et al. [10] and Walsh and Partin [35]; as parapelvic fascia by Graefen et al. [36] and Budaus et al. [37]; and Menon et al. [38] and Secin et al. [39] have used the term prostatic fascia.

This fascia is not a discrete single-layered structure stretching over the lateral surface of the prostate. Often it is multilayered structure over the prostate, consisting of both collagenous and adipose tissue elements. Walz has done an excellent review on the pelvic fascias and their relationship to the NVB [40]. Similarly, for ease of review, we will use the term periprostatic fascia (PPF) to signify all fascias on the prostate that are external to the prostate capsule. The PPF covering the prostate can now be subdivided into three basic elements according to location.

Anterior Periprostatic Fascia (Visceral Endopelvic Fascia)

This represents the visceral endopelvic fascia discussed earlier in this section. It is associated with the anterior surface of the prostate from approximately the 10-o'clock to 11-o'clock positions to the 1-o'clock to 2-o'clock positions, where it covers the detrusor apron, dorsal vascular complex (DVC), and is fused in the midline with the anterior fibromuscular stroma of the prostate.

Lateral Periprostatic Fascia

Once the endopelvic fascia is opened lateral to the fascial tendinous arch of the pelvis and the levator ani muscle is deflected laterally, the outermost fascial layer on the lateral surface of the prostate is the levator ani fascia (LAF).

Under this layer lies the prostatic fascia. The PF is fused anteriorly with the puboprostatic

ligaments/dorsal venous complex, coming into intimate contact with the prostate pseudocapsule more laterally [21].

Both of these layers (LAF and PF) constitute PPF for the operating surgeon. The outer LAF covers the underlying, laterally distributed levator ani muscle and therefore forms the lateral boundary of the axial triangular space occupied by the bulk of the cavernous nerves and vessels, and varying amounts of fat. It extends posteriorly over the muscle fibres and continues over the lateral aspect of the rectum to form the so-called pararectal fascia (separating the rectum from the levator ani). The medial boundary of this triangle is formed by the inner PF and underlying prostate pseudocapsule and the posterior boundary by Denonvilliers' fascia [15].

The relationship between the prostate capsule and the lateral PF may differ depending on interindividual variations (Fig. 1.10). Kiyoshima et al. found that in 52 % of all cases, the LAF, which they called "lateral pelvic fascia," does not adhere to their prostate "capsule" [17]. In the cases just cited, the apparent space consisted of loose connective and adipose tissue referred to as areolar tissue. Furthermore, in such cases the NVB could not be identified as a distinct structure but was spread out over the lateral prostatic surface. In the remaining 48 %, LAF was fused with their prostate capsule, and no areolar tissue was seen between the layers. An exception to this fusion was only seen at the posterolateral angle of the prostate, and the NVB was identified there as a distinct bundle.

Posterior Prostatic Fascia and Seminal Vesicles Fascia (Denonvilliers' Fascia)

Denonvilliers' fascia (DF) (first described in 1837 [41]) is a continuous layer of posterior prostatic fascia (pPF) and seminal vesicles fascia (SVF), that closely covers the posterior surface of the prostate and the seminal vesicles. This fascia is also known as fascia rectoprostatica, septum rectovesicale, prostatoseminal vesicular fascia.

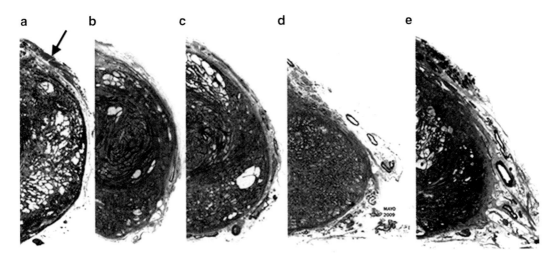

Fig. 1.10 Variation of prostate capsule to prostatic fascia (PF) on the lateral surface of the prostate. Masson-trichrome staining: fascia stains *bright blue*; smooth muscle stains *red*. (**a**) Capsule present but no PF visible (*arrow*: fascial tendinous arch of pelvis); (**b**) PF fused to capsule; (**c**) capsule fused to PF; very fine levator ani fascia lateral to vessels; (**d**) fascia-capsular interface, variable and poorly defined; (**e**) relatively thick PF present but no capsule visible. Reprinted from Walz J et al. A critical analysis of the current knowledge of surgical anatomy related to optimization of cancer control and preservation of continence and erection in candidates for radical prostatectomy. Eur Urol. 2010 Feb;57(2):179–92, by permission of Mayo Foundation for Medical Education and Research. All rights reserved

The origin of DF is controversial. While some authors support the theory of fusion of the anterior and posterior sheaths of the embryological cul-de-sac, others simply propose that DF originates from condensation of loose areolar tissue [42].

The pPF/SVF extends from the caudal end of the rectovesical pouch, to the prostate apex to end at the prostatourethral junction in a terminal plate in continuity with the central perineal tendon [32]. Histologically, it has a double-layered quality which is *not identifiable intraoperatively*. The fascia extends from the deepest point of the interprostatorectal peritoneal pouch to the pelvic floor and, contrary to the theory of Villers et al. [43], does not lie forward of the anterior wall of the pouch. The often described posterior layer does not exist and is actually the rectal fascia propria [44, 45].

The mesorectum is a fatty layer covered by the fascia propria of the rectum. Dissection between the rectal fascia propria and Denonvillers' fascia [45] is the plane that should be followed during RP in order to minimize the risk of injuring the pelvic plexuses and NVB [46], and avoid having a positive surgical margin at the posterior aspect of the prostate (Fig. 1.11).

There is a commonly held misconception that there is a separate anterior layer of Denonvillers' fascia interposed between the posterior bladder neck and the anterior aspect of the SV and vasa deferentia [47]. These are actually posterior longitudinal fibres of the detrusor running in between and behind the ureteral orifices (called vesicoprostatic muscle by Dorschner and colleagues [48], or posterior longitudinal fascia of detrusor muscle by Secin et al. [47]). This was confirmed by Secin et al. [47] who found histologically that this fascia represents the fusion of two separate tissue layers, an inner lamella composed of longitudinally disposed smooth muscle fibres in continuation with the longitudinal fascia of the bladder detrusor (medial fascicle of the detrusor running in between the ureters) and an outer lamella composed of fibroadipose tissue in continuation with the bladder adventitia.

Vesical remnants of these posterior longitudinal fibres of the detrusor are what Rocco and colleagues term the residual DF [49], which they suture to the posterior median raphe during their posterior

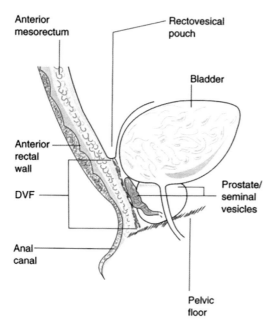

Anterior mesorectum

Rectovesical pouch

Bladder

Anterior rectal wall

DVF

Prostate/ seminal vesicles

Anal canal

Pelvic floor

Fig. 1.11 Lateral view of DF and its relations. Reprinted from Lindsey I, Guy R J, Warren B F, et al. Anatomy of Denonvilliers' fascia and pelvic nerves, impotence, and implications for the colorectal surgeon. Br J Surg, 2000; 87(10): 1288–99, with permission from John Wiley and Sons

reconstruction of the rhabdosphincter, prior to performing the urethrovesical anastomosis.

Denonvilliers' fascia is very often fused with the prostate capsule at the centre of the posterior prostatic surface. Towards the posterolateral aspect of the prostate, DF has no significant adherence to the prostatic capsule, and the triangular space between DF and the capsule is once again filled by areolar tissue and the NVB.

Denonvillier's fascia is significant in that it presents a barrier to the spread of prostate cancer posteriorly. Incomplete excision of this fascia can lead to positive margins [43].

Prostate Capsule

As taught by pathologists, the prostate has no real capsule. The outermost part of the prostate is often composed of variable layers of condensed fibromuscular fascicles inseparable from the prostatic stroma [50]. This pseudocapsule is almost absent at the anterior aspect of the pros-

tate, where the anterior fibromuscular stroma is identified. In addition, the pseudocapsule is absent at the apex of the gland and at the prostate base, where the gland fuses with the urinary sphincter and the bladder neck, respectively.

Despite extensive research in the field of prostate anatomy, the exact anatomy of the fascias surrounding the prostate remains controversial. We are in agreement with Walz's [40] simplification of recognizing the PPF as outer LAF and inner PF, the latter covering the prostate capsule and with the neurovascular structures found merged into or sandwiched between LAF and PF with some interindividual variation with respect to the NVB.

Surgical Planes of Dissection

Intrafascial Dissection

Intrafascial dissection of the NVB is considered a dissection that follows a plane on the prostate capsule, remaining medial to the PF at the anterolateral and posterolateral aspect of the prostate and remaining anterior to pPF/SVF [34, 40].

The intrafascial approach allows a whole-thickness preservation of the lateral PF left laterally and therefore a complete preservation of the NVB because it remains covered by and lateral to the PF. At the end of the procedure, the prostate capsule will be bare of both PF and that portion of the pPF/SVF at the posterolateral and lateral surfaces where the NVB resided. Intrafascial dissection carries the greatest risk of violating the prostate capsule [51].

Interfacial Dissection

Interfacial dissection of the NVB is considered a dissection lateral to the PF at the anterolateral and posterolateral aspects of the prostate combined with a dissection medial to the NVB at the 5-o'clock and 7-o'clock positions or the 2-o'clock and 10-o'clock positions of the prostate in axial section. This is done by moving the intact NVB off the prostate, so that the posterolateral prostate still remains covered with fascia. Lateral PF stays on the prostate rather than staying attached to the NVB, and the pPF/SVF remains on the posterior surface of the prostate. This approach allows a greater tissue buffer to surround the prostate in contrast to the intrafascial dissection, presumably resulting in an oncologically safer approach [32, 33, 35].

Depending on anatomic variations, the NVB might be more prone to partial resection with this technique because this dissection will not necessarily allow the preservation of all of the nerve fibres dispersed on the anterolateral surface of the prostate.

Extrafascial Dissection

The dissection is carried out posterior to the NVB and out laterally to the LAF. The prostate is removed with all layers of visceral fibrofatty sheath present on the specimen (wide resection), partially sparing the lateral part of the NVB within the angle between the LAF and pPF/SVF. This approach results in the largest amount of tissue surrounding the prostate compared with the intra- and interfascial dissections. It is therefore an oncologically safer dissection but carries with it a higher chance of erectile dysfunction [32, 33, 35].

Non-nerve-Sparing Dissection

This is a wide dissection, taking the LAF and the pPF/SVF, and would result in complete excision of the NVB, and probable erectile dysfunction [29] (Fig. 1.12).

Vascular Anatomy

Arterial Supply of the Prostate

The principal arterial supply to the prostate is from the inferior vesical branch of the anterior division of the internal iliac artery. Smaller contributions are given by the middle rectal and pudendal branches of the internal iliac artery. The inferior vesical artery originates near the

upper margin of the greater sciatic notch. It travels forward to the bladder base, which it also supplies. It also sends branches to the seminal vesicles, including a relatively constant branch to the tip of the seminal vesicle that needs to be controlled during radical prostatectomy. It then divides into urethral and prostatic branch groupings. The urethral branches penetrate the prostate substance at the prostatovesical junction posterolaterally. These then travel perpendicular to the urethra and approach the bladder neck mainly at the 5 and 7 o'clock positions. These vessels then course parallel to the urethra and are named the arteries of Flocks [52]. These supply the urethra, the transition zone, and the periurethral glands and are responsible for arterial bleeding during TURP. The capsular branch of the prostatic artery runs posterolaterally between the levator fascia and prostatic fascia. It is accompanied by the cavernous nerves and contributes to the NVB.

The NVB may be tethered to the prostatic apex by fine vascular branches (micropedicles), and neural elements are particularly at risk of damage during dissection of the prostatic apex. The capsular branch gives perpendicular branches that penetrate the capsule to supply the glandular tissue and terminate by supplying the pelvic floor with small vessels.

Accessory Pudendal Arteries (APA)

Accessory or aberrant pudendal arteries are arteries superior to the pelvic diaphragm passing posterior to the pubic bone to finally enter the penile hilum. They may originate from the internal or external iliac or obturator arteries as opposed to the small arteries present within the DVC [53–56].

APA Can Be Divided into Two Categories: Apical APA or Lateral APA

Lateral Accessory Arteries

Lateral APA run along the fascial tendinous arch of the pelvis in the groove between the bladder, prostate and pelvic sidewall (Fig. 1.13).

a 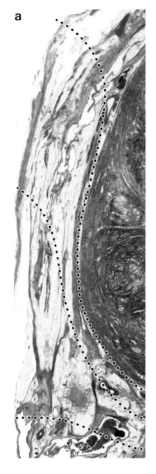   b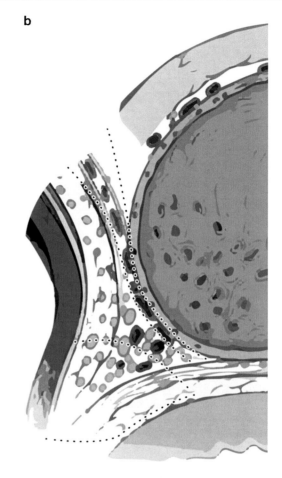

Fig. 1.12 Nerve-sparing grades. (**a**) Transverse sections. Masson-trichrome staining. Intra-, inter- and extrafascial dissections are shown. (**b**) Schematic of nerve-sparing grades. Reprinted from Hinata N, Sejima T and Takenaka A. Progress in pelvic anatomy from the viewpoint of radical prostatectomy. Int J Urol 2012 Nov 26. With permission from John Wiley and Sons

Another variation enters laterally below the pubic bone. All run either above or below the endopelvic fascia. Those running above the endopelvic fascia usually branch off from either the inferior vesical or internal iliac artery, whereas those running below usually emanate from an obturator artery or external iliac artery [57].

Apical Accessory Arteries

Apical APA are found inferior and lateral to the puboprostatic/pubovesical ligaments, in proximity to the anterolateral aspect of the prostate apex (Fig. 1.13). They usually pass through the levator ani muscle and emerge laterally. They then approach the apex tangentially and may extend to the apex before running parallel into the DVC and toward the penis [57]. They are likely to originate from the obturator artery or infralevator pudendal artery. Large apical APA may represent aberrant pudendal arteries, whereas smaller ones often provide only minor arterial supply to the corpora cavernosa.

The incidence of APA has been reported from 4 % in an open prostatectomy series [58] and 7 % with the use of conventional angiography [53]. Previous studies on laparoscopic RP suggest that endoscopic magnification results in a six- to sevenfold increase in the APA detection

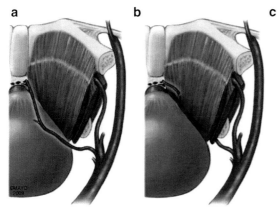

Fig. 1.13 Aberrant and accessory pudendal arteries: (**a**) aberrant lateral supralevator pudendal artery branching from internal iliac artery; (**b**) accessory apical pudendal artery branching from infralevator pudendal artery; (**c**) accessory lateral pudendal artery branching from obturator artery; (**d**) accessory pudendal artery branching from external iliac artery with aberrant obturator and infravesi- cal branches. Reprinted from Walz J et al. A critical analy- sis of the current knowledge of surgical anatomy related to optimization of cancer control and preservation of con- tinence and erection in candidates for radical prostatec- tomy. Eur Urol. 2010 Feb;57(2):179–92, by permission of Mayo Foundation for Medical Education and Research. All rights reserved

rate of (26–30 %) [57, 59]. Investigators from Korea found a similarly high incidence of APA with multidetector-row CT angiography [60].

APA provide unilaterally or bilaterally arterial blood supply to the corpora cavernosa [61]. Nehra and colleagues showed an incidence of APA of 35 % in their series of selective pudendal pharmacoangiograms in men with erectile dys- function, of which in 54 %, the APA represented the dominant blood supply to the penis [62]. Droupy found APA in 17 of 20 cadavers, of which in 3, the APA was the sole blood supply to the penis [63].

Must We Preserve the APA?

Post radical prostatectomy erectile dysfunction in men with preserved NVBs is a result of a combi- nation of neuropraxia (from traction), arterial insufficiency and venous leak.

The hemodynamic changes in APA and cav- ernous arteries during penile erection are similar, providing evidence of a functional role for APA in penile tumescence [61].

Between 1987 and 1994 the group from Johns Hopkins found APA in only 4 % of 835 patients undergoing open radical prostatectomy. APA preservation was possible in 19 of 24 patients (79 %). On assessment there was little difference in erectile function between the 12 men (67 %) in whom APA were preserved and the 10 (50 %) in whom they were not. At that time the investiga- tors concluded that the presence of APA was rare and that, although preservation was possible in most patients, it was associated with excessive dorsal vein complex bleeding and, because no significant difference in potency rates was seen with preservation, routine APA preservation may not be productive [58].

Nine years later the same group compared potency outcomes between patients who under- went nerve-sparing RP with and without APA preservation. Compared with excision, preserva- tion of APA more than doubled the probability of remaining potent and was associated with a shorter time to regain potency (6 months vs. 12 months). This effect was particularly strong in men with unilateral accessory arteries (91 % vs. 50 %) and in men younger than 60 years old. These effects achieved statistical significance. However, in men with bilateral APA, 100 % of men were potent regardless of whether APA was preserved or ligated [54].

The functional significance of APA can be variable, depending on the size of the APA and whether the APA represents the sole blood supply to the penis.

Thus whenever feasible, every effort should be made to preserve these arteries during prostatectomy to avoid erectile dysfunction caused by penile arterial insufficiency.

We hypothesize that APA division may contribute to the penile shrinkage reported by some patients after radical prostatectomy.

Dorsal Vascular Complex (DVC)

The dorsal venous complex or Santorini's plexus covers the prostate and the urethral sphincter ventrally, comprises the deep dorsal vein of the penis entering the retropubic space through Buck's fascia below the pubic arch into three major branches: one superficial (pre-prostatic) branch and two lateral venous plexuses.

It is important to look out for this superficial branch during the initial exposure of the vesical visceral fascia in the retropubic radical prostatectomy, as disruption of this vein can lead to serious blood loss if the vein is large. Several anatomical variations of these superficial preprostatic veins have been reported by Myers [64]. Although the most common finding (in nearly 60 % of cases) is a single midline vein, in another 20 % of cases there is a bifurcation that originates right or left pelvic sidewall branches. The third most common distribution is a single vein to the pelvic sidewall without vesicovenous plexus anastomosis and, finally, in about 10 % of cases the vein is completely absent.

The lateral venous plexuses form a network of veins lying immediately underneath the puboprostatic ligaments and the endopelvic fascia. While traversing posterolaterally, they usually originate branches that communicate with pudendal, obturator and vesical plexuses. Near the puboprostatic ligaments, small branches may penetrate the pelvic sidewall musculature and communicate with the internal pudendal veins. An increased number of branches, as well as anatomical variations in the veins' course are frequent also at the deep venous plexus level and may account for the unpredictable and sometimes

unavoidable troublesome bleeding during radical prostatectomy [65].

With the advent of laparoscopic and robotic technology, the increased intra-abdominal pressure afforded by CO_2 insufflation has allowed surgeons to divide the DVC safely without initial ligation. This anatomical view provides a unique opportunity to further characterize the DVC. Specifically, previously undescribed small arteries have been identified within the complex. These arteries are often located near the midline. They are commonly encountered during division of the DVC and are probably either a terminal branch of the internal pudendal artery or a small branch of the prostatic capsular artery [66].

Therefore, the dorsal vein complex is in essence a DVC [67].

Ventrally, the DVC is covered by extensions of the visceral endopelvic fascia and the detrusor apron. At the prostatourethral junction, an avascular plane is present between the prostate and the DVC, forming a landmark for DVC control [67].

If there is significant anterolateral BPH expansion of the prostate at the apex and a broad commissure, the venous plexus rides up, leaving an accessible, relatively avascular space for the insertion of a right angle for the purpose of venous ligation [68].

If there is no BPH, there will be relatively little space; the venous plexus will come off the urethra and enter the vesicovenous plexus after passing a narrow prostate commissure. In this situation, imprecise passage of a right angle forceps or vascular stapler could lead to tremendous bleeding from disruption of the venous complex at the prostatourethral junction. Also, the external striated sphincter is subject to damage [30] (Fig. 1.14).

Urethral–Sphincter Complex

Just like the anatomy of the NVB, that of the male urethral sphincters is controversial. However, findings from recent studies have shed more light on this subject.

The urethral sphincter comprises of two muscle layers—an outer striated muscle layer commonly known as the external urethral sphincter or

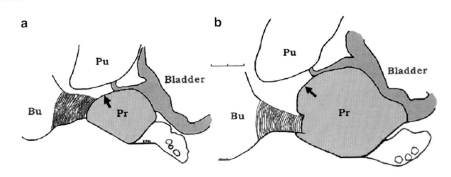

Fig. 1.14 Avascular plane. Variable distance in sagittal plane from detrusor apron's pubic attachment to prostateurethral junction: (**a**) 1.3-cm avascular plane (*arrow*) of small prostate contrasted with (**b**) 2.5-cm avascular plane (*arrow*) of 90-g prostate with BPH. Scaled reconstruction from sagittal magnetic resonance images with inset 2-cm ruler between images. *Bu* bulb, *Pr* prostate, *Pu* pubis. Reprinted from Myers RP. Detrusor apron, associated vascular plexus, and avascular plane: relevance to radical retropubic prostatectomy—anatomic and surgical commentary. Urology 2002;59(4):472–9, with permission from Elsevier

rhabosphincter, and an inner smooth muscle layer known as the internal urethral sphincter or *lissosphincter.*

External Urethral Sphincter (EUS)

The striated external urethra sphincter has been described as horseshoe or omega shaped. This is nicely illustrated in the 3D reconstructions in foetal cadavers by Wallner et al. [69]. They showed that at the prostate level, the superior part of the striated EUS is largely confined to the anterior side of the urethra and prostate. Inferior to the prostate, the EUS is horseshoe-shaped with the opening on the dorsal side. The dorsal muscle fibres of the left and right sides approach the midline and sometimes cross it.

Initially, it was thought that the EUS composed solely of slow twitch fibres, indicating that the external urethral sphincter is functionally adapted to maintain tone over prolonged periods, which suggests a passive function in urinary continence [70]. However, later work by Schroder [71], then Tokunaka [72] have shown that while type 1 slow twitch fibres predominate in the EUS, fast twitch fibres can constitute up to 61 % of muscle fibres.

Koratim proposes that the external urethral sphincter has a dual genitourinary function [73]. He proposed that fast twitch muscles (which are only capable of briefly sustained activity lasting only a few seconds) predominate at the caudal part of the EUS and are thus responsible for rapid forceful urethral closure during active continence, as they contract against the fixed posterior median raphe, resulting in collapse of the anterior urethral wall against the posterior wall. The rigid posterior plate comprised of Denonvilliers' fascia and the rectourethralis muscle, against which compression of the anterior urethral wall might increase the surface area of coaptation; thus, creating a higher urethral resistance.

On the other hand, the arrangement of muscle fibres on the anterior aspect of the prostate would only allow a side to side compression of the prostatic urethra, which is not sufficient to produce continence but could result in antegrade propulsion of semen in the presence of a closed vesical orifice (Fig. 1.15).

Inner Urethral Sphincter (IUS)

The IUS is an inner layer of smooth involuntary muscle that is thickest at the bladder neck and is thins out as courses distally in the urethra. It forms a complete cylinder of circular muscle fibres around the urethra and lies between the urethral mucosa and the striated external urethral muscle, making up the bulk of the urethral wall with connective and elastic tissue. It consists of a

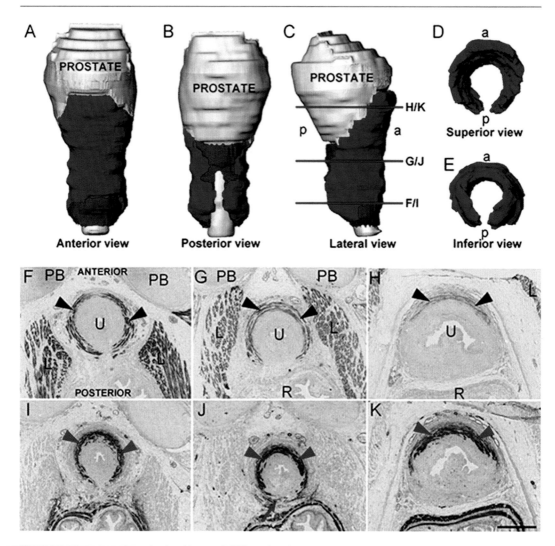

Fig. 1.15 The external urethral sphincter (EUS) and internal urethral sphincter (IUS) in a male foetus (12-week gestation). Three-dimensional reconstruction in (**a**) anterior view, (**b**) posterior view, (**c**) right-lateral view, (**d**) superior view and (**e**) inferior view. The EUS is shown in *blue*, and the IUS is shown in *pink*. The urethra and prostate are shown in *light grey*. Anterior and posterior directions are represented by the letters "a" and "p." Immunohistochemically stained sections: Sections from inferior (**f**) to superior (**h**) stained immunohistochemically for striated muscle, showing the EUS (*black arrowheads*). Panels (**i**) through (**k**) are from same level as sections (**f**) through (**h**), stained immunohistochemically for smooth muscle, showing the IUS (*red arrowheads*). Note the smooth muscle tissue at the dorsal side of the urethra, where the striated muscle of the external sphincter is lacking; see *red arrow* in (**j**). *Red lines* in (**c**) illustrate the level of the sections as seen in (**f**) through (**h**). L = levator ani muscle, PB = pubic bone, R = rectum, U = urethra, bar = 0.5 mm. Reprinted from Wallner C, Dabhoiwala NF, DeRuiter MC, et al. The anatomical components of urinary continence. Eur Urol 2009; 55:932–943, with permission from Elsevier

distinct layer of longitudinal smooth muscle surrounded by a wider layer of circular smooth muscle. The lissosphincter maintains continence at rest by contraction of its circular muscle fibres, resulting in closure of the vesical orifice and concentric narrowing of the posterior urethra. Maximum closure may be assumed to be at the level of the vesical orifice, where the lissosphincter is thickest, and in the membranous urethra, where the urethra is most narrow. Contraction of the longitudinal fibres widens the urethra during the evacuation of urine [73].

Complete preservation is not necessary for continence, as passive continence may be accomplished by preserving a minimal length of smooth muscle sphincter postoperatively as demonstrated in patients after posterior urethroplasty [74] or prostatectomy [75], respectively.

This could be a second rationale for better continence results after RP hypothesized in patients with longer membranous urethras.

Relationship of Sphincters to Pelvic Floor

Wallner et al. [69] investigated the relationship of the external urinary sphincter with the muscular pelvic floor in male foetal and adult cadaveric pelves and found that the striated sphincter has no attachments to the levator ani muscle. Yucel and Baskin in their earlier work on three-dimensional reconstructions of male foetal anatomy also showed that the levator ani does not completely encircle the urethra [76]. They showed that while the rectourethralis muscle and the aperture of the horseshoe-shaped external urinary sphincter were in juxtaposition, the levator ani muscles were separated from the external urinary sphincter muscle by a distinct layer of connective tissue.

Both sets of investigators hypothesized that the continence mechanism in the male is based on the external sphincter complex in isolation, without any support of the levator ani muscle. These observations support the principle that as much sphincter tissue as possible should be preserved during radical prostatectomy to improve postoperative continence outcomes.

This hypothesis is supported by observations published previously that showed better continence results in patients with longer postoperative urethral length [77].

The Urogenital Diaphragm Does Not Exist

Many anatomy and surgical textbooks propagate the concept of an external sphincter contained within the urogenital diaphragm, consisting of two aponeuroses containing the deep transverse perineal muscle. Mirilas and Skandalakis have reviewed the history behind this erroneous concept and the reassessment disproving it [78]. Dorscher using histomorphology and MRI studies proved that the so-called deep transverse perineal muscle does not exist and that the external sphincter is an independent anatomical unit completely separated from the surrounding musculature of the pelvic floor by connective tissue [79].

Innervation of the Membranous Urethra

Autonomic Innervation of the IUS

It is generally accepted that the smooth muscle of the IUS has an autonomic innervation from the pelvic plexus. Karam et al. have confirmed this with their histologic and immunohistologic 3D reconstruction of the nerves of the male urethra [80]. They showed that unmyelinated fibres (indicating autonomic postganglionic fibres) and some myelinated nerves (possible sensory afferents) innervated the submucosal and smooth muscles of the IUS.

Somatic Innervation of the EUS

Hollabaugh [8] and Song [6] have shown that the rhabdosphincter received dual somatic innervation via the extrapelvic perineal/dorsal penile nerve and the intrapelvic branch of the pudendal nerve.

Takenaka [10] and Narayana [7] estimated a 3–13 mm distance from the prostatic apex to the point where the nearest pudendal neural branch enters the sphincter. These branches penetrate the rhabdosphincter laterally at 3 and 9 o'clock [9].

Preserving these branches may be important for postoperative urinary continence, thus, it seems prudent to limit the distal dissection of the membranous urethra [81].

Does the Rhabdosphincter Have Autonomic Innervation?

There is controversy in the literature regarding whether there is an autonomic component to the innervation of the rhabdosphincter.

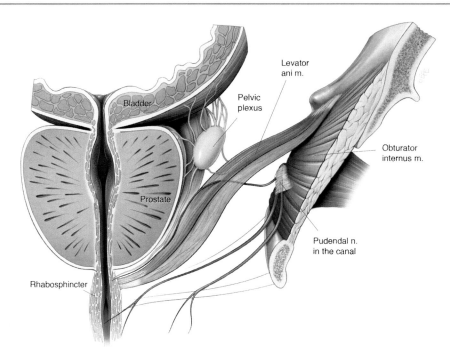

Fig. 1.16 Branches from the pelvic plexus and pudendal nerve supplying the rhabdosphincter

Some groups have found that it is innervated by autonomic branches of the pelvic plexus. These autonomic nerves run partly in close proximity to the NVB [6] and partly along branches of the pudendal nerve [8] (Fig. 1.16).

Unlike the nerve sparing for potency, in which the NVB is deliberately dissected away from the prostate, these nerves to the rhabdosphincter are spared by avoiding injury to them during the prostate apical dissection and the vesicourethral anastomosis [82].

We did not find similar branches in our cadaveric dissections [15]. Furthermore, in the same experiment described earlier, Karam et al. [80] showed that the rhabdosphincter was innervated solely by myelinated fibres, the majority of which entered at the 3 and 9 o'clock positions—thus precluding postganglionic autonomic innervation.

More importantly, since autonomic nerves do not control striated muscles, any autonomic supply to the rhabosphincter is likely sensory in nature. However, preservation of sensation is important as shown by a group from Brazil [83].

They performed prospective neurophysiological studies of men who underwent nerve-sparing radical prostatectomies. All the men had preserved afferent and efferent pudendal innervation. Autonomic afferent denervation at the membranous urethra mucosa was found in more than 90 % of men with urinary incontinence. In comparison, 80 % of men who were continent had preserved autonomic afferent innervation. Afferent innervation to the urethra is essential for its guarding reflex activity. Thus the authors hypothesized that patients with denervated membranous urethral mucosa were unable to detect urine drops which reached the membranous urethra to trigger the rhabdosphincter reflex contraction to prevent urinary leakage via the guarding reflex, which is a hypogastric-pelvic autonomic nervous system reflex. After urine reaches the intact sensory innervation at the bulbar urethra patients become aware of the imminent leakage, which triggers a voluntary sphincter contraction. However, at this point urine has crossed the functional sphincteric urethral area and cannot be contained, manifesting as occasional urine leakage. Thus, preservation of the autonomic urethral innervation correlates with the nonexistence of occasional urine leakage.

There is controversy in the literature in relation to the role of NVB preservation in recovery of urinary continence [84, 85]. Although it is unclear whether preservation of the NVBs themselves or the meticulous dissection required to dissect the nerves from the apex of the prostate is responsible for the improvement in continence after "nerve-sparing" surgery, every effort should be made to preserve those nerve fibres as long as oncologic safety is not compromised.

Pubovesical (Puboprostatic) Ligaments

The popularly known puboprostatic ligaments are in reality pubovesical ligaments. As in the woman, detrusor muscle in the man extends to its pubic attachment within pubovesical ligaments. In men, as the prostate grows, the pubovesical ligaments take on the appearance of puboprostatic ligaments. This illusion is especially so with the emergence of BPH [30].

The bladder does not end at the bladder neck but continues as the detrusor apron draping the anterior prostate. Dorschner and associates demonstrated histologically this smooth muscle extension of the bladder to the pubis anterior to the prostate, thus confirming the continuity of ligaments with the bladder not prostate [86]. Because there is demonstrable anatomic continuity with the bladder, pubovesical (puboprostatic) sparing retropubic prostatectomy previously meant that the puboprostatic ligaments were disconnected proximally closer to the prostate instead of disarticulation at their junction with the pubis [87]. However, Gaston [88] and Stolzenburg [89] have shown that truly pubovesical ligament sparing retropubic prostatectomy is possible and may improve continence outcomes.

In the perineal operation, the prostate can be dissected out from underneath the overlying detrusor apron and venous plexus, thereby entirely avoiding these ligaments [90, 91].

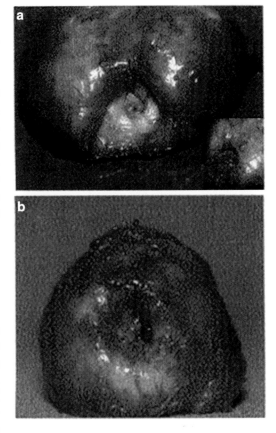

Fig. 1.17 Contrasting prostate apices. (**a**) Apical notch of cadaveric "croissant" prostate. Note veru. Same prostate with urethra intact to show its insertion into the notch (*Inset*). (**b**) "Doughnut," or toroidal, apex of radical prostatectomy specimen with no notch configuration. Reprinted from Myers RP. Practical Surgical Anatomy for Radical Prostatectomy. Urologic Clinics of North America 2001; 28(3), with permission from Elsevier

Variability of Prostate Apex and Impact on Preservation of Urethral Length

The prostate apex is the location with the highest incidence of margin positivity after radical prostatectomy. However aggressive apical dissection may compromise urethral length and consequent continence outcomes.

The shape of the prostate at the apex may vary substantially, directly influencing the length of the urethra after emerging from the apex. Myers described two basic prostatic shapes, distinguished by the presence or absence of an anterior apical notch [92] (Fig. 1.17).

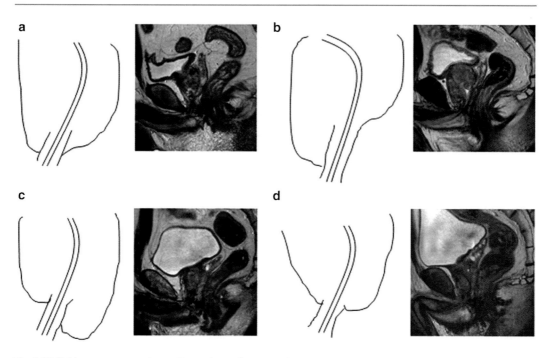

Fig. 1.18 Subjects were grouped according to shape of prostatic apex observed on mid-sagittal MRI scan: (**a**) apex overlapping membranous urethra both anteriorly and posteriorly; (**b**) apex overlapping membranous urethra anteriorly; (**c**) apex overlapping membranous urethra posteriorly; and (**d**) no overlapping observed between apex and membranous urethra. Reprinted from Lee SE, Byun SS, Lee HJ, et al. Impact of variations in prostatic apex shape on early recovery of urinary continence after radical retropubic prostatectomy. Urology 2006;68:137–41, with permission from Elsevier

Lee et al. observed circumferential overlap of the apex observed in 38 % of all cases, anterior overlap in 25 %, posterior overlap in 22 % and no overlap in 15 % (Fig. 1.18). Importantly, they noted the group with no overlap had a better rate of early return of continence (83.3 %) compared to the other groups with overlap (66.7 %) [93].

The shape of the prostate apex and overlap with the membranous urethra should be considered during apical dissection in order to preserve maximal urethral length without compromising oncological outcomes.

References

1. Schwalenberg T, Hohenfellner R, Neuhaus J, Winkler MH, Liatsikos EN, Stolzenburg JU. Surgical anatomy for radical prostatectomy. In: Stolzenburg JU, Gettman MT, Liatsikos EN, editors. Endoscopic extraperitoneal radical prostatectomy. Berlin Heidelberg: Springer; 2007. p. 12–9.
2. Mauroy B, Demondion X, Drizenko A, Goullet E, Bonnal JL, Biserte JAC. The inferior hypogastric plexus (pelvic plexus): its importance in neural preservation techniques. Surg Radiol Anat. 2003;25(1): 6–15.
3. Baader B, Herrmann M. Topography of the pelvic autonomic nervous system and its potential impact on surgical intervention in the pelvis. Clin Anat. 2003;16(2):119–30.
4. Hruby S, Ebmer J, Dellon AL, Aszmann OC. Anatomy of pudendal nerve at urogenital diaphragm-new critical site for nerve entrapment. Urology. 2005;66(5):949–52.
5. Yucel S, Baskin LS. Neuroanatomy of the male urethra and perineum. BJU Int. 2003;92(6):624–30.
6. Song LJ, Lu HK, Wang JP, Xu YM. Cadaveric study of nerves supplying the membranous urethra. Neurourol Urodyn. 2010;29(4):592–5.
7. Narayan P, Konety B, Aslam K, Aboseif S, Blumenfeld W, Tanagho E. Neuroanatomy of the external urethral sphincter: implications for urinary continence preservation during radical prostate surgery. J Urol. 1995; 153(2):337–41.
8. Hollabaugh R, Dmochowski R, Steiner M. Neuroanatomy of the male rhabdosphincter. Urology. 1997;49(3):426–35.
9. Shafik A, Doss S. Surgical anatomy of the somatic terminal innervation to the anal and urethral sphincters: role in anal and urethral surgery. J Urol. 1999;161(1):85–9.

10. Takenaka A, Hara R, Soga H, Murakami G, Fujisawa M. A novel technique for approaching the endopelvic fascia in retropubic radical prostatectomy, based on an anatomical study of fixed and fresh cadavers. BJU Int. 2005;95(6):766–71.

11. Gillitzer R, Hampel C, Wiesner C, Pahernik S, Melchior SW, Thüroff JW. Pudendal nerve branch injury during radical perineal prostatectomy. Urology. 2006;67(2):423.e1–3.

12. Benoit G, Droupy S, Quillard J, Paradis V, Giuliano F. Supra and infralevator neurovascular pathways to the penile corpora cavernosa. J Anat. 1999;195(Pt 4): 605–15.

13. Yucel S, Baskin LS. Identification of communicating branches among the dorsal, perineal and cavernous nerves of the penis. J Urol. 2003;170(1):153–8.

14. Alsaid B, Moszkowicz D, Peschaud F, Bessede T, Zaitouna M, Karam I, et al. Autonomic-somatic communications in the human pelvis: computer-assisted anatomic dissection in male and female fetuses. J Anat. 2011;219(5):565–73.

15. Costello AJ, Brooks M, Cole OJ. Anatomical studies of the neurovascular bundle and cavernosal nerves. BJU Int. 2004;94(7):1071–6.

16. Walsh PC, Donker PJ. Impotence following radical prostatectomy: insight into etiology and prevention. J Urol. 1982;128(3):492–7.

17. Kiyoshima K, Yokomizo A, Yoshida T, Tomita K, Yonemasu H, Nakamura M, et al. Anatomical features of periprostatic tissue and its surroundings: a histological analysis of 79 radical retropubic prostatectomy specimens. Jpn J Clin Oncol. 2004;34:463–8.

18. Eichelberg C, Erbersdobler A, Michl U, Schlomm T, Salomon G, Graefen M, et al. Nerve distribution along the prostatic capsule. Eur Urol. 2007;51(1): 105–11.

19. Lunacek A, Schwentner C, Fritsch H, Bartsch G, Strasser H. Anatomical radical retropubic prostatectomy: 'curtain dissection' of the neurovascular bundle. BJU Int. 2005;95(9):1226–31.

20. Takenaka A, Murakami G, Soga H, Han SH, Arai Y, Fujisawa M. Anatomical analysis of the neurovascular bundle supplying penile cavernous tissue to ensure a reliable nerve graft after radical prostatectomy. J Urol. 2004;172(3):1032–5.

21. Menon M, Shrivastava A, Kaul S, Badani KK, Fumo M, Bandari M, et al. Vattikuti Institute prostatectomy: contemporary technique and analysis of results. Eur Urol. 2007;51(3):648–58.

22. Costello AJ, Dowdle BW, Namdarian B, Pedersen J, Murphy DG. Immunohistochemical study of the cavernous nerves in the periprostatic region. BJU Int. 2010;107(8):1210–5.

23. Yucel S, Erdogru T, Baykara M. Recent neuroanatomical studies on the neurovascular bundle of the prostate and cavernosal nerves: clinical reflection on radical prostatectomy. Asian J Androl. 2005;7(4): 339–49.

24. Takenaka A, Murakami G, Matsubara A. Variation in course of cavernous nerve with special reference to details of topographic relationships near prostatic apex: histological study using male cadavers. Urology. 2005;65(1):136–42.

25. Clarebrough EE, Challacombe BJ, Briggs C, Namdarian B, Weston R, Murphy DG, et al. Cadaveric analysis of periprostatic nerve distribution: an anatomical basis for high anterior release during radical prostatectomy? J Urol. 2011;185(4):1519–25.

26. Ganzer R, Blana A, Gaumann A, Stolzenburg JU, Rabenalt R, Bach T, et al. Topographical anatomy of periprostatic and capsular nerves: quantification and computerised planimetry. Eur Urol. 2008;54(2): 353–60.

27. Ganzer R, Stolzenburg JU, Wieland WF, Brundl J. Anatomic study of periprostatic nerve distribution: immunohistochemical differentiation of parasympathetic and sympathetic nerve fibres. Eur Urol. 2012; 62(6):1150–6.

28. Kaiho Y, Nakagawa H, Saito H, Ito A, Ishidoya S, Saito S, et al. Nerves at the ventral prostatic capsule contribute to erectile function: initial electrophysiological assessment in humans. Eur Urol. 2009;55(1): 148–55.

29. Hinata N, Sejima T, Takenaka A. Progress in pelvic anatomy from the viewpoint of radical prostatectomy. Int J Urol. 2013;20(3):260–70.

30. Myers RP. Practical surgical anatomy for radical prostatectomy. Urol Clin North Am. 2001;28(3):473–90.

31. Secin FP, Touijer K, Karanikolas NT, Raj GV, Guillonneau B. Laparoscopic radical prostatectomy: lessons learned in surgical technique. Eur Urol. 2006;5:942–9.

32. Myers RP, Villers A. Anatomic considerations in radical prostatectomy. In: Kirby RS, Partin AW, Feneley M, Parsons JK, editors. Prostate cancer; principles and practice, vol. 1. Abingdon, UK: Taylor & Francis; 2006. p. 701–13.

33. Stolzenburg JU, Schwalenberg T, Horn LC, Neuhaus J, Constantinides C, Liatsikos EN. Anatomical landmarks of radical prostatectomy. Eur Urol. 2007;51(3): 629–39.

34. Tewari A, Peabody JO, Fischer M, Sarle R, Vallancien G, Delmas V, et al. An operative and anatomic study to help in nerve sparing during laparoscopic and robotic radical prostatectomy. Eur Urol. 2003;43(5): 444–54.

35. Walsh PC, Partin AW. Anatomic radical retropubic prostatectomy. In: Wein AJ, Kavoussi LR, Peters CA, Novick AC, Partin AW, editors. Campbell-walsh urology, vol. 3. Philadelphia, PA: Elsevier Health Sciences; 2006. p. 2956–78.

36. Graefen M, Walz J, Huland H. Open retropubic nerve-sparing radical prostatectomy. Eur Urol. 2006;49(1): 38–48.

37. Budaüus L, Isbarn H, Schlomm T, Heinzer H, Haese A, Stueber T, et al. Current technique of open intrafascial nerve-sparing retropubic prostatectomy. Eur Urol. 2009;56(2):317–24.

38. Menon M, Kaul S, Bhandari A, Shrivastava A, Tewari A, Hemal A. Potency following robotic radical

prostatectomy: a questionnaire based analysis of outcomes after conventional nerve sparing and prostatic fascia sparing techniques. J Urol. 2005;174(6): 2291–6.

39. Secin FP, Serio A, Bianco Jr FJ, Karanikolas NT, Kuriowa K, Vickers A, et al. Preoperative and intraoperative risk factors for side-specific positive surgical margins in laparoscopic radical prostatectomy for prostate cancer. Eur Urol. 2007;51(3):764–71.

40. Walz J, Burnett AL, Costello AJ, Eastham JA, Graefen M, Guillonneau B, et al. A critical analysis of the current knowledge of surgical anatomy related to optimization of cancer control and preservation of continence and erection in candidates for radical prostatectomy. Eur Urol. 2010;57(2):179–92.

41. Denonvilliers C. Propositions et observation d'anatomie, de physiologie at de pathologie. These De l'Ecole De Medicine. 1837;285:23.

42. Fritsch H, Lienemann A, Brenner E, Ludwikowski B. Clinical anatomy of the pelvic floor. Adv Anat Embryol Cell Biol. 2004;175:III–IX. 1–64.

43. Villers A, McNeal JE, Freiha FS, Boccon-Gibod L, Stamey TA. Invasion of Denonvilliers' fascia in radical prostatectomy specimens. J Urol. 1993;149: 793–8.

44. Lindsey I, Warren BF, Mortensen NJ. Denonvilliers' fascia lies anterior to the fascia propria and rectal dissection plane in total mesorectal excision. Dis Colon Rectum. 2005;48(1):37–42.

45. Lindsey I, Guy RJ, Warren BF, Mortensen NJ. Anatomy of Denonvilliers' fascia and pelvic nerves, impotence, and implications for the colorectal surgeon. Br J Surg. 2000;87(10):1288–99.

46. Kinugasa Y, Murakami G, Uchimoto K, Takenaka A, Yajima T, Sugihara K. Operating behind Denonvilliers' fascia for reliable preservation of urogenital autonomic nerves in totalmesorectal excision: a histologic study using cadavericspecimens, including a surgical experiment using fresh cadaveric models. Dis Colon Rectum. 2006;49(7):1024–32.

47. Secin FP, Karanikolas N, Gopalan A, Bianco FJ, Shayegan B, Touijer K, et al. The anterior layer of Denonvilliers' fascia: a common misconception in the laparoscopic prostatectomy literature. J Urol. 2007; 177(2):521–5.

48. Dorschner W, Stolzenburg JU. A new theory of micturition and urinary continence based on histomorphological studies. The two parts of the musculus sphincter urethrae: physiological importance for continence in rest and stress. Urol Int. 1994;52(4): 185–8.

49. Rocco F, Carmignani L, Acquati P, Gadda F, Dell'Orto P, Rocco B, et al. Restoration of posterior aspect of rhabdshpincter shortens continence time after radical retropubic prostatectomy. J Urol. 2006;175(6): 2201–6.

50. Ayala AG, Ro JY, Babaian R, Troncoso P, Grignon DJ. The prostatic capsule: does it exist? Its importance in the staging and treatment of prostatic carcinoma. Am J Surg Pathol. 1989;13(1):21–7.

51. Savera AT, Kaul S, Badani K, Stark AT, Shah NL, Menon M. Robotic radical prostatectomy with the "veil of Aphrodite" technique: histologic evidence of enhanced nerve sparing. Eur Urol. 2006;49:1065–74.

52. Flocks RH. The arterial distribution within the prostate gland: its role in transurethral prostate resection. J Urol. 1937;37:524–48.

53. Rosen MP, Greenfield AJ, Walker TG, Grant P, Guben JK, Dubrow J, et al. Arteriogenic impotence: findings in 195 impotent men examined with selective internal pudendal angiography. Radiology. 1990;174(3pt2): 1043–8.

54. Rogers CG, Trock BP, Walsh PC. Preservation of accessory pudendal arteries during radical retropubic prostatectomy: surgical technique and results. Urology. 2004;64(1):148–51.

55. Secin FP, Karanikolas N, Touijer AK, Salamanca JI, Vickers AJ, Guillonneau B. Anatomy of accessory pudendal arteries in laparoscopic radical prostatectomy. J Urol. 2005;174(2):523–6.

56. Mulhall JP, Slovick R, Hotaling J, Aviv N, Valenzuela R, Waters WB, et al. Erectile dysfunction after radical prostatectomy: hemodynamic profiles and their correlation with the recovery of erectile function. J Urol. 2002;167(3):1371–5.

57. Secin FP, Touijer K, Mulhall J, Guillonneau B. Anatomy and preservation of accessory pudendal arteries in laparoscopic radical prostatectomy. Eur Urol. 2007;51(5):1229–35.

58. Polascik TJ, Walsh PC. Radical retropubic prostatectomy: the influence of accessory pudendal arteries on the recovery of sexual function. J Urol. 1995;154(1): 150–2.

59. Matin SF. Recognition and preservation of accessory pudendal arteries during laparoscopic radical prostatectomy. Urology. 2006;67(5):1012–5.

60. Park BJ, Sung DJ, Kim MJ, Cho SB, Kim YH, Chung KB, et al. The incidence and anatomy of accessory pudendal arteries as depicted on multidetector-row CT angiography: clinical implications of preoperative evaluation for laparoscopic and robot-assisted radical prostatectomy. Korean J Radiol. 2009;10(6):587–95.

61. Droupy S, Hessel A, Benoit G, Blanchet P, Jardin A, Giuliano F. Assessment of the functional role of accessory pudendal arteries in erection by transrectal color Doppler ultrasound. J Urol. 1999;162(6): 1987–91.

62. Nehra A, Kumar R, Ramakumar S, Myers RP, Blute ML, McKusick MA. Pharmacoangiographic evidence of the presence and anatomical dominance of accessory pudendal artery(s). J Urol. 2008;179(6): 2317–20.

63. Droupy S, Benoit G, Guliano F, Jardin A. Penile arteries in humans – origins, distribution, variations. Surg Radiol Anat. 1997;19(3):161–7.

64. Myers RP. Anatomical variation of the superficial preprostatic veins with respect to radical retropubic prostatectomy. J Urol. 1991;145(5):992–3.

65. Gontero P, Marchioro G, Maso G, Tizzani A, Frea B. Cadaveric anatomy of structures related to the prostate.

In: Kirby R, Montorsi F, Gontero P, Smith Jr JA, editors. Radical prostatectomy: from open to robotic. UK: Informa Healthcare; 2007. p. 11–22.

66. Power NE, Siberstein JL, Kulkarni GS, Laudone VP. The dorsal venous complex (DVC): dorsal venous or dorsal vasculature complex? Santorini's plexus revisited. BJU Int. 2011;108(6):930–2.

67. Myers RP. Detrusor apron, associated vascular plexus, and avascular plane: relevance to radical retropubic prostatectomy—anatomic and surgical commentary. Urology. 2002;59(4):472–9.

68. Reiner WG, Walsh PC. An anatomical approach to the surgical management of the dorsal vein and Santorini's plexus during radical retropubic surgery. J Urol. 1979;121(2):198–200.

69. Wallner C, Dabhoiwala NF, DeRuiter MC, Lamers WH. The anatomical components of urinary continence. Eur Urol. 2009;55(4):932–43.

70. Gosling JA, Dixon JS, Critchley HO, Thompson SA. A comparative study of the human external sphincter and periurethral levator ani muscles. Br J Urol. 1981;53(1):35–41.

71. Schroder HD, Reske-Nielsen E. Fiber types in the striated urethral and anal sphincters. Acta Neuropathol. 1983;60(3–4):278–82.

72. Tokunaka S, Okamura K, Fujii H, Yachiku S. The proportions of fiber types in human external urethral sphincter: electrophoretic analysis of myosin. Urol Res. 1990;18(5):341–4.

73. Koraitim MM. The male urethral sphincter complex revisited: an anatomical concept and its physiological correlate. J Urol. 2008;179(5):1683–9.

74. Koraitim MM, Atta MA, Fattah GA, Ismail HR. Mechanism of continence after repair of post-traumatic posterior urethral strictures. Urology. 2003;61(2):287–90.

75. Gudziak MR, McGuire EJ, Gormley EA. Urodynamic assessment of urethral sphincter function in post-prostatectomy incontinence. J Urol. 1996;156(3):1131–4.

76. Yucel S, Baskin LS. An anatomical description of the male and female urethral sphincter complex. J Urol. 2004;171(5):1890–7.

77. Paparel P, Akin O, Sandhu JS, Otero JR, Serio AM, Scardino PT, et al. Recovery of urinary continence after radical prostatectomy: association with urethral length and urethral fibrosis measured by preoperative and postoperative endorectal magnetic resonance imaging. Eur Urol. 2009;55(3):629–37.

78. Mirilas P, Skandalakis JE. Urogenital diaphragm: an erroneous concept casting its shadow over the sphincter urethrae and deep perineal space. J Am Coll Surg. 2004;198(2):279–90.

79. Dorschner W, Biesold M, Schmidt F, Stolzenburg JU. The dispute about the external sphincter and the urogenital diaphragm. J Urol. 1999;162(6):1942–5.

80. Karam I, Droupy S, Abd-Alsamad I, Korbage A, Uhl JF, Benoit G, et al. The precise location and nature of the nerves to the male human urethra: histological and immunohistochemical studies with three-dimensional reconstruction. Eur Urol. 2005;48(5):858–64.

81. Burnett AL, Mostwin JL. In situ anatomical study of the male urethral sphincteric complex: relevance to continence preservation following major pelvic surgery. J Urol. 1998;160(4):1301–6.

82. Steiner MS. Continence-preserving anatomic radical retropubic prostatectomy. Urology. 2000;55(3):427–35.

83. Catarin MV, Manzano GM, Nóbrega JA, Almeida FG, Srougi M, Bruschini H. The role of membranous urethral afferent autonomic innervation in the continence mechanism after nerve sparing radical prostatectomy: a clinical and prospective study. J Urol. 2008;180(6):2527–31.

84. Burkhard FC, Kessler TM, Fleischmann A, Tharmann GN, Schumacher M, Studer UE. Nerve sparing open radical retropubic prostatectomy—does it have an impact on urinary continence? J Urol. 2006;176(1):189–95.

85. Marien TP, Lepor H. Does a nerve-sparing technique or potency affect continence after open radical retropubic prostatectomy? BJU Int. 2008;102(11):1581–4.

86. Dorschner W, Stolzenburg JU, Leutert G. A new theory of micturition and urinary continence based on histomorphological studies. 1. The musculus detrusor vesicae: occlusive function or support of micturition? Urol Int. 1994;52(2):61–4.

87. Poore RE, McCullough DL, Jarow JP. Puboprostatic ligament sparing improves urinary continence after radical retropubic prostatectomy. Urology. 1998;51(1):67–72.

88. Asimakopoulos AD, Annino F, D'Orazio A, Pereira CF, Mugnier C, Hoepffner JL, et al. Complete periprostatic anatomy preservation during robot-assisted laparoscopic radical prostatectomy (RALP): the new pubovesical complex-sparing technique. Eur Urol. 2010;58(3):407–17.

89. Stolzenburg JU, Liatsikos EN, Rabenalt R, Do M, Sakelaropoulos G, Horn LC, et al. Nerve sparing endoscopic extraperitoneal radical prostatectomy–effect of puboprostatic ligament preservation on early continence and positive margins. Eur Urol. 2006;49(1):103–11.

90. Hinman F,editor. Total perineal prostatectomy. In: Atlas of urologic surgery. USA: WB Saunders; 1998. p. 451–64.

91. Wimpissinger TF, Tschabitscher M, Feichtinger MH, Stackl W. Surgical anatomy of the puboprostatic complex with special reference to radical perineal prostatectomy. BJU Int. 2003;92(7):681–4.

92. Myers RP, Goellner JR, Cahill DR. Prostate shape, external striated urethral sphincter and radical prostatectomy: the apical dissection. J Urol. 1987;138(3):543–50.

93. Lee SE, Byun SS, Lee HJ, Song SH, Chang IH, Kim YJ, et al. Impact of variations in prostatic apex shape on early recovery of urinary continence after radical retropubic prostatectomy. Urology. 2006;68(1):137–41.

Anesthetic Considerations: Open Versus Minimally Invasive Surgery

Anahita Dabo-Trubelja and Eric R. Kelhoffer

Preoperative Evaluation

As the age of patients undergoing urology procedures increases, there is increased morbidity and mortality [1–4]. A preanesthesia evaluation is a basic component of anesthesia care and has multiple purposes. This includes gathering the patient's history and physical examination, prior medical records, and preoperative testing. In addition, a detailed cardiac risk assessment, airway and pulmonary risks, metabolic, endocrine, infectious and anticoagulation risks are obtained, along with the anesthesia risk classification and an underlying specific procedure related risks, as that will influence the choice of anesthesia technique [5, 6].

The preoperative assessment represents a specific opportunity to identify a medical/anesthetic issue that should be further evaluated with a specific diagnostic test and intervention which if not performed would impact outcome. In a low-risk patient group it is extremely difficult to link the value of a preoperative test to morbidity and mortality [7]. Therefore, we look in this low-risk patient population at the benefit of more testing and for general outcomes such as costs, resource utilization, hospital length of stay, and patient

satisfaction [8]. In the high-risk population, however, we have a number of studies to better assess anesthetic risk that directly affect outcomes such as MI, stroke, death, and length of stay. The merit of preoperative testing rests in compiling and analyzing data to improve the efficacy of the perioperative process [2]. The ultimate goal of preoperative testing is to reduce perioperative morbidity and mortality and have the patient back to a normal routine as soon as possible. We should ask ourselves what tests should be ordered, is the patient in optimal medical condition for surgery, and what can be done to improve the patient's medical status to improve outcomes? Does the patient need further testing? What are the risks of anesthesia and surgery for the patient? Guidelines for preoperative evaluation help us identify which patients are at increased risk for preoperative morbidity and mortality independent of those associated with surgery and for the future new paradigms which would decrease additional preoperative risks [9–11].

Preoperative History and Physical Examination

Preoperative evaluation should begin with a history and physical examination several weeks prior to surgery. The indication for surgery should be noted as this determines the urgency of the surgery, the risks associated with the particular surgery, as well as the risk to the patient in relation to the patient's acute and chronic

A. Dabo-Trubelja, M.D. • E.R. Kelhoffer, M.D. (✉)
Anesthesiology and Critical Care, Memorial Sloan Kettering Cancer Center, Weil Cornell Medical College, 1275 York Ave., C330, New York, NY 10065, USA
e-mail: kelhoffe@mskcc.org

medical conditions. The patient's history regarding prior anesthetics should be obtained in order to determine the presence of a difficult airway, any prior problems with anesthesia, a history of malignant hyperthermia, and the patient's individual response to the surgical stress in the preoperative period. Whenever possible the patient's prior anesthesia records should be reviewed. Allergies to medications and their reactions should be noted. The history should also include the patient medications in order to best define a preoperative regimen: doses may need to be adjusted and potential drug interactions need to be considered. Functional status should be evaluated as well as the patient's social support and need for assistance once discharged from the hospital. Once we have identified all these issues, we can focus on specific organ systems [1, 12].

Cardiac Evaluation

Cardiovascular disease remains the leading cause of death in the United States. Cardiac patients experience more overall perioperative complications with cardiac issues the most common complications that threaten a patient's life and prolonged patient's hospital length of stay. A detailed cardiovascular history is critical to the appropriate preoperative assessment of a patient's surgical risk.

The ASA classification of physical status stratifies risk based on the patient's medical history. The ASA classification of physical status was first developed in 1941 by Drs. Saklad and Rovenstine and modified in 1963 to its present day classification [11, 13–16] (Table 2.1).

Risk factors for cardiac complications have long been known. In 1977, Lee Goldman, M.D. attempted to stratify cardiac risk for patients undergoing non-cardiac surgery. He evaluated patients based on risk factors known as the Goldman Cardiac Risk Index or CRI and assigned each a point. Adding up the total points assesses the probability of risk for perioperative cardiac morbidity and mortality. Subsequent studies have shown that some surgical procedures carry minimal risk, while others have excessive

Table 2.1 ASA physical classification system [14]

ASA physical status 1—A normal healthy patient

ASA physical status 2—A patient with mild systemic disease

ASA physical status 3—A patient with severe systemic disease

ASA physical status 4—A patient with severe systemic disease that is a constant threat to life

ASA physical status 5—A moribund patient who is not expected to survive without the operation

ASA physical status 6—A declared brain-dead patient whose organs are being removed for donor purposes

risk which this index does not take into account. The American Cardiology College (ACC) and American Heart Association (AHA) have expanded this assessment to include risk associated with a particular surgical procedure as well as patient characteristics that influence perioperative cardiac morbidity and mortality [17–19] (Fig. 2.1 and Tables 2.2, 2.3, and 2.4).

The approach to the patient's cardiac assessment includes a detailed history of previous diagnoses of coronary artery disease (CAD), any prior cardiac interventions including previous cardiac testing, current therapies, symptoms associated with angina, or congestive heart failure and if the patient has a pacemaker and/or implantable cardioverter defibrillator [20]. It is important to identify any new or change in symptoms which may require a change in or initiation of new management that would be the cause of delay or cancellation of non-elective surgeries. Perioperative morbidity related to non-cardiac surgical procedures ranges from 1 to 5 % [20, 21].

Patient risk for CAD should be evaluated. Diabetics have a higher probability of CAD than nondiabetics. It is important in these patients to determine the length of disease and the degree of end-organ dysfunction as they have a higher association of silent myocardial ischemia and myocardial infarction. Diabetes has been shown to be an independent risk factor for cardiac morbidity in the perioperative period [22, 23].

Hypertension has also been associated with cardiac morbidity in the perioperative period. An EKG that shows left ventricular hypertrophy with a strain pattern suggests a chronic ischemic state.

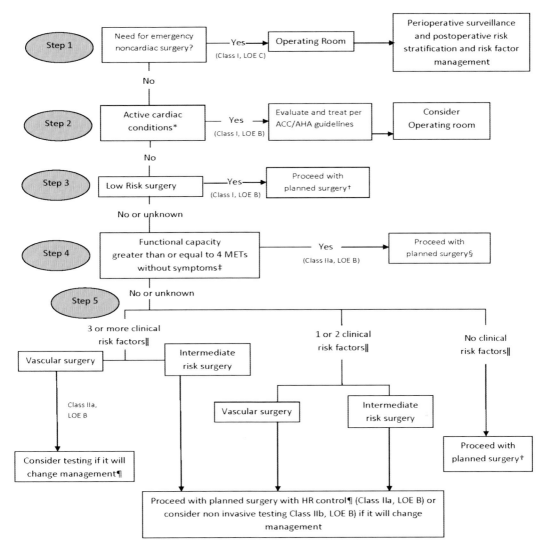

Fig. 2.1 Cardiac evaluation and care. ACC/AHA indicates American College of Cardiology and American Heart Association, *HR* heart rate, *LOE* level of evidence, and *MET* metabolic equivalent. From Fleisher et al. [19]. Reprinted with permission from Wolters Kluwer Health

Therefore, these patients are considered at a higher risk for perioperative cardiac morbidity. Hypertension should be aggressively treated as this has been shown to improve long-term risk [5, 24].

Assessing the need for further cardiac evaluation is based on the patient's clinical risk predictive factors gathered from the preoperative evaluation and the risk associated with the particular surgery [25]. Possible intervention is based on the recommendation that only if the patient would benefit regardless of any planned non-cardiac surgery [23, 26].

Pulmonary Evaluation

Pulmonary dysfunction is the most common perioperative complication. A thorough assessment of the pulmonary status of the patient prior to surgery is essential as the impact on respiratory dysfunction is predictable. The failure to recognize patients who are at increased risk of perioperative pulmonary dysfunction may have significant morbidity and mortality. Failure to recognize can impact patient care intraoperatively;

Table 2.2 Goldman revised cardiac risk index [17, 19]

1. History of ischemic heart disease
2. History of congestive heart failure
3. History of cerebrovascular disease (stroke or transient ischemic attack)
4. History of diabetes requiring preoperative insulin use
5. Chronic kidney disease (creatinine >2 mg/dL)
6. Undergoing suprainguinal vascular, intraperitoneal, or intrathoracic surgery

Risk for cardiac death, nonfatal myocardial infarction, and nonfatal cardiac arrest: 0 predictors = 0.4 %, 1 predictor = 1 %, 2 predictors = 2.4 %, ≥3 predictors = 5.4 %
From Fleisher et al. [19]. Reprinted with permission from Wolters Kluwer Health
And from McGuirt JK [17]. Reprinted with permission from Elsevier Limited

Table 2.3 Cardiac risk stratification for non-cardiac surgery

High (reported cardiac risk often greater than 5 %)
• Emergent major operations, particularly in the elderly
• Aortic and other major vascular surgery
• Peripheral vascular surgery
• Anticipated prolonged surgical procedures associated with large fluid shifts and/or blood loss
Intermediate (reported cardiac risk generally less than 5 %)
• Carotid endarterectomy
• Head and neck surgery
• Intraperitoneal and intrathoracic surgery
• Orthopedic surgery
• Prostate surgery
Low (reported cardiac risk generally less than 1 %)
• Endoscopic procedures
• Superficial procedure
• Cataract surgery
• Breast surgery

From Eagle et al. [23]. Reprinted with permission from Wolters Kluwer Heath

Table 2.4 Estimated energy requirements for various activities

Estimated energy	Activity
1 MET	Self-care
	Eating, dressing, or using the toilet
	Walking indoors and around the house
	Walking one to two blocks on level ground at 2–3 mph
4 METs	Light housework (e.g., dusting, washing dishes)
	Climbing a flight of stairs or walking up a hill
	Walking on level ground at 4 mph
	Running a short distance
	Heavy housework (e.g., scrubbing floors, moving heavy furniture)
	Moderate recreational activities (e.g., golf, dancing, doubles tennis, throwing a baseball or football)
Greater than 10 METs	Strenuous sports (e.g., swimming, singles tennis, football, basketball, skiing)

MET metabolic equivalent, *mph* miles per hour
From Fleisher et al. [19]. Reprinted with permission from Wolters Kluwer Health

the patient may develop bronchospasm, atelectasis, and pneumonia and may require postoperative mechanical ventilation.

The pulmonary evaluation should encompass a detailed history of the patient's pulmonary disease, type and severity, and possible reversibility. An account of the current medications used as well as steroid use, can be used to determine the proper perioperative regimen, and change in medication if necessary. The ASA has listed potential patient-related factors for the development of postoperative pulmonary complications. These include smoking, chronic obstructive pulmonary disease (COPD), obesity, ASA class >II, age >70, and prolonged general anesthesia >3 h. The patient should also be evaluated for obstructive sleep apnea and treatment instigated if necessary. This condition is associated with intermittent airway obstruction and increased difficult airway. Some patients have their own continuous positive airway pressure (CPAP) machine at home which they should bring for use in the postoperative setting. Patients should be evaluated for symptoms of cough, wheezing, dyspnea, productive sputum, as these patients may require further pulmonary testing. These may include chest radiograph, pulmonary function testing, arterial blood gas, and a preoperative pulmonary consult. There are no guidelines that define the degree of pulmonary function impairment that would prohibit surgery, except for lung resection. The pulmonary function tests that are associated with increased pulmonary complication in the perioperative period include; FEV1 <2 L, MVV <50 %, of predicted value, PEF <100 or 50 % of predicted value, pCO_2 ≥45 mmHg, and pO_2 ≤50 mmHg. Patients with known pulmonary disease should have their pulmonary function optimized before surgery. Careful consideration should be given to the choice of anesthesia, general vs. regional [5, 27].

Smoking is well known to increase risk in the perioperative period. The value for smoking cessation preoperatively has been evaluated. Cessation for 24 h prior to surgery has been shown to correlate with an improvement in hemoglobin, reduction in carbon monoxide, and improvement in oxygenation. Smoking cessation for more than 6 weeks has been shown to restore ciliary function back to baseline as well as improve oxygenation [9].

The patient with a recent upper respiratory infection poses a dilemma. If surgery is urgent or emergent then it should proceed. If surgery is elective the infection should be treated and surgery postponed. However the risk of delaying surgery should be weighed against the risk of proceeding with surgery at an increased risk of perioperative complications. The patient should be educated on the importance of smoking cessation and well as taught lung expansion maneuvers using incentive spirometry as risk reduction strategies in the preoperative period.

failure include congestive heart failure, altered platelet function, hyperkalemia and other electrolyte disturbances, and chronic anemia. Patients must be evaluated for coagulation disorders as appropriate treatment may be instituted in the perioperative period and medications which may alter platelet function such as nonsteroidal anti-inflammatory drugs (NSAIDs) should be avoided. Those patients with thyroid disease may benefit from an adjustment in medication prior to surgery as hypothyroidism or hyperthyroidism may have a significant impact on perioperative morbidity. Surgery may need to be postponed until medication is adjusted, and thyroid function test is within normal limits [1, 28].

Nutritional assessment is an important part of the preoperative evaluation. Malnourished patients are at an increased risk for perioperative morbidity and mortality [29]. Risk factors for malnutrition should be evaluated especially in the elderly population. Risk factors such as chronic disease, poor dentition, limited financial resources, social isolation, depression, and chronic constipation–diarrhea are common in the elderly and are associated with poor nutrition status [30]. In addition anxiety related to surgery can lead to increased periods of non-eating and can further increase the malnourished state. An albumin level <3.2 g/dL is associated with malnutrition, and a lymphocyte count <3,000 µg/L is associated with increased postoperative complications [29–31].

Other Organ Systems

The patient should be evaluated for organ dysfunction that can have an impact in the perioperative period. Liver disease may impact the clearance of anesthetic drugs. Coagulation factors are produced in the liver and hepatic dysfunction may impact coagulation in the perioperative period. Renal disease can severely impact the perioperative period as many anesthetic drugs are cleared via the kidneys. Chronic renal failure can impact clearance of anesthetic drugs as well as fluid management. Patients with chronic renal failure may need hemodialysis in the perioperative period. Complications from chronic renal

Reducing the Risk of Perioperative Infection

Antibiotic prophylaxis in the perioperative period is an important modality in preventing surgical site infections [32]. This is of great importance to the anesthesiologist as urologic procedures involve deep surgical sites which if manipulated while infected can induce urosepsis within a few minutes and place the patient in a life-threatening situation [33]. The timing of antibiotic administration has been greatly debated over the years, and studies have demonstrated significant variability in the timing of prophylactic antibiotic administration. Postoperative infections are associated with high morbidity and mortality and add significantly to health care costs [34]. Specific antibiotic prophylaxis is required in patients with implantable devices such as prosthetic heart valves, coronary stents, automatic implantable cardiac defibrillator (AICD), and cosmetic implants. Prophylactic antibiotics administration is best given 1 h prior to surgical incision. This has shown to best correlate with reduction in the incidence of postoperative infections [34–36].

Patients taking anticoagulant therapy for chronic atrial fibrillation, prosthetic valves, coronary stents, and those who are at increased risk of developing thromboembolic events are at increased risk of bleeding during surgery. Warfarin, which decreases the synthesis of vitamin K dependent factors, should ideally be stopped 5–7 days before surgery. The day of surgery coagulation studies should be repeated and if normal surgery may proceed. Warfarin may be reversed with vitamin K administration, FFP, cryoprecipitate, or rFVII [37, 38]. Clopidogrel is an antiplatelet agent, which blocks amplification of platelet activation by released ADP. It should be stopped ideally 3–5 days before surgery. The effect of clopidogrel can be reversed with platelet transfusion, and there have been case reports that methyl prednisolone is effective as well [37, 39].

Fondaparinux is a synthetic pentasaccharide Factor Xa inhibitor and forms the high affinity binding site for the anticoagulant factor antithrombin III (ATIII). It does not inhibit thrombin, has a lower risk for heparin-induced thrombocytopenia (HIT) than low molecular weight heparin (LMWH), and is contraindicated in patients with renal dysfunction and in patients with body weight less than 50 kg [40]. There have been case reports of fondaparinux being used to anticoagulate patients with established HIT. Fondaparinux has been shown to be similar to enoxaparin in reducing the risk of ischemic events at 9 days and to improve long-term morbidity and mortality [41]. The therapeutic effect of fondaparinux can be monitored with a factor Xa assay. There is no known reversal agent for fondaparinux. In the event of overdosage associated with bleeding complications, the drug should be discontinued and supportive care provided.

The mean half-life of fondaparinux is 17–21 h. Fresh frozen plasma is ineffective in reversal and should not be used for this purpose [40, 42].

LMWH include Lovenox (Enoxaparin) and Fragmin (Dalteparin). They act by binding to, and enhancing the activity of, antithrombin III, thereby inhibiting the activity of activated clotting factors including thrombin (factor IIa) and activated factor X (factor Xa). Both medications preferentially inhibit Factor Xa while only slightly affecting clotting time. LMWH is dosed by weight and is contraindicated in patients with a body weight of less than 50 kg. Monitoring of LMWH is not necessary. However, if there is a concern for bleeding, or there is uncertainty about the therapeutic level, an LMWH blood assay is available. The therapeutic interval ranges between 0.5 and 1.1 U/mL. Hemorrhagic complications of therapy can generally be treated by stopping the medication. The mean half-lives for Lovenox and Fragmin are 4.5 and 2.2 h, respectively. Protamine sulfate can be used to reverse the effects of LMWH. The recommended dose is 1 mg protamine for every 1 mg Lovenox or 1 mg protamine for every 100 anti-Xa IU of Fragmin. Fresh frozen plasma is ineffective in reversal of LMWH to achieve hemostasis and should not be used for this purpose [43].

A new class of oral anticoagulants was approved by the FDA in 2010, as an alternative to warfarin in terms of dosing, monitoring, dietary concerns, drug interaction, and variability of response. Dabigatran (Pradaxa) and rivaroxaban (Xarelto) are direct thrombin inhibitors [44, 45]. These drugs target the tissue factor/Factor VIIa complex (Factors IXa or Xa, or their respective coenzymes, Factors VIIIa and Va), preventing the initiation of coagulation. They do not require frequent blood tests for international normalized ratio monitoring and offer similar results in terms of efficacy [46]. Dabigatran and rivaroxaban are contraindicated in patients with a creatinine clearance less than 30 mL/min. No specific modality exists to reverse the anticoagulant effect of both drugs in case of a major bleeding event [47, 48]. However, in the event of overdose within 2 h, activated charcoal may be given to reverse its effect. In the event of severe bleeding, dabigatran and rivaroxaban should be discontinued and supportive measure should be instituted: control of bleeding site, IVF, and blood monitoring with aPTT and TT. Monitoring with aPTT is used as a negative predictive value, where a normal value suggests little anticoagulant activity. TT monitoring is a sensitive tool and a normal value denotes no presence of anticoagulant [49, 50]. The administration of prothrombin complex concentrate (PCC) and rFVIIa should be used as a last resort. In renal failure patients, dabigatran's half-life is prolonged to more than 24 h and may be eliminated up to 60 % with hemodialysis. Rivaroxaban is highly protein bound and is not eliminated with hemodialysis. Dabigatran and rivaroxaban should be discontinued 3–5 days before surgery. Patients requiring anticoagulation therapy may be admitted to the hospital and bridged with heparin infusion, which may be stopped 3–4 h prior to surgery [39, 44, 46, 51].

Preoperative Testing

The goal of preoperative testing is to detect asymptomatic disease processes not apparent on a history and physical examination. In the latter half of the twentieth century this was performed routinely in otherwise healthy individuals. The widespread use of laboratory testing was thought to detect those individuals who had latent disease processes and treat them before surgery in order to minimize morbidity and mortality in the perioperative period. Clinical effectiveness and cost effectiveness were not evaluated [52–54].

In the 1980s, several studies showed that routine preoperative testing was not cost-effective and did not influence perioperative management nor decrease perioperative morbidity and mortality [55]. Subsequent studies have shown that the majority of preoperative testing was done without any clear indications and that only a small percentage of patients had abnormal test results. This however, did not influence nor change their perioperative management. The problem lies in the ability of such tests to detect disease processes in otherwise healthy persons in whom the prevalence of such illnesses is low [56].

In patients who are more than 70 years of age, there is increased morbidity and mortality and increased hospital length of stay. However, in this age group there is also a greater incidence of comorbid conditions, and it remains unclear if the increased morbidity and mortality is secondary to age or to the comorbid conditions [7, 8].

The current recommendations for preoperative testing are based on specific indications in a patient. This greatly reduces the number of tests ordered. The following summarizes the recommended preoperative laboratory testing based on findings from the history and physical examination [52, 56, 57].

In healthy patients ≤40 years of age a baseline hemoglobin should be performed. In patients >40 year of age add an ECG and blood glucose (age ≥45 years) should be checked.

In patients with a history of cardiovascular disease, an ECG, chest radiograph, hemoglobin, serum electrolytes, BUN, and creatinine should be performed.

In patients with a recent MI (≤6 weeks), unstable angina, decompensated chronic heart failure (CHF), significant arrhythmias, severe valvular disease, and a cardiology consultation should be obtained [22]. If the patient suffered an MI more than 6 weeks ago or has a history of mild stable angina, compensated CHF, and/or diabetes mellitus, a stress test is indicated. If the patient has low functional capacity, consider echocardiography to assess left ventricular function [24, 58].

In patients with a history of pulmonary disease, the following should be obtained: chest radiographs hemoglobin, glucose (age ≥45 years), and ECG (age >40 years). Patients should be provided instructions for incentive spirometry or deep-breathing exercises. In asthmatics consider pulmonary function testing or peak flow rate to assess disease status. In patients with COPD consider pulmonary function testing and arterial blood gas analysis for assessment of disease severity. Any patient with a cough or dyspnea should be evaluated for etiology of symptoms. Patients who are current smokers should be counseled to stop smoking 4–8 weeks before surgery and provided with instructions for incentive spirometry or deep-breathing exercises. If malnutrition is suspected an albumin and lymphocyte count should be obtained; if malnutrition is severe, consider postponing surgery and providing preoperative supplementation [52–54, 57].

Intraoperative Management

Anesthetic Concerns

The anesthetic concerns regarding prostate surgery relate to positioning and ensuing hemodynamic changes. Whether the procedure is an open radical prostatectomy or performed as a minimally invasive surgery (MIS; laparoscopy with or without robotic assistance) ensuing physiologic changes that the patient encounters can significantly impact intraoperative management and perioperative morbidity [59, 60].

The decision as to the type of anesthesia given is first determined by the surgical procedure itself. Open RP may be performed under general anesthesia, regional anesthesia with sedation, or a combined general/regional technique. Regional anesthesia has been associated with less intraoperative blood loss, lower incidence of postoperative thromboembolic events, less incidence of postoperative nausea and vomiting (PONV), faster postoperative recovery, less postoperative mortality, and lower cancer recurrence rate [61]. Advocates of general anesthesia consider better airway control, greater intraoperative comfort, less intraoperative hemodynamic and pulmonary compromise, and less anesthesia time. When comparing general versus regional anesthesia, there is no difference in postoperative morbidity and no difference in outcome 3 months post-surgery [61–63].

Laparoscopic- and robotic-assisted RP (subsequently referred to as MIS) are preferably performed under general anesthesia, as under regional anesthesia, there is referred pain from the diaphragm that is not blocked using a regional technique. MIS surgery reduces blood loss and thus requires less intraoperative fluid replacement related to the increased risk in regards to positioning issues. In the post-anesthesia care

unit (PACU), the immediate recovery period is noted for lower pain scores utilizing the ten point pain scale, less opioids administration, less PONV, and decrease PACU length of stay. The period after PACU discharge is significant for less postoperative complications, better hematocrit and platelet scores on discharge from the hospital, as well as decreased hospital length of stay. The laparoscopy approach has shown as well to be less stressful for the patient [3, 58–60].

The patient should have the standard monitors for general anesthesia. Additional intravenous access and placement of an arterial line should be a consideration depending on the patient's comorbid condition. This is a concern especially in the elderly and the high-risk patient.

Open RP has the potential for rapid blood loss especially from the dorsal vein complex [64]. Our preference is to perform low-volume general anesthesia in which intravenous fluid administration is kept to a minimum until the prostate is removed in order to keep venous pressure low. Once the prostatectomy is completed fluids are given to replace blood and insensible fluid losses. Fluid restriction may also be helpful in MIS to reduce orbital, pharyngeal and laryngeal edema that may occur due to the Trendelenburg position. MIS has less blood loss than open RP with minimal insensible or third spaces losses. As such, MIS patients typically receive low volumes of fluid replacement. One concern, however, is decreased renal perfusion caused not only by restricted fluid replacement but also increased intra-abdominal pressure from the pneumoperitoneum and from activation of the sympathetic nervous system which causes an increased release of catecholamines and vasoconstriction of the afferent vessels to the glomeruli. This may increase creatinine levels measured in the postoperative period. In the absence of renal disease this is transient and has not shown to affect hospital length of stay and discharge [65]. On the other hand, the resultant oliguria may be interpreted as volume depletion and fluid may be given too generously. This can have a significant impact leading to pulmonary edema even in healthy patients. In the cardiac patient especially, this is a great concern as heart failure can develop acutely. Fluid replacement should be given cautiously is this patient population.

Additional anesthetic concerns with MIS are related to the effects of pneumoperitoneum and steep Trendelenburg position that affects homeostasis of most organ systems of the body.

Cerebral Effects

The cerebral perfusion pressure (CPP) is the driving pressure for brain perfusion and can be expressed as CCP = MAP (mean arterial pressure)—(CVP) central venous pressure. The head down position in steep Trendelenburg increases arterial and central venous pressure (CVP), thus impending venous flow from the brain and increasing hydrostatic pressure within the brain vasculature [66]. There is an increase in perivascular edema and the extracellular water content of the dependent tissues which may lead to cerebral edema. The resultant increase in intracranial pressure (ICP) can increase cerebrovascular resistance and reduce blood flow. In patients with cerebrovascular disorders these changes can lead to impaired tissue oxygenation, impaired perfusion and diffusion, and disastrous consequences. The brain is also very sensitive to CO_2. Hypercarbia causes direct vasodilation which also increases ICP. Slight elevations can cause direct cortical depression and decrease the threshold for seizure activity. This hypersensitivity is enhanced by hypercarbia-induced stimulation of the hypothalamus from catecholamines released from the medulla of the adrenal gland. Increased intraabdominal pressure causes increased intrathoracic pressure which causes a direct increase in ICP by the mechanisms described above. The added hypercarbia contributes as well to increase ICP, but hyperventilation will not cause a decrease in intracranial pressure until the abdominal pressure is released. Although all these various factors described contribute to an increase in intracranial pressure, this is well tolerated by the ASA class I or ASA class II patient. The use of a cerebral oxygen monitor during steep Trendelenburg position has shown that there is a slight increase in regional cerebral oxygen saturation with increased CO_2 in healthy patients. Consequently, the $PaCO_2$ should be maintained within normal ranges during the steep Trendelenburg position [66, 67].

Cardiovascular Effects

Pneumoperitoneum can have significant circulatory effects. The Trendelenburg position can cause acute cardiac decompensation especially in patients with cardiac disease. With initial insufflation, there is vagal stimulation that can cause severe bradycardia and even asystole. Insufflation should be discontinued until the patient is stabilized and re-insufflation accomplished at a much slower rate to allow the patient to adjust to these new physiologic changes. Healthy patients are less likely to have hemodynamic compromise but patients with a cardiac history are more likely to undergo these dramatic changes. Both in healthy patients and in patients with cardiac disease the head down position with pneumoperitoneum causes an increase in mean arterial pressure (MAP) by up to 20 %, CVP up to 50 %, and pulmonary capillary wedge pressure (PCWP) >18 mmHg. Even in healthy patients these changes can reach heart failure levels. Cardiac output is unaffected or decreased. The stroke volume (SV) remains unchanged, whereas the heart rate (HR) and systemic vascular resistance (SVR) increase by as much as 20 %. The strain of the heart as measured by right-sided and left-sided stroke work index increase as much as twofold. These changes have been mostly studied in patients with class ASA I and ASA II. In patients with cardiac disease there is an increase in myocardial oxygen demand that can precipitate heart failure [68]. Hypercarbia stimulates the sympathetic system which can lead to increased blood pressure, heart rate, and risk of arrhythmias, especially in the presence of hypoxemia. These effects may last well into the postoperative period. Increasing the respiratory rate in an attempt to decrease the hypercarbia may lead to an increase in intrathoracic pressure which can further impede venous return and increase PCWP to heart failure levels (>18 mmHg).

In patients with cardiac disease this can lead to acute decompensation. It is unclear whether the use of MIS requiring the Trendelenburg position with pneumoperitoneum is suitable in patients with cardiac disease. Clinical implications are significant, and reports of acute adverse events including heart failure and death have been reported. At present there is no set of specific risks in the preoperative period that can be identified in this patient population. The physiology of the closed chest in steep Trendelenburg, and the interaction of the intra-abdominal, intrathoracic pressures, blood volume and cardiac pressures and ventilatory pressures have yet to be elaborated. Further studies in healthy patients as well as those with significant cardiac disease and the use of 3D echocardiography to measure the pressure and volume changes in steep Trendelenburg position are needed to identify the physiology that might enlightened the preoperative risks for this patient population [9, 59, 68].

Pulmonary Effects

During the steep Trendelenburg position and insufflation of pneumoperitoneum, the abdominal content and the mediastinal content shift the diaphragm cephalad. This has a significant impact on pulmonary function. There is a decrease in the compliance of the lungs, decreased functional residual capacity, which predisposes to atelectasis. Increased peak inspiratory pressure causes a ventilation/perfusion mismatch and pulmonary shunting and results in decreased arterial oxygenation. This is seen as decreased oxygen saturation level on digital pulse oximetry. With insufflation pressures greater than 15 mmHg, peak inspiratory pressures greater than 50 % from baseline have been recorded. This can severely impact compliance, as high as a 68 % decrease has been noted. The compromised ventilation also increases the risk of barotrauma as seen in patients with peak airway pressures greater than 50 cmH$_2$O. Therefore, insufflation pressures should be kept at ≤15 mmHg. In order to overcome the increase airway pressure different modes of ventilation may be tried, the patient may tolerate pressure control ventilation better, in order to maintain constant minute ventilation, and permissive hypercarbia should be allowed. In comparing modes of ventilation, volume control versus pressure control, pressure control has less peak airway pressure and better compliance while maintaining minute ventilation. Both modes of ventilation may be applied, as there is no difference in outcome between the two modes [69]. Pulmonary gas exchange is well preserved with both modes of ventilation. Responses may vary as one mode may be better tolerated by an individual patient. This is especially true with pressure regulated ventilation in patient with COPD or other forms of pulmonary disease. These patients experience greater intraoperative ventilation problems, and it may be more difficult to maintain adequate ventilation [70]. As long as oxygen requirements of the patient are met, a high CO$_2$ concentration is well tolerated. During the initial insufflation CO$_2$ rapidly increases for the first 35 min. Despite continued insufflation there is a leveling of end tidal CO$_2$ seen on the ventilator monitor because of the draining of CO$_2$ into storages sites. The body stores CO$_2$ in different tissues. During MIS fat and bone serve as storage sites for CO$_2$. CO$_2$ has a diffusion capacity twenty times greater than oxygen and is dependent on the pressure gradient across the membranes. Patients who are overweight in the steep Trendelenburg position experience significant pulmonary dysfunction intraoperatively [27]. Arterial oxygenation, oxygen diffusion capacity, and decreases in functional residual capacity are seen. Difficulty with ventilation in respect to airway pressures and maintaining minute ventilation are frequent occurrences. It is occasionally necessary to maintain the patient is less steep Trendelenburg position, 30° vs. 45°, for the duration of the surgery [6, 71, 72].

Positioning Concerns in Steep Trendelenburg

Positioning in steep Trendelenburg is a major concern for the Anesthesiologist, as serious consequences can develop and manifest in the postoperative period [67]. Restricted access to the patient because of positioning and the mass of equipment placed over the patient can delay response in case of emergency and make it difficult to conduct regular safety checks on the patient intraoperatively [73]. It is recommended to place a second intravenous line after induction of anesthesia. Carbon dioxide is the preferred drug of choice for MIS as even 200 mL injected into a vein is not life-threatening because of its solubility. Air in the amount of 20 mL can cause significant harm and may be lethal. Carbon dioxide is 24 times more soluble than oxygen and has a diffusion capacity 20 more times than oxygen. The diffusion capacity is directly proportional to its solubility in water and inversely to its weight. The ability for carbon dioxide to move across different membranes and organs and eventually be excreted by the lungs is related to the pressure gradient across two membranes. The storage site for carbon dioxide in the body is immense. Well perfused organs can store extra carbon dioxide and serve as buffers and wait until the extra carbon dioxide is removed from the body via the lungs. The body produces about 200 mL of carbon dioxide per minute and can be excreted at a rate 800 times its basic metabolic rate when maximum demands of the body are needed. The disadvantage of carbon dioxide is that it affects the body physiologically. It causes direct peritoneal irritation and pain. If the patient is anemic, the absence of red blood cells makes carbon dioxide less soluble; therefore, it can remain in its gaseous state in the peritoneum well after into the postoperative period and incite referred pain in the shoulder. Hypercarbia and respiratory acidosis can ensue. In the patient with COPD, hypercarbia can cause respiratory compromise in the postoperative period. Systemic effects of carbon dioxide are wide ranging: hypertension, tachycardia, cerebral vasodilation, increased cardiac output, hypercarbia, and respiratory acidosis. If the procedure is especially long or complicated, an arterial line should be considered as the carbon dioxide equilibrium is interrupted. This can cause a significant arterial to end tidal CO_2 gradient and disrupt the normal relationship. The measured end tidal CO_2 can be overestimated or underestimated. As a consequence, the patient may experience a greater metabolic and physiologic effect from the hypercarbia, and those patients with cardiac disease are especially sensitive and may experience more pronounced hemodynamic compromise and decompensation. The endocrine effects of pneumoperitoneum are related to increase intra-abdominal pressure and hypercarbia. The sympathetic system is activated, and epinephrine and norepinephrine are released from the adrenal medulla of the adrenal gland. Cortisol, renin, aldosterone, and antidiuretic hormone (ADH) hormones are also released. Atrial natriuretic peptide is decreased as this hormone is released following stretch of the atrium; therefore low levels suggest decreased venous return resulting from insufflation of the abdomen.

Complications of Steep Trendelenburg and Pneumoperitoneum

Complications resulting from the steep Trendelenburg position and pneumoperitoneum often manifest in the postoperative period. A common complication seen in 4% of laparoscopic surgery is carbon dioxide subcutaneous emphysema observed in the upper thorax and head and neck area. The carbon dioxide passes along anatomical paths under increased pressure from insufflation to cause subcutaneous emphysema, pneumothorax, pneumomediastinum, and pneumopericardium. This usually presents when end tidal carbon dioxide levels are greater than 50 mmHg, with more than six operative port sites, longer surgery, and older patients [75]. This is a transient complication that worsens with the patient in the upright sitting position. In severe cases of hypercarbia there may be edema of the airway and airway obstruction. It is recommended to keep the patient ventilated at the end of surgery until hypercarbia is resolved. There have been some case reports of life-threatening pneumothorax, pneumomediastinum, and pneumopericardium intraoperatively which have quickly resolved with the cessation of insufflation [74].

Hypercarbia, as well as stretching of the peritoneum by insufflation, is responsible for PONV.

Carbon dioxide insufflation is known to be associated with venous gas embolism which can be a potential life-threatening complication. There have been case reports of lethal massive carbon dioxide gas embolism. The incidence of venous gas embolism has been reported as high as 17 %. The size of the bubble is less important than the rate at which the carbon dioxide is absorbed into the circulation. There are two phases where this complication may occur, at the beginning of insufflation through a broken vein and during the dissection of the deep dorsal venous complex. It occurs more commonly during the dissection of the deep dorsal vein. At the beginning of the procedure insufflation is slow and the absorption through a broken vein is slow and constant. The carbon dioxide is slowly diffused, has a high solubility rate in the blood, and is cleared faster by the lungs than it is absorbed through the broken vein. During dissection of the deep dorsal vein, the operative site is higher than the heart, which creates a gradient between the dorsal vein complex and the heart and venous gas entrapment can easily occur. In open RP the entrained gas is air and is more readily entrapped than carbon dioxide [75]. Air is not readily absorbed like carbon dioxide in blood and can pass down passively into an open, non-collapsible vein by negative intrathoracic venous pressure. A pressure gradient as little as 5 cmH_2O is sufficient to entrap air. This entrapment can lead to life-threatening situations due to hemodynamic and respiratory changes. The clinical signs of air embolism are not consistent. Tachycardia, cardiac arrhythmias, hypotension, desaturation, or electrocardiographic changes may occur independently, in combination or altogether. If suspicion is high the most definitive test for detection of air emboli is transesophageal echocardiogram. On auscultation a precordial rumbling is heard. The incidence of venous gas embolism is higher in open prostatectomy surgery than in MIS. Most embolic events occur during transection of the deep dorsal vein complex and are undetected. In healthy patients there may not be any hemodynamic compromise, but in patients with a history of cardiac disease hemodynamic instability can be life threatening [76, 77].

Ocular injuries are also a major concern following the steep Trendelenburg position. They range from corneal abrasions to retinal detachment to perioperative visual loss caused by ischemic optic neuropathy. Corneal abrasions have an incidence rate from 3 to 13 %. The patient should be warned of the risk of corneal abrasion following prostate surgery whether performed as open or MIS. Ischemic optic neuropathy has been described in a variety of surgical cases. Most often it is associated with cardiac surgery or spine surgery, especially in the prone position [78]. There is a lack of controlled studies, a limited understanding of the pathophysiology and risk factors involved in the mechanism of development of ischemic optic neuropathy. Most knowledge is from individual case reports and the American Society of Anesthesiologist (ASA) Visual Loss Data Registry. The ASA task force for the prevention of perioperative blindness has published recommendation for surgical cases performed in the prone position. There have been reports of ischemic optic neuropathy in open RP and MIS [79]. The effect of steep Trendelenburg position on increased intraocular pressure (IOP) has been proposed as a possible mechanism for ischemic optic neuropathy [80]. There are a variety of perioperative variables that have been proposed as significant predictors of ischemic optic neuropathy. Initially, the steep Trendelenburg position causes an increase in CVP which leads to increased orbital venous pressure and increased IOP. Over time, however different mechanisms come into play. The increased end tidal carbon dioxide level from continuous carbon dioxide insufflation from the pneumoperitoneum can lead to vasodilation and also increased IOP. The continuous production of aqueous fluid by the ciliary body of the eye also contributes to increase IOP during surgery. This aqueous fluid accumulates and there is impendence of outflow from the eye due to increased CVP and increased peak airway pressure. Factors such as the length of surgery, body position, and CO_2 insufflation, duration in steep Trendelenburg position and sustained increase in IOP more than 4 h have all been proposed to have influence in the development of ischemic optic neuropathy. The patient's comorbid states also need to be considered. The presence of glaucoma or other ocular diseases have not shown to be a predictable risk factor. The presence of ischemic optic neuropathy in previously healthy patients undergoing open or MIS in relation to specific variables related to these procedures and position in steep Trendelenburg are not known. The significant predictors of IOP over time are peak airway pressure, mean arterial pressure, end tidal carbon dioxide level, and surgical duration. Further studies are need to evaluate these significant predictors over time in relation to increase IOP and the development of ischemic optic neuropathy [79].

Lower extremity neuropathy has been reported in patients in the postoperative period following RP. The mechanism for development of this injury is related to the split leg position in stirrups which hyperextend the hip and places the femoral nerve at risk. In the lithotomy position, extension cause common peroneal nerve neuropathies. Symptoms appear in the immediate postoperative period and can appear up to 7 days post operatively, and include lower extremity weakness, numbness, and paresthesias in the femoral nerve distribution. Most symptoms are self-limited and resolve within a few weeks. The most significant risk factor associated with the development of lower extremity neuropathy is the duration of surgery more than 4 h. Secondary risk factors include a history of neuropathy, a BMI less than 20, and smoking [81].

Compartment syndrome is a rare but well-described complication of the lithotomy position. The ensuing rhabdomyolysis and possible renal failure may result in limb loss if the condition is not recognized in a timely fashion. The limbs in the lithotomy position and in stirrups are elevated and are not well perfused [82]. There is ensuing ischemia of the muscles of the lower extremities. The lumbar and pelvic muscles are compressed by the severe Trendelenburg position which may also lead to limb hypoperfusion. The risk significantly increases at about 5 h of duration of surgery. Other factors that contribute to decreased perfusion in the lower limbs are the use of compression devices on the lower extremities in stirrups in the lithotomy position, hypotension, the use of vasoactive drugs, preexisting myopathies, the use of fibrate monotherapy for hyperlipidemia, and a BMI greater than 25 [82]. The risk of developing compartment syndrome may be avoided by careful patient selection for the proposed surgery, limiting lithotomy and the Trendelenburg position, limiting duration of surgery, and avoidance of compression devices on the lower extremities that in stirrups decrease limb perfusion [83].

In the PACU, the patient is monitored for postoperative complications. General postoperative concerns include physiologic changes that affect multiple organ systems. Pain management is a great concern. The patient is assessed based on the 0–10 pain scale and given narcotics for pain control as needed. The patient may also receive ketorolac (Toradol) intravenously and intravenous acetaminophen (Tylenol). These non-opioids significantly reduced the requirements for narcotic pain control and may alleviate the side effects seen with narcotic use. These agents, however, are limited if the patient has renal or liver impairment. Whether the patient has undergone open RP or MIS non-opioid adjunct to pain control is a good choice in the immediate postoperative period [62]. Intravenous fluid in the postoperative period should be adjusted to maintenance fluid and intravenous boluses may be given depending on the patient's hemodynamic and renal function. Some patients after laparoscopy experience EKG changes. Approximately 3 % of patients undergoing laparoscopy have EKG changes even if the individual is healthy. These include new onset of left ventricular strain, atrial fibrillation, right bundle branch block, and ST segment depression. These changes do not correlate to a prior history of cardiac disease. In healthy individuals with new EKG changes after laparoscopy in the postoperative period, a monitored setting with telemetry for the next 24 h is required until the EKG reverts to baseline. Electrolytes should be checked and repleted as needed as electrolyte disturbances may contribute to cardiac sensitivity in the postoperative period [9, 28].

Patients with a history of cardiac disease may experience hemodynamic effects of prolonged hypercarbia, such as tachycardia, hypertension, which increase oxygen demand and may lead to cardiac compromise and demise. These patients may need to be transferred to the intensive care unit for further work up and management [84].

Patients with preexisting pulmonary disease may experience respiratory disturbances in the postoperative period, especially if the patient has undergone MIS. There may have been difficulty in ventilation and maintaining of minute ventilation intraoperatively and the patient with pulmonary disease is at increased risk of developing atelectasis, hypoventilation, and hypoxemia in the postoperative period. This can lead to pneumonia, which further compromises the patient, and may lead to respiratory compromise and increase length of hospital stay [85]. The patient should be listened to for wheezing and treated accordingly if present. If the patient has asthma or COPD, signs of exacerbation should be looked for and treatment instituted immediately. The use of steroids should also be considered. The patient should be encouraged to use incentive spirometry to reduce atelectasis and the chance of developing pneumonia. The patient with obstructive sleep apnea who uses a CPAP machine at home may need to do so in the immediate postoperative period [86]. The use of pain medication in the patient recovering from anesthesia may cause worsening of sleep apnea. A chest X-ray is indicated in the postoperative period if the patient is in respiratory distress, if subcutaneous emphysema is noted, if pneumothorax is noted or suspected, if the patient is oliguric despite adequate fluid resuscitation, and if the patient has a history of cardiac or pulmonary disease. Urine volumes should be recorded and diuresis expected at 0.5 mL/kg/h [9]. PONV is greater in patients who have undergone MIS than open RP. The incidence can be as high as 40 %. This is the most important factor in prolonged hospital length of stay in ambulatory surgery and overnight admission, as well as short stay surgery. The cause of nausea and vomiting is related to the overdistention of the peritoneum by insufflation, a reflex that is activated by the splanchnic neurogenic pathway. Medication for PONV should be given during surgery and may be repeated in the PACU [87].

Shivering and hypothermia may occur in the postoperative period as a result of intraoperative hypothermia or from the effects of volatile anesthetic agents. The incidence is directly related to the duration of surgery and the concentration of inhaled anesthetic agents. The cause of shivering is from the redistribution of heat from the core to the peripheral compartment of the body. The shivering may at times be so intense as to cause hyperthermia to 38–39 °C and metabolic acidosis. Meperidine in small doses 10–50 mg intravenously has been effective in decreasing the shivering and stopping it. Shivering in the immediate postoperative period is important as it increases oxygen consumption. In the patient with cardiac disease this increase in oxygen consumption can lead to myocardial ischemia [85].

In order for the patient to leave the recovery room or PACU a set of discharge criteria needs to be met by the patient. The patient should be evaluated by an Anesthesiologist before being discharged from the PACU. There is a wide variety of discharge scoring systems available. The basic assessment includes: vital signs, they should be stable and within 20 % of preoperative level, activity level, whether a patient is able to ambulate on his own, how well the patient's pain is controlled, assessing nausea and vomiting, and assessing surgical bleeding. These are generally used in short stay surgery or ambulatory surgery and fast tracking the patient to home. Other factors to be taken into consideration, especially if the patient has had a complex procedure and/or has multiple comorbidities include: the level of consciousness, respiratory status, medications administered, time spent in the PACU, adverse events in the PACU, urine output per hour, and whether the patient has taken any fluids by mouth. These different scoring systems have been adapted by the PACU nurse at the bedside to determine whether the patient is ready for discharge to the floor, from the intensive care unit, to PACU phase II ambulatory department, or directly to home [9, 84–87].

References

1. Cima RR, Lackore KA, Nehring SA, Cassivi SD, Donohue JH, Deschamps C, et al. How best to measure surgical quality? Comparison of the Agency for Healthcare Research and Quality Patient Safety Indicators (AHRQ-PSI) and the American College of Surgeons National Surgical Quality Improvement Program (ACS-NSQIP) postoperative adverse events at a single institution. Surgery. 2011;150(5):943–9. PubMed PMID: 21875734.

2. Figueroa AJ, Stein JP, Dickinson M, Skinner EC, Thangathurai D, Mikhail MS, et al. Radical cystectomy for elderly patients with bladder carcinoma: an updated experience with 404 patients. Cancer. 1998;83(1):141–7. PubMed PMID: 9655304.

3. Trinh QD, Sammon J, Sun M, Ravi P, Ghani KR, Bianchi M, et al. Perioperative outcomes of robot-assisted radical prostatectomy compared with open radical prostatectomy: results from the nationwide inpatient sample. Eur Urol. 2012;61(4):679–85. PubMed PMID: 22206800.

4. Grewal K, Wijeysundera DN, Carroll J, Tait G, Beattie WS. Gender differences in mortality following noncardiovascular surgery: an observational study. Can J Anaesth. 2012;59(3):255–62.

5. Maddox TM. Preoperative cardiovascular evaluation for noncardiac surgery. Mt Sinai J Med. 2005;72(3):185–92. PubMed PMID: 15915313.

6. Halachmi S, Katz Y, Meretyk S, Barak M. Perioperative morbidity and mortality in 80 years and older undergoing elective urology surgery - a prospective study. Aging Male. 2008;11(4):162–6. PubMed PMID: 19172546.

7. Froehner M, Hentschel C, Koch R, Litz RJ, Hakenberg OW, Wirth MP. Which comorbidity classification best fits elderly candidates for radical prostatectomy? Urol Oncol. 2013;31(4):461–7. PubMed PMID: 21498089.

8. Djokovic JL, Hedley-Whyte J. Prediction of outcome of surgery and anesthesia in patients over 80. JAMA. 1979;242(21):2301–6. PubMed PMID: 490827.

9. Miller RD. Miller's anesthesia. 7th ed. Philadelphia, PA: Churchill Livingstone/Elsevier; 2010.

10. Hightower CE, Riedel BJ, Feig BW, Morris GS, Ensor Jr JE, Woodruff VD, et al. A pilot study evaluating predictors of postoperative outcomes after major abdominal surgery: physiological capacity compared with the ASA physical status classification system. Br J Anaesth. 2010;104(4):465–71. PubMed PMID: 20190255. Pubmed Central PMCID: 2837548.

11. Owens WDMD, Felts JAMD, Spitznagel ELJPD. ASA physical status classifications: a study of consistency of ratings. Anesthesiology. 1978;49:239–43. (0003–3022). PubMed PMID: 00000542-197810000-00003.

12. Fitz-Henry J. The ASA, classification and perioperative risk. Ann R Coll Surg Engl. 2011;93(3):185–7. PubMed PMID: 21477427. Pubmed Central PMCID: 3348554.

13. Saklad MMD. Grading of patients for surgical procedures. Anesthesiology. 1941;2(0003–3022):281–3. PubMed PMID: 00000542-194105000-00004.

14. Dripps R. New classification of physical status. Anesthesiology. 1963;24:111.

15. Daabiss M. American society of anaesthesiologists physical status classification. Ind J Anaesth. 2011;55(2):111–5. PubMed PMID: 21712864. Pubmed Central PMCID: 3106380.

16. Thomas M, George NA, Gowri BP, George PS, Sebastian P. Comparative evaluation of ASA classification and ACE-27 index as morbidity scoring systems in oncosurgeries. Indian J Anaesth. 2010;54(3):219–25. PubMed PMID: 20885868. Pubmed Central PMCID: 2933480.

17. McGuirt JK. Goldman criteria of cardiac risk for noncardiac surgery. Am J Cardiol. 1994;74(3):307. PubMed PMID: 8037150.

18. Arora V, Velanovich V, Alarcon W. Preoperative assessment of cardiac risk and perioperative cardiac management in noncardiac surgery. Int J Surg. 2011;9(1):23–8. PubMed PMID: 20934543.

19. Fleisher LA, Beckman JA, Brown KA, Calkins H, Chaikof E, Fleischmann KE, et al. ACC/AHA 2007 guidelines on perioperative cardiovascular evaluation and care for noncardiac surgery: executive summary: a report of the American College of Cardiology/American Heart Association Task Force on Practice Guidelines (Writing Committee to Revise the 2002 Guidelines on Perioperative Cardiovascular Evaluation for Noncardiac Surgery): developed in collaboration with the American Society of Echocardiography, American Society of Nuclear Cardiology, Heart Rhythm Society, Society of Cardiovascular Anesthesiologists, Society for Cardiovascular Angiography and Interventions, Society for Vascular Medicine and Biology, and Society for Vascular Surgery. Circulation. 2007;116(17):1971–96. PubMed PMID: 17901356.

20. Froehlich JB, Fleisher LA. Noncardiac surgery in the patient with heart disease. Anesthesiol Clin. 2009;27(4):649–71. PubMed PMID: 19942172.

21. Iglesias JF, Sierro C, Aebischer N, Vogt P, Eeckhout E. [Preoperative cardiac assessment before noncardiac surgery: cardiac risk stratification]. Rev Med Suisse. 2010;6(251):1110–4, 6. PubMed PMID: 20572353. Evaluation cardiologique preoperatoire avant chirurgie non cardiaque: stratification du risque cardiovasculaire.

22. Hollenberg M, Mangano DT, Browner WS, London MJ, Tubau JF, Tateo IM. Predictors of postoperative myocardial ischemia in patients undergoing noncardiac surgery. The Study of Perioperative Ischemia Research Group. JAMA. 1992;268(2):205–9. PubMed PMID: 1535109.

23. Eagle KA, Berger PB, Calkins H, Chaitman BR, Ewy GA, Fleischmann KE, et al. ACC/AHA Guideline Update for perioperative Cardiovascular Evaluation for Noncardiac Surgery—Executive Summary. A report of the American College of Cardiology/

American Heart Association Task Force on Practice Guidelines (Committee to update the 1996 guidelines on perioperative cardiovascular evaluation for noncardiac surgery). Anesth Analg. 2002;94(5):1052–64. PubMed PMID: 11973163.
24. Mangano DT, Browner WS, Hollenberg M, Li J, Tateo IM. Long-term cardiac prognosis following noncardiac surgery. The Study of Perioperative Ischemia Research Group. JAMA. 1992;268(2):233–9. PubMed PMID: 1608143.
25. Kheterpal S, O'Reilly M, Englesbe MJ, Rosenberg AL, Shanks AM, Zhang L, et al. Preoperative and intraoperative predictors of cardiac adverse events after general, vascular, and urological surgery. Anesthesiology. 2009;110(1):58–66. PubMed PMID: 19104171.
26. Eagle KA, Rihal CS, Mickel MC, Holmes DR, Foster ED, Gersh BJ. Cardiac risk of noncardiac surgery: influence of coronary disease and type of surgery in 3368 operations. CASS Investigators and University of Michigan Heart Care Program. Coronary Artery Surgery Study. Circulation. 1997;96(6):1882–7. PubMed PMID: 9323076.
27. Dindo D, Muller MK, Weber M, Clavien PA. Obesity in general elective surgery. Lancet. 2003;361(9374):2032–5. PubMed PMID: 12814714.
28. Barash PG. Handbook of clinical anesthesia. 6th ed. Philadelphia: Wolters Kluwer Health/Lippincott Williams & Wilkins; 2009. xiv, p 1180.
29. Heys SD, Ogston KN. Peri-operative nutritional support: controversies and debates. Int J Surg Investig. 2000;2(2):107–15. PubMed PMID: 12678508.
30. McClave SA, Snider HL, Spain DA. Preoperative issues in clinical nutrition. Chest. 1999;115(5 Suppl):64S–70. PubMed PMID: 10331336.
31. Francon D, Chambrier C, Sztark F. Nutritional assessment of patients before surgery. Ann Fr Anesth Réanim. 2012;31(6):506–11. PubMed PMID: 22483754. Evaluation nutritionnelle a la consultation d'anesthesie.
32. Shapiro M. Perioperative prophylactic use of antibiotics in surgery: principles and practice. Infect Control. 1982;3(1):38–40. PubMed PMID: 6915901.
33. Matsumoto M, Shigemura K, Yamamichi F, Tanaka K, Nakano Y, Arakawa S, et al. Prevention of infectious complication and its risk factors after urological procedures of the upper urinary tract. Urol Int. 2012;88(1):43–7. PubMed PMID: 22005053.
34. Wilson SE, Turpin RS, Kumar RN, Itani KM, Jensen EH, Pellissier JM, et al. Comparative costs of ertapenem and cefotetan as prophylaxis for elective colorectal surgery. Surg Infect (Larchmt). 2008;9(3):349–56. PubMed PMID: 18570576.
35. Ho VP, Barie PS, Stein SL, Trencheva K, Milsom JW, Lee SW, et al. Antibiotic regimen and the timing of prophylaxis are important for reducing surgical site infection after elective abdominal colorectal surgery. Surg Infect (Larchmt). 2011;12(4):255–60. PubMed PMID: 21790479.

36. Grabe M, Botto H, Cek M, Tenke P, Wagenlehner FM, Naber KG, et al. Preoperative assessment of the patient and risk factors for infectious complications and tentative classification of surgical field contamination of urological procedures. World J Urol. 2012;30(1):39–50. PubMed PMID: 21779836.
37. Reynolds MW, Fahrbach K, Hauch O, Wygant G, Estok R, Cella C, et al. Warfarin anticoagulation and outcomes in patients with atrial fibrillation: a systematic review and metaanalysis. Chest. 2004;126(6):1938–45. PubMed PMID: 15596696.
38. Ansell J, Hirsh J, Poller L, Bussey H, Jacobson A, Hylek E. The pharmacology and management of the vitamin K antagonists: the Seventh ACCP Conference on Antithrombotic and Thrombolytic Therapy. Chest. 2004;126(3 Suppl):204S–33. PubMed PMID: 15383473.
39. Eerenberg ES, Kamphuisen PW, Sijpkens MK, Meijers JC, Buller HR, Levi M. Reversal of rivaroxaban and dabigatran by prothrombin complex concentrate: a randomized, placebo-controlled, crossover study in healthy subjects. Circulation. 2011;124(14):1573–9. PubMed PMID: 21900088.
40. Turpie AG, Bauer KA, Eriksson BI, Lassen MR. Fondaparinux vs enoxaparin for the prevention of venous thromboembolism in major orthopedic surgery: a meta-analysis of 4 randomized double-blind studies. Arch Intern Med. 2002;162(16):1833–40. PubMed PMID: 12196081.
41. Turpie AG, Bauer KA, Caprini JA, Comp PC, Gent M, Muntz JE, et al. Fondaparinux combined with intermittent pneumatic compression vs. intermittent pneumatic compression alone for prevention of venous thromboembolism after abdominal surgery: a randomized, double-blind comparison. J Thromb Haemost. 2007;5(9):1854–61. PubMed PMID: 17723125.
42. Peters RJ, Joyner C, Bassand JP, Afzal R, Chrolavicius S, Mehta SR, et al. The role of fondaparinux as an adjunct to thrombolytic therapy in acute myocardial infarction: a subgroup analysis of the OASIS-6 trial. Eur Heart J. 2008;29(3):324–31. PubMed PMID: 18245119.
43. Cella G, Girolami A, Sasahara AA. Platelet activation with unfractionated heparin at therapeutic concentrations and comparison with low-molecular-weight heparin and with a direct thrombin inhibitor. Circulation. 1999;99(25):3323. PubMed PMID: 10385510.
44. Lepic K, Crowther M. New anticoagulants for the prevention of thromboembolism. Curr Pharm Des. 2010;16(31):3472–4. PubMed PMID: 20858184.
45. Weitz JI, Bates SM. New anticoagulants. J Thromb Haemost. 2005;3(8):1843–53. PubMed PMID: 16102051.
46. Douketis JD, Berger PB, Dunn AS, Jaffer AK, Spyropoulos AC, Becker RC, et al. The perioperative management of antithrombotic therapy: American College of Chest Physicians Evidence-Based Clinical

Practice Guidelines (8th Edition). Chest. 2008;133(6 Suppl):299S–339. PubMed PMID: 18574269.

47. Stangier J, Rathgen K, Stahle H, Gansser D, Roth W. The pharmacokinetics, pharmacodynamics and tolerability of dabigatran etexilate, a new oral direct thrombin inhibitor, in healthy male subjects. Br J Clin Pharmacol. 2007;64(3):292–303. PubMed PMID: 17506785. Pubmed Central PMCID: 2000643.

48. Di Nisio M, Middeldorp S, Buller HR. Direct thrombin inhibitors. New Engl J Med. 2005;353(10):1028–40. PubMed PMID: 16148288.

49. Kubitza D, Haas S. Novel factor Xa inhibitors for prevention and treatment of thromboembolic diseases. Expert Opin Investig Drugs. 2006;15(8):843–55. PubMed PMID: 16859389.

50. Fifth Organization to Assess Strategies in Acute Ischemic Syndromes Investigators, Yusuf S, Mehta SR, Chrolavicius S, Afzal R, Pogue J, et al. Comparison of fondaparinux and enoxaparin in acute coronary syndromes. N Engl J Med. 2006;354(14):1464–76. PubMed PMID: 16537663.

51. Bates SM, Weitz JI. The status of new anticoagulants. Br J Haematol. 2006;134(1):3–19. PubMed PMID: 16803562.

52. Kaplan EB, Sheiner LB, Boeckmann AJ, Roizen MF, Beal SL, Cohen SN, et al. The usefulness of preoperative laboratory screening. JAMA. 1985;253(24):3576–81. PubMed PMID: 3999339.

53. Narr BJ, Hansen TR, Warner MA. Preoperative laboratory screening in healthy Mayo patients: cost-effective elimination of tests and unchanged outcomes. Mayo Clin Proc. 1991;66(2):155–9. PubMed PMID: 1899710.

54. Macpherson DS, Snow R, Lofgren RP. Preoperative screening: value of previous tests. Ann Intern Med. 1990;113(12):969–73. PubMed PMID: 2240920.

55. Smetana GW, Macpherson DS. The case against routine preoperative laboratory testing. Med Clin North Am. 2003;87(1):7–40. PubMed PMID: 12575882.

56. Turnbull JM, Buck C. The value of preoperative screening investigations in otherwise healthy individuals. Arch Int Med. 1987;147(6):1101–5. PubMed PMID: 3592875.

57. Narr BJ, Warner ME, Schroeder DR, Warner MA. Outcomes of patients with no laboratory assessment before anesthesia and a surgical procedure. Mayo Clin Proc. 1997;72(6):505–9. PubMed PMID: 9179133.

58. Gardner TA, Bissonette EA, Petroni GR, McClain R, Sokoloff MH, Theodorescu D. Surgical and postoperative factors affecting length of hospital stay after radical prostatectomy. Cancer. 2000;89(2):424–30. PubMed PMID: 10918175.

59. Gainsburg DM, Wax D, Reich DL, Carlucci JR, Samadi DB. Intraoperative management of robotic-assisted versus open radical prostatectomy. JSLS. 2010;14(1):1–5. PubMed PMID: 20529522. Pubmed Central PMCID: 3021297.

60. D'Alonzo RC, Gan TJ, Moul JW, Albala DM, Polascik TJ, Robertson CN, et al. A retrospective comparison of anesthetic management of robot-assisted laparoscopic radical prostatectomy versus radical retropubic prostatectomy. J Clin Anesth. 2009;21(5):322–8. PubMed PMID: 19700296.

61. Biki B, Mascha E, Moriarty DC, Fitzpatrick JM, Sessler DI, Buggy DJ. Anesthetic technique for radical prostatectomy surgery affects cancer recurrence: a retrospective analysis. Anesthesiology. 2008;109(2):180–7. PubMed PMID: 18648226.

62. Liu SS, Wu CL. The effect of analgesic technique on postoperative patient-reported outcomes including analgesia: a systematic review. Anesth Analg. 2007;105(3):789–808. PubMed PMID: 17717242.

63. Bhandari A, Mc Intire L, Kaul SA, Hemal AK, Peabody JO, Menon M. Perioperative complications of robotic radical prostatectomy after the learning curve. J Urol. 2005;174(3):915–8.

64. Ead DN, Koch M, Smith JA. Is invasive anesthetic monitoring necessary during radical prostatectomy? Prostate Cancer Prostatic Dis. 1999;2(5/6):282–4. PubMed PMID: 12497175.

65. Piegeler T, Dreessen P, Schläpfer M, Schmid DM, Beck-Schimmer B. Impact of intraoperative fluid management on outcome in patients undergoing robotic-assisted laparoscopic prostatectomy - a retrospective analysis: 6AP1-6. Eur J Anaesthesiol. 2011;28:81.

66. Kalmar AF, Dewaele F, Foubert L, Hendrickx JF, Heeremans EH, Struys MM, et al. Cerebral haemodynamic physiology during steep Trendelenburg position and CO(2) pneumoperitoneum. Br J Anaesth. 2012;108(3):478–84. PubMed PMID: 22258202.

67. Park EY, Koo BN, Min KT, Nam SH. The effect of pneumoperitoneum in the steep Trendelenburg position on cerebral oxygenation. Acta Anaesthesiol Scand. 2009;53(7):895–9. PubMed PMID: 19426238.

68. Lestar M, Gunnarsson L, Lagerstrand L, Wiklund P, Odeberg-Wernerman S. Hemodynamic perturbations during robot-assisted laparoscopic radical prostatectomy in 45 degrees Trendelenburg position. Anesth Analg. 2011;113(5):1069–75. PubMed PMID: 21233502.

69. Choi EM, Na S, Choi SH, An J, Rha KH, Oh YJ. Comparison of volume-controlled and pressure-controlled ventilation in steep Trendelenburg position for robot-assisted laparoscopic radical prostatectomy. J Clin Anesth. 2011;23(3):183–8.

70. Hong JY, Oh YJ, Rha KH, Park WS, Kim YS, Kil HK. Pulmonary edema after da Vinci-assisted laparoscopic radical prostatectomy: a case report. J Clin Anesth. 2010;22(5):370–2. PubMed PMID: 20650386.

71. Meininger D, Zwissler B, Byhahn C, Probst M, Westphal K, Bremerich DH. Impact of overweight and pneumoperitoneum on hemodynamics and oxygenation during prolonged laparoscopic surgery. World J Surg. 2006;30(4):520–6. PubMed PMID: 16568232.

72. Schrijvers D, Mottrie A, Traen K, De Wolf AM, Vandermeersch E, Kalmar AF, et al. Pulmonary gas exchange is well preserved during robot assisted

surgery in steep Trendelenburg position. Acta Anaesthesiol Belg. 2009;60(4):229–33. PubMed PMID: 20187485.

73. Fuller A, Pautler SE. Complications following robot-assisted radical prostatectomy in a prospective Canadian cohort of 305 consecutive cases. Can Urol Assoc J. 2012;2:1–6.

74. Chatti C, Corsia G, Yates DR, Vaessen C, Bitker MO, Coriat P, et al. Prevention of complications of general anesthesia linked with laparoscopic access and with robot-assisted radical prostatectomy. Prog Urol. 2011;21(12):829–34. PubMed PMID: 22035907. Complications de l'anesthesie generale inherentes a la voie laparoscopique et a la prostatectomie totale robot-assistee.

75. Hong JY, Kim JY, Choi YD, Rha KH, Yoon SJ, Kil HK. Incidence of venous gas embolism during robotic-assisted laparoscopic radical prostatectomy is lower than that during radical retropubic prostatectomy. Br J Anaesth. 2010;105(6):777–81. PubMed PMID: 20880950.

76. Park EY, Kwon JY, Kim KJ. Carbon dioxide embolism during laparoscopic surgery. Yonsei Med J. 2012;53(3):459–66. PubMed PMID: 22476987. Pubmed Central PMCID: 3343430.

77. Hewer CL. The physiology and complications of the Trendelenburg position. Can Med Assoc J. 1956;74(4):285–8. PubMed PMID: 13293598. Pubmed Central PMCID: 1824068.

78. Berg KT, Harrison AR, Lee MS. Perioperative visual loss in ocular and nonocular surgery. Clin Ophthalmol. 2010;4:531–46. PubMed PMID: 20596508. Pubmed Central PMCID: 2893763.

79. Roth S. Perioperative visual loss: what do we know, what can we do? Br J Anaesth. 2009;103 Suppl 1:i31–40. PubMed PMID: 20007988. Pubmed Central PMCID: 2791856.

80. Awad H, Santilli S, Ohr M, Roth A, Yan W, Fernandez S, et al. The effects of steep trendelenburg positioning on intraocular pressure during robotic radical prostatectomy. Anesth Analg. 2009;109(2):473–8. PubMed PMID: 19608821.

81. Koc G, Tazeh NN, Joudi FN, Winfield HN, Tracy CR, Brown JA. Lower extremity neuropathies after robot-assisted laparoscopic prostatectomy on a split-leg table. J Endourol. 2012;26(8):1026–9. PubMed PMID: 22515378.

82. Ankichetty S, Angle P, Margarido C, Halpern SH. Case report: rhabdomyolysis in morbidly obese patients: anesthetic considerations. Can J Anaesth. 2012. PubMed PMID: 23161100. Presentation de cas: rhabdomyolyse chez les patients obeses morbides: considerations anesthesiques.

83. Galyon SW, Richards KA, Pettus JA, Bodin SG. Three-limb compartment syndrome and rhabdomyolysis after robotic cystoprostatectomy. J Clin Anesth. 2011;23(1):75–8.

84. Filippou DK, Triga A, Rizos S, Grigoriadis E, Shipkov CD, Nissiotis AS. Electrocardiographic changes after laparoscopic cholecystectomy. Folia Med. 2004;46(4):37–41. PubMed PMID: 15962814.

85. Aust H, Eberhart LH, Kranke P, Arndt C, Bleimuller C, Zoremba M, et al. [Hypoxemia after general anesthesia]. Anaesthesist. 2012;61(4):299–309. PubMed PMID: 22526741. Hypoxamie nach Allgemeinanasthesie.

86. Scott B. Airway management in post anaesthetic care. J Perioper Pract. 2012;22(4):135–8. PubMed PMID: 22567765.

87. Tinsley MH, Barone CP. Preventing postoperative nausea and vomiting: refresh your knowledge of how to recognize and respond to this common complication. Plast Surg Nurs. 2012;32(3):106–11. PubMed PMID: 22929197.

Patient Positioning; Incision/Port Placement

Elias S. Hyams and Edward M. Schaeffer

Abbreviations

RALRP   Robotic-assisted laparoscopic radical prostatectomy

RRP   Radical retropubic prostatectomy

Positioning

Positioning for RALRP

After anesthesia is induced, the patient is placed in a low dorsal lithotomy position (Fig. 3.1). Legs are placed in yellowfin stirrups or a split leg attachment depending on surgeon preference (Fig. 3.2). It is critical that pressure points are adequately padded to avoid continuous pressure on the calf muscle or the peroneal nerve. If stirrups are used, pressure should be distributed to the heel rather than the calf. Egg crates or other padding can be used to cushion the lateral aspect of the lower leg to protect the peroneal nerve. With positioning, the hip and thigh should be in anatomic position without extension to decrease

E.S. Hyams, M.D. (✉)
Section of Urology, Dartmouth-Hitchcock Medical Center, One Medical Center Drive, Lebanon, NH 03756, USA
e-mail: elias.s.hyams@hitchcock.org

E.M. Schaeffer, M.D., Ph.D.
Brady Urological Institute, Johns Hopkins Medical Institution, Baltimore, MD, USA

risk of femoral nerve injury. The patient's arms are secured at his side. Padding of the elbows is critical to avoid ulnar neuropathy. Also it is important to ensure the hands are padded and wrapped to avoid inadvertent trauma. The "foot" of the bed may be detachable or motorized; in the latter case, it is critical to ensure the hands are in view during bed movement to ensure they are not injured. It is critical that the entire surgical team (surgeon, anesthesia, nursing staff) attend to positioning and padding, and voice any concerns prior to final prepping and draping.

Securing the patient to the table can be safely performed in various ways. The patient's chest may be strapped to the table either transversely or in a crossing "X" fashion. Alternatively, an inflatable bean bag can be secured around the patient including above the shoulders to prevent movement during positioning (Fig. 3.1). As the patient's arms are tucked at the patient's side, it is important that pulse oximetry, blood pressure cuff placement, and secure intravenous access be established prior to final positioning.

Trendelenburg positioning is necessary to ensure the bowel falls gravitationally out of the pelvis during the procedure (Fig. 3.2). Trendelenburg positioning is generally the extreme of the table, between 30 and 45°. Less Trendelenburg may be utilized depending on a patient's ability to tolerate the positioning from a cardiopulmonary standpoint. In general, maximal Trendelenburg of a table will allow for correct positioning; however measurement of angulation using a nautical inclinometer was been employed [2].

J.A. Eastham and E.M. Schaeffer (eds.), *Radical Prostatectomy: Surgical Perspectives*,
DOI 10.1007/978-1-4614-8693-0_3, © Springer Science+Business Media New York 2014

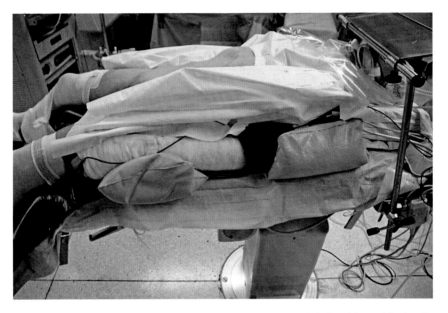

Fig. 3.1 Patient positioned in low lithotomy position with a split leg attachment. The arms are positioned anatomically alongside the body and carefully secured. The vacuum mattress is inflated for cushioning. From John H. et al. Atlas of Robotic Prostatectomy. 2013;19–26. With permission from Springer Science + Business Media, LLC

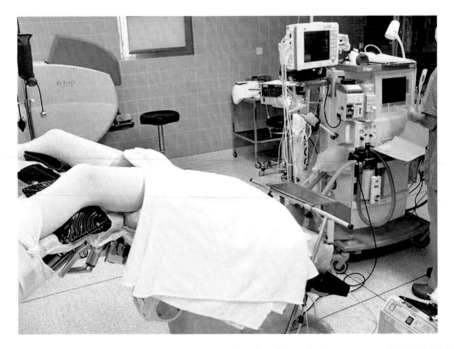

Fig. 3.2 Steep Trendelenburg positioning. From John H. et al. Atlas of Robotic Prostatectomy. 2013;19–26. With permission from Springer Science + Business Media, LLC

Trendelenburg position is associated with numerous physiological effects about which the surgeon and anesthesiologist should be aware. These effects may impair cerebrovascular, respiratory, and hemodynamic function and may be exacerbated by pneumoperitoneum [4]. Cerebrovascular effects of Trendelenburg include increased intracranial pressure, which may be dangerous in patients with cerebral ischema or cerebrovascular disorders. However, overall there have been conflicting findings regarding the impact of Trendelenburg on cerebral oxygenation. Respiratory effects with Trendelenburg and pneumoperitoneum include mechanical pressure on the diaphragm, reducing functional reserve capacity and compliance, and predisposing patients to atelectasis. Difficulty ventilating may necessitate relieving some pneumoperitoneum or decreasing bed tilt. Hypercarbia may occur from CO_2 insufflation and necessitate adjustments in minute and tidal volumes and/or adjustments of insufflation pressure by the surgeon. Effects on dead-space ventilation and oxygenation are thought to be small and are not typically an obstacle to positioning [3].

Hemodynamic effects occur with Trendelenburg in concert with pneumoperitoneum as well. Mean arterial pressure and systemic vascular resistance increase when pneumoperitoneum is initiated; adding Trendelenburg may return systemic vascular resistance to baseline but not change mean arterial pressure [6]. While central venous pressure, mean pulmonary arterial pressure, and pulmonary capillary wedge pressure do not change with insufflation, adding steep positioning may cause a significant increase in these values [6]. Heart strain may increase with Trendelenburg positioning as well. In general, patients with normal cardiac function tolerate these perturbations; however, those with compromised heart function may be at risk for heart failure from preload increase with positioning [6]. Finally, bradycardia may be induced as a vagal response to pneumoperitoneum; this generally subsides with relief of intraabdominal pressure. It is prudent for patients with a history of significant cardiopulmonary disease to consult with cardiology and/or

pulmonology prior to surgery to address the safety of Trendelenburg positioning.

Additional risks of steep Trendelenburg include facial, pharyngeal, and laryngeal edema, associated with venous congestion, facial swelling, and increased intracranial pressure. Restricting fluids and minimizing operative time may help to minimize perioperative edema.

Patient movement during Trendelenburg positioning should be avoided, in particular to avoid instability of the head and neck. Obese patients may be at greater risk for migration on the table. Generally, however, the patient remains stable after docking of the robot. Meticulous attention in securing the patient prior to bed tilt is essential to minimize patient movement.

A potential complication with steep Trendelenburg positioning is compartment syndrome and/or rhabdomyolysis, which may be life threatening. Longer operative times and high body mass index may be risk factors for this complication [12]. In patients with longer case duration, particularly for obese patients, there should be a higher index of suspicion for rhabdomyolysis, and surveillance serum creatine kinase measurements and aggressive postoperative hydration should be considered [12]. Gluteal and calf fasciotomies have been required for compartment syndrome in isolated reports [5, 8].

Patients with a history of glaucoma are at theoretical risk for exacerbation of their disease with Trendelenburg positioning. Studies of intraocular pressure have demonstrated that surgical duration and end-tidal CO_2 are significant predictions of intraocular pressure increase in the Trendelenburg position [1]. However, the precise risks of positioning in these patients are unclear. While it is thought that RALRP is safe in patients with controlled glaucoma, patients with severe or uncontrolled disease should consult with ophthalmology prior to surgery. Additionally, there has been one reported case of ischemic optic neuropathy during RALRP, with prolonged positioning, substantial intravenous fluids, and substantial blood loss [10]. Ultimately, avoidance of protracted positioning is physiologically advantageous to the patient and an expeditious procedure is likely to minimize risk of ocular and other complications.

Positioning for Radical Retropubic Prostatectomy

For standard positioning, the patient is placed in the supine position. Traditionally the patient is placed with his hip on the break of the table, and the table is flexed to increase the distance between pubis and umbilicus. However, flexion of the table is not universally performed. If the table is flexed (i.e., hyperlordotic positioning), the kidney rest may be elevated to increase puboumbilical distance to improve exposure. However, while this is the classical approach to positioning, there have been reports of femoral and sciatic nerve injuries, and rhabdomyolysis with acute renal failure in this position [9]. Obese patients may be at increased risk for rhabdomyolysis and nerve palsy syndromes with RRP, thus require extra care with positioning. Another concern with hyperlordotic positioning is that with severe lumbar stenosis, extension of the spine may compress neural elements and potentially cause spinal cord trauma [9]. Thus the authors generally recommend supine positioning without table flexion.

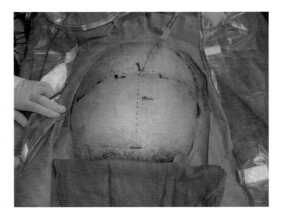

Fig. 3.3 Measurements for placement of camera, robotic, and assistant ports

Incisions

Port Placement for RALRP

Initial access to the abdomen is performed with Veress or Hassan technique at the surgeon's discretion. The authors' preference is Veress access as Hassan access is more time consuming, has not been systematically shown to be safer, and there is an increased likelihood of air leak during the case. The Veress needle is generally placed transumbilically, however when there has been prior periumbilical surgery (e.g., hernia repair, prior laparoscopy) the needle should be placed in a remote quadrant of the abdomen. If the abdomen does not insufflate normally, it is important to remove the needle promptly and reattempt with consideration of placement elsewhere in the abdomen. When the abdomen is insufflated to 15 mmHg, a vertical incision is made at the midline for camera port access. In patients with standard body habitus, the camera port can be placed

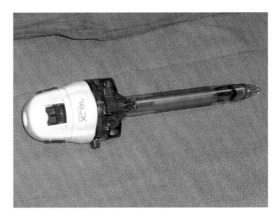

Fig. 3.4 10 mm Optiview trocar (Ethicon, Somerville, NJ)

supraumbilically. The distance from the pubis to the camera port should be approximately 15 cm (Fig. 3.3). In taller patients, it may be helpful to measure this distance and place the camera port infraumbilically to ensure that the robotic instruments reach the membranous urethra. The initial camera port is a 10 mm port and can be placed using various techniques including with an Optiview trocar (Ethicon, Somerville, NJ) (Fig. 3.4) and 0° lense under vision or with the Visiport (Covidien, Mansfield, MA) device. In patients with no prior abdominal surgery, blind access can be considered using a bladeless Step trocar device (Covidien, Mansfield, MA).

Robotic ports are customarily placed 1 cm inferiorly and 8 cm laterally to the camera port

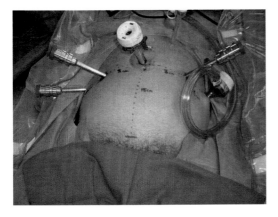

Fig. 3.5 Six-port technique including camera port, three robotic working ports, and two assistant ports

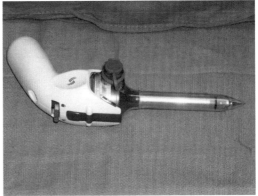

Fig. 3.6 10 mm Assistant trocar (Airseal) (Surgiquest, Orange, CT)

(Fig. 3.3). At least 8 cm should separate the ports to ensure that the external arms of the robot do not clash. In taller patients, there may be concern about the ability of robotic arms to reach the membranous urethra. Thus robotic arms should be no more than 18 cm from the pubic bone [7]. The fourth robotic arm can be placed on the left or right side of the abdomen depending on surgeon and assistant preference. However, the assistant will stand on the side opposite the fourth robotic arm, as the primary assistant port will be placed contralaterally.

A six port technique is typically utilized for RALRP, with a camera port, three working robotic ports, and two assistant ports (Fig. 3.5). The primary assistant port (10 mm) is placed at least 8 cm laterally to the first arm, and at least 1 cm superior to the anterior superior iliac spine. Careful placement of this port is important to avoid clashing of assistant and robotic instruments. Various types of assistant ports can be utilized, though an Airseal port (Surgiquest, Orange, CT) may be useful to reduce abdominal desufflation during suctioning (Fig. 3.6). Obese patients present an added challenge as pannus may hinder angulation of assistant instruments. A second (5 mm) assistant port is placed in the upper abdomen on the side of assistant (Fig. 3.7). A triangle is created cranially from the camera and robotic ports to the upper abdomen, to a site equidistant from these ports (Fig. 3.8). This port primarily accommodates the suction/irrigator,

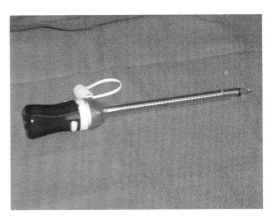

Fig. 3.7 5 mm Assistant trocar (Ethicon, Somerville, NJ)

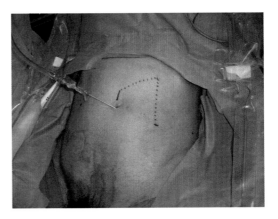

Fig. 3.8 Triangulation between camera and robotic port sites for placement of 5 mm assistant trocar

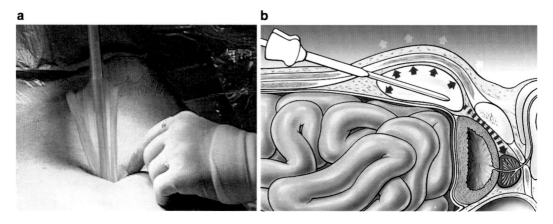

Fig. 3.9 Balloon dilation of the extraperitoneal space. From John H. et al. Atlas of Robotic Prostatectomy. 2013;19–26. With permission from Springer Science + Business Media, LLC

while surgical clips are placed through the primary assistant port.

Different types of assistant trocars can be utilized. Step trocars are radially dilating and do not require closure of the fascia; however, they can migrate and need to be secured to the skin with a suture. Ribbed trocars do not require suturing to the skin; however, fascial entries 1 cm or greater do require fascial closure at the conclusion of the case.

In patients with prior lower abdominal surgery, adhesions may be present and entry into the abdomen should be performed with extra care. In patients with prior umbilical herniorrhaphy, Veress access should be performed remote from the prior surgical site, e.g., in the right upper quadrant, or Hassan access can be performed. In patients with a current umbilical hernia, some authors recommend placement of a 5 mm camera port in the upper abdomen, as an assistant port, with a 5 mm laparoscopic camera to enable visualization and reduction of the hernia from a remote site [11]. The camera port is subsequently placed under vision through the fascial defect, which is closed transversely at the end of the case. This approach of remote access with a 5 mm trocar can be utilized in patients with prior midline or contralateral abdominal surgery to survey the abdomen and enable safe access for adhesiolysis. A spinal needle can be used to assess the trajectory of trocar placement and precise entry site prior to placement of the trocar.

After initial access, the abdomen is surveyed to ensure no signs of injury to visceral contents and to survey any possible adhesions. Then, additional ports are placed under vision.

While positioning is similar for extraperitoneal RALRP compared with the transperitoneal approach, port placement for extraperitoneal surgery initially differs. A 1.5 cm incision is made transversely below the umbilicus, and the anterior rectus sheath is exposed. This is incised vertically for 1 cm, the rectus muscle is divided and the posterior rectus sheath is exposed. With blunt finger dissection, a space is created anterior to the posterior rectus sheath. A balloon dilator is advanced along the posterior rectus sheath to the pubis (Fig. 3.9). The balloon trocar is insufflated to develop the space of Retzius under laparoscopic vision using 10–15 pumps. Additional trocars are then placed under vision with the technique elaborated above.

Incision for RRP

Incision for RRP is generally a vertical, lower abdominal incision extending from the pubis 8 cm toward the umbilicus. This enables extraperitoneal access for prostatectomy. Alternatively, a transverse incision above the pubis (i.e., Pfannenstiel incision) can be made for thin patients. The anterior fascia is exposed and incised vertically in the midline, and the rectus muscles are split. Transversalis fascia is sharply incised to give access to the space of Retzius. A self-retaining Balfour retractor is placed and the prostatectomy is performed. Alternative retractors may be used at the discretion of the surgeon.

References

1. Awad H, Santilli S, Ohr M, et al. The effects of steep trendelenburg positioning on intraocular pressure during robotic radical prostatectomy. Anesth Analg. 2009;109(2):473–8.
2. Cestari A, Buffi NM, Scapaticci E, et al. Simplifying patient positioning and port placement during robotic-assisted laparoscopic prostatectomy. Eur Urol. 2010;57:530–3.
3. Chrijvers D, Mottri A, Traen K, et al. Pulmonary gas exchange is well preserved during robot assisted surgery in steep Trendelenberg position. Acta Anaesthesiol Belg. 2009;60(4):229–33.
4. Gainsburg DM. Anesthetic concerns for robotic-assisted laparoscopic radical prostatectomy. Minerva Anestesiol. 2012;78(5):596–604.
5. Keene R, Froelich JM, Milbrandt JC, et al. Bilateral gluteal compartment syndrome following robotic-assisted prostatectomy. Orthopedics. 2010;33(11):852.
6. Lestar M, Gunnarsson L, Lagerstrand L, et al. Hemodynamic perturbations during robot-assisted laparoscopic radical prostatectomy in 45 degree Trendelenburg position. Anesth Analg. 2011;113:1069–75.
7. Pick DL, Lee DI, Skarecky DW, et al. Anatomic guide for port placement for da Vinci robotic radical prostatectomy. J Endourol. 2004;18:572–5.
8. Rosevear HM, Lightfoot AJ, Zahs M, et al. Lessons learned from a case of calf compartment syndrome after robot-assisted laparoscopioc prostatectomy. J Endourol. 2010;24(10):1597–601.
9. Roth JV. Bilateral sciatic and femoral neuropathies, rhabdomyolysis, and acute renal failure caused by positioning during radical retropubic prostatectomy. Anesth Analg. 2007;105:1747–8.
10. Weber ED, Colyer MH, Lesser RI, et al. Posterior ischemic optic neuropathy after minimally invasive prostatectomy. J Neuroophthalmol. 2007;27:285–7.
11. Kim W, Abdelshehid C, Lee HJ et al. Robotic-assisted laparoscopic prostatectomy in umbilical hernia patients: University of California, Irvine, technique for port placement and repair. Urology 2012;79:1412.e1–1412.e3.
12. Mattei A, DiPierro GB, Rafeld V, et al. Positioning injury, rhabdomyolysis and serum creatinine kinase-concentration course in patients undergoing robot-assisted radical prostatectomy and extended pelvic lymph node dissection. J Endourol 2013;27(1):45–51.

Pelvic Lymph Node Dissection for Prostate Cancer

4

Jonathan L. Silberstein and Vincent P. Laudone

Abbreviations

CT	Computerized tomography
EAU	European Association of Urology
MRI	Magnetic resonance imaging
PLND	Pelvic lymph node dissection
PSA	Prostate-specific antigen
ROC	Receiver operating characteristic
RP	Radical prostatectomy
SPECT/CT	Single-photon emission CT

Introduction

Pelvic lymph node dissection (PLND) is a critical yet controversial aspect of the surgical treatment of prostate cancer. The aim of PLND at the time of radical prostatectomy (RP) is twofold: to properly stage the disease and to provide therapeutic benefit. Much like prostate cancer itself, these aims have evolved over time and the role of PLNDs in the management of prostate cancer must be considered in this context.

PLND is performed in order to acquire the most accurate staging information regarding disease extent. Decades ago, PLND was routinely done either as a separate procedure or in combination with intended RP. If nodal involvement was found, the RP was aborted, as this was considered an ominous prognostic sign [1–3]. More recently, the incidence of nodal involvement has declined, largely due to stage migration as a result of widespread prostate-specific antigen (PSA) testing. Despite this, PLND continues to provide important staging information. Even in current series, between 3 and 26 % of patients without radiographic evidence of regional spread will be found to harbor metastatic pelvic lymph nodes [4–7]. This wide variation reflects not only the heterogeneity of the patient population undergoing RP but also the varying extents of PLNDs being performed.

In addition to the accurate staging information provided by PLND, multiple studies in the more recent era (the "PSA era") have also demonstrated a therapeutic benefit. In older series, nodal involvement was associated with rapid progression to bony metastasis, with 40 % of patients dying of prostate cancer within 5 years [8]. Most patients in these series were generally understaged and often had gross nodal involvement. More recent series have demonstrated that a subset of patients with limited nodal metastasis and favorable pathologic features are curable with a combination of RP and PLND, without the need for additional treatment [4, 9, 10].

Despite the totality of evidence demonstrating the significant advantages associated with PLND, not every patient who undergoes RP receives a

J.L. Silberstein, M.D.
Urology Service, Department of Surgery, Memorial Sloan-Kettering Cancer Center, New York, NY, USA

V.P. Laudone, M.D. (✉)
Sidney Kimmel Center for Prostate and Urologic Cancers, Memorial Sloan-Kettering Cancer Center, 353 East 68th Street, New York, NY 10065, USA
e-mail: laudonev@mskcc.org

J.A. Eastham and E.M. Schaeffer (eds.), *Radical Prostatectomy: Surgical Perspectives*,
DOI 10.1007/978-1-4614-8693-0_4, © Springer Science+Business Media New York 2014

concurrent PLND. In fact, there has been an increasing trend away from PLND [11, 12]. Stage migration in the PSA era has resulted in earlier detection and treatment of prostate cancer and a decreased risk of nodal positivity for many patients. Additionally, more accurate tools, such as nomograms, have emerged that can assess an individual's risk for node positivity. Together these factors have contributed to a decline in the proportion of patients who receive PLND. This has been accentuated by the increased use of minimally invasive surgery, in particular the rapid adoption of robotic surgery [11]. Furthermore, even when practitioners do perform PLND, both the extent and yield of PLND have also declined [13]. This is particularly important because the value of a PLND is dependent on the adequacy of the dissection. Omitting key nodes or nodal packets limits both the staging accuracy and therapeutic value of the procedure.

This chapter reviews these issues, describe techniques for performing a robotic-assisted PLND, and highlight the most common complications and management of complications associated with PLND.

Prostatic Lymphatic Drainage, Preoperative Imaging, and the Sentinel Node

Until the 1970s, lymphatic drainage of the prostate was defined based on autopsy dissections. Since then, a variety of radiographic imaging approaches have been utilized in an attempt to better define the drainage in situ [14]. However, because of a variety of obstacles—including the redundancy, variability, complexity, and crossover of the prostatic lymphatic drainage for a given prostatic tumor—the lymphatic drainage of the prostate, or perhaps more importantly for a given prostate tumor, is still not as clearly defined as in other organs such as the testis [15, 16]. Generally, the prostate gland drains first into the periprostatic subcapsular network from which three main drainage routes—the ascending, lateral, and posterior groups—extend. The ascending

ducts drain into the external iliac lymph nodes, the lateral ducts drain into the hypogastric node chain, and the posterior ducts drain from the caudal prostate to the subaortic lymph nodes of the sacral promontory [7].

Imaging studies that are frequently obtained in patients undergoing RP—such as computerized tomography (CT) or magnetic resonance imaging (MRI) with or without an endorectal coil—are relatively insensitive for the detection of lymph node metastasis [17]. This may be due, in part, to the fact that these imaging modalities primarily use size criteria to identify suspicious nodes. In current surgical series, most nodal metastases are limited to a single node and are small, often less than one centimeter [6]. Newer developments, such as sentinel node lymphoscintigraphy, allow identification of sentinel nodes by injecting the prostate with radioactive or fluorescent imaging agents that are detectable with single-photon emission CT/CT (SPECT/CT), gamma probes [18], near-infrared fluorescence guidance, or a combination of these modalities using a hybrid radiocolloid [19]. Regardless of the modality, however, this method requires direct injection of the prostate prior to RP and is limited by a lack of cancer specificity.

Combining superparamagnetic particles of iron oxide with traditional or MRI-weighted imaging may allow preoperative radiographic detection of normal-size malignant nodes. However, more than two decades after the initial animal studies [20], and 10 years since a promising report of their use in patients with prostate cancer [21], these agents have failed to win Food and Drug Administration approval for use in clinical practice in the USA. A very recent study in Switzerland of ultra-small superparamagnetic particles of iron oxide and MRI in both prostate and bladder cancer reported an overall diagnostic accuracy of 77 %, with the majority of missed metastases being smaller than 5 mm [22]. For the time being there is no reliable imaging modality to detect lymph node metastases, and a meticulous PLND remains the most accurate diagnostic tool and the gold standard for prostate cancer staging.

Table 4.1 Nomenclature of pelvic lymph node dissection

| Description of dissection | Nomenclature | | |
	Historic definition	Zones of dissection	Current MSKCC definition
External iliac vein	Limited	1	Limited
External iliac vein and obturator fossa	Standard	1, 2	Limited
External iliac vein, obturator fossa, and hypogastric vessels	Extended	1, 2, 3	Standard
External iliac vein, obturator fossa, hypogastric vessels, and common iliac to ureteral crossing	Super-extended	1, 2, 3, 4	Extended

Extent of Pelvic Lymph Node Dissection

Crucial to any discussion of the appropriate extent of a PLND is clarification of the nomenclature used to define it. Frequently, well-meaning investigators use terms such as "limited" or "extended" without a complete description of the anatomic parameters involved. Furthermore, in the era of PSA screening, as the risk of nodal invasion has diminished and the frequency and extent of PLND has decreased [11, 12], some commonly held definitions have changed. Such definitions are used for simplicity but may not be universal and may create confusion. For clarification purposes, Table 4.1 lists frequently used terminology and the commonly interpreted explanation of the extent of dissection.

Regardless of the definition, the extent of the template that should be used for a PLND remains controversial. Many practitioners perform a limited nodal sampling, as evidenced by the low overall nodal yields recorded in population-based databases such as the Surveillance, Epidemiology, and End Results (SEER) registries. In 2006, according to SEER, the median number of lymph nodes removed during PLND was six, indicating a substantial decline over the previous two decades [13]. While the reasons for these disturbing trends are not altogether clear, it may be that practitioners are unconvinced by data indicating the therapeutic nature of PLND, or there is lack of clarity regarding which nodes to remove, or perhaps because more-extended PLNDs require more time, effort, and skill, with a concurrent increase in the risk of complications associated with the procedure [23]. In an effort to determine the appropriate template for PLND, a few small, randomized trials have compared limited with more extended templates, but because of their small size and single-institution design, they have failed to resolve the issue [24, 25].

Despite these uncertainties, there are some principles that can provide clarity. First, and perhaps most important, the more nodes removed, the higher the probability of discovering a positive node. Because a positive node can only be detected if it has been resected, a negative PLND will only be truly negative if a positive node has not been inadvertently omitted at the time of resection. PLNDs with small nodal yields have higher false-negative rates than dissections with greater numbers of nodes removed. Briganti et al. [26] eloquently demonstrated this principle by creating receiver operating characteristic (ROC) curves demonstrating that the ability to detect a positive node is dependent on the number of nodes removed. They found that 28 nodes need to be removed and examined to achieve a 90 % probability of detecting a positive node, whereas the probability is less than 10 % when ten or fewer nodes are removed.

Unfortunately, measuring lymph node yield as a surrogate for discerning adequacy of dissection has limitations. There may be significant variation in nodal yield from one patient to the next, even when the same PLND template is performed by the same surgeon and analyzed by the same group of pathologists in the same manner [27]. This variation may reflect differences in the number of nodes in the individual patient or subtle differences in either the collection or processing of the specimen. Lymph nodes smaller than 1 cm are difficult to detect in bulky or en bloc specimens, whereas individually labeled, less bulky packets are easier for pathologists to dissect. Methods to increase nodal yield (which usually also increases the cost of the procedure) may include sending separate nodal packets to pathology rather than sending en bloc specimens [28].

Packeted dissections may provide higher nodal yield, but perhaps more importantly they allow surgeons to attribute nodal metastases to a specific anatomic location. Bader et al. performed packeted dissections on 365 patients, dividing the PLND into external iliac, obturator, and internal iliac packets based on the anatomic boundaries of the dissection [5]. The authors found nodal positivity in 88 patients; positive nodes were located along the internal iliac artery in more than half of these patients (58 %) and exclusively in this location in 19 % of patients. A more recent study by another group of investigators reported similar findings. Of 642 consecutive patients, 35 were found to have nodal metastasis; of them, 80 % had only one (49 %) or two (31 %) positive lymph nodes. Isolated nodal positivity was found more commonly in either the obturator or hypogastric fossa than the external iliac fossa [6]. Most important, the authors demonstrated that a PLND limited to the external iliac area would have identified and removed positive nodes in only a third of the patients actually found to have node positivity on a full PLND. Multiple other studies have confirmed these findings, indicating that positive nodal tissue is often found exclusively below the obturator nerve or along the hypogastric artery [7, 29]. Together these investigators have clearly established that, at minimum, a PLND should include all the tissue from the iliac bifurcation cranially to Cooper's ligament caudally, from the pelvic sidewall laterally to the urinary bladder medially, and from the external iliac vein superiorly to the pelvic floor inferiorly, exposing the hypogastric vein and skeletonizing the obturator vessels. Minimal templates should include zones 1, 2, and 3 (referred to at MSKCC as a "standard dissection"), but for patients with higher risk tumors these templates are often expanded to include zone 4 or beyond (referred to at MSKCC at an "extended PLND").

Many have suggested that PLND templates should be expanded to include tissue cephalad to the iliac bifurcation—along the common iliac up to or above the ureteric crossing—or include tissue medial to this region in the presacral area [29–31]. These extended or superextended templates have been advocated by some investigators, either because of lymphoscintigraphy studies demonstrating they capture a greater proportion of the prostate's primary landing zone or because isolated positive nodes have been identified in these regions. Templates above the aortic bifurcation have also been attempted but have revealed that nodal positivity is only found above this region when multiple nodes (five or greater) are positive within the pelvis [32]. Because lymph node dissection only provides durable therapeutic benefit when limited numbers of nodes are positive, *the benefit of a PLND extending above the aortic bifurcation must be questioned until there is clear evidence to the contrary* [9, 10]. (See "Therapeutic Benefit of PLND," below.)

Can Adequate PLND be Performed Using a Robotic Approach?

The surgical technique of RP has changed dramatically since 2001, when the da Vinci surgical platform was first introduced. Currently there are more than 2,500 robotic systems installed worldwide [33]. In the USA, robot-assisted laparoscopic RP was rapidly adopted and is now the most commonly used technique for performing RP [34]. Unfortunately, population-based studies have demonstrated that the probability of receiving a PLND at the time of RP is lower when the surgery is performed using the robotic technique [11]. The exact cause for this disparity is not completely clear but likely stems from (1) the lack of formal robotic and/or oncologic training by most early adopters of robotic techniques, and (2) concern regarding the potential difficulty in addressing major vascular complications with robotic systems.

Many of the largest published series establishing the robotic approach as a viable alternative to open RP have included little to no information regarding PLND [35]. Consequently, questions remain regarding the proportion of patients who receive a concurrent PLND, the extent of the templates used, or typical lymph node yields or density. Several published reports comparing outcomes after open and robotic approaches for RP and/or PLND have failed to show that an equivalent PLND dissection can be performed robotically; and each of these studies has been limited in various ways (Table 4.2). However, recent studies have begun to establish that when attention and focus is placed on R-PLND by experienced surgeons, an equivalent number of positive nodes can be obtained and equivalent oncologic outcomes can be achieved [36]. Nodal yields, like biochemical recurrence and margin status, ultimately depend more on the surgeon than on the surgical approach [36–38].

Complications

Complications directly attributable to PLND during RP are rare, but the true number is difficult to ascertain because undergoing a simultaneous RP is more likely to cause complications [42, 43]. The most common complication resulting from PLND is leakage of the lymphatic fluid into the space surrounding the transected lymphatic channels. Ideally, at the time of PLND all open lymphatic channels will be ligated and sealed, but there is a risk of some open channels remaining and subsequent leakage. This lymphatic fluid may leak into the peri-lymphatic space and, rarely, cause problems. Symptoms depend on the size, location, and potential for this fluid collection to get secondarily infected. Symptomatic lymphoceles can result in abdominal or pelvic distention, pain, deep venous thrombosis by compressing on the iliac veins and disrupting laminar blood flow, potential disruption of the urethral anastomosis, or superinfection. Because lymphoceles are detected only when they are symptomatic, their true incidence is underestimated but has been reported to be as high as 26–51 % when routine imaging is performed [44, 45]. The rate of symptomatic lymphoceles is widely variable and reported to range from 5–15 % [45, 46]. The wide

variation likely reflects differences in surgical technique, patient characteristics, and detection methods. While surgical technique is the most prominent causative factor of lymphocele, other influencing factors include the extent of dissection [46], presence of lymph node invasion, use of heparin [47], use of cautery, or prior radiation. Various strategies have been suggested for mitigating lymphocele formation, including use of preoperative heparin in an upper rather than lower extremity [48] or use of fibrin sealants to the operative bed [49, 50]. Meticulous surgical technique that includes careful dissection and generous use of clips to ligate all transected lymphatic channels likely has the greatest impact in preventing this complication.

While surgical technique may be critical in the prevention of lymphocele formation, surgical approach may not be. The hypothesis that transperitoneal laparoscopic approaches may be associated with lower rates of lymphocele formation due to the ability of the lymphatic fluid to drain into the peritoneum for reabsorption may be unfounded. In one study, routine CT following PLND in 76 patients noted lymphoceles in 51 % of patients, with 15 % being clinically symptomatic [45].

When a lymphocele does become symptomatic and treatment is required, percutaneous drainage is the most common technique utilized. Once a drain is placed, the fluid is aspirated and tested for creatinine to rule out a urine leak, and bacterial cultures are obtained to direct appropriate antibiotic therapy. Simple drainage may not resolve the issue alone, and continued lymphatic drainage may require injection of a sclerosing solution to seal the open lymphatic. Multiple sclerosing agents have been used, including tetracycline, doxycycline, bleomycin, ethanol, povidone iodine, and sodium amidotrizoate [51]. Alternatively, the lymphatic collection maybe treated with open drainage or marsupialized within the peritoneal cavity. Both practices are reported to have greater success rates than percutaneous drainage, but with greater levels of intervention and higher rates of morbidity [52].

Most patients undergoing RP and PLND are considered to be at high risk for the development

Table 4.2 Comparative studies of lymph node yields for open and robotic pelvic lymph node dissection during radical prostatectomy

Study	Institution	Number of patients	Nodal yield			Limitations
			Open	RALP	P value	
Zorn et al. [39]	University of Chicago Medical Center	767	Mean 15.0	12.5	<0.01	Contemporary RALP series was compared to historical open series
Cooperberg et al. [40]	University of California, San Francisco, Cancer Center	524	Mean 14.4	9.3	<0.01	Only a small fraction of patients received PLND
Truesdale et al. [41]	Columbia University Medical Center	316	Mean 7.5	6.3	0.06	Open group was at greater risk of lymph node involvement
Silberstein et al. [36]	Memorial Sloan-Kettering Cancer Center	323	Median 20.0	16.0	0.01	Differences between surgeons were greater than differences between techniques

RALP robot-assisted laparoscopic radical prostatectomy

of thromboembolic events by virtue of their age (typically >50 years), known malignancy, and pelvic surgery [53]. However, because thrombo-embolic events are rare and may go undetected, determining the impact that PLND has on potentiating this risk is challenging [39, 53]. Lymphocele formation has been demonstrated to be associated with greater risk of deep venous thrombosis formation, again highlighting the need for meticulous ligation of all lymphatic channels [46].

Though rare, injuries to nerves within the pelvis, most notably the obturator nerve, can occur during PLND. The obturator nerve enters the pelvis behind the iliac vessels, runs laterally along the pelvic sidewall, and exits through the obturator foramen. The nerve provides motor innervation of the adductor muscles of the thigh and sensory innervation to the skin on the medial aspect of the proximal thigh. The fibrofatty tissue removed during PLND completely surrounds the nerve, obscuring its visualization at the start of the dissection. This tissue needs to be carefully dissected off the nerve, and during this process the nerve may be subject to partial or complete transection, or stretch, thermal, or crush injury. If transected, the nerve may be approximated with fine non-absorbable suture.

During PLND, particularly when an extended template dissection is performed with dissection of tissue along the course of the common iliac vessels, there is risk of injury to the ureters as they enter the pelvis. Depending on the extent of the injury, ureteral reimplantation or stenting may be required. A detailed understanding of the pelvic anatomy and the relationship between the various structures is necessary to avoid neural, vascular, or ureteric injury during PLND.

Of the possible intraoperative complications that can occur during a robot-assisted operation, the most challenging and potentially life threatening is sudden hemorrhage that is not controllable with the robotic platform. A major vascular complication during open PLND can usually be controlled by tamponading the bleeding vessel with a sponge stick or a vascular clamp. In the case of a robotic procedure, the situation can be more difficult. Immediate conversion to an open procedure may be necessary to achieve vascular control as quickly as possible. This process is impeded by several factors, including the primary surgeon not being at the bedside, the robot blocking access to the patient, and standard robotic instruments being inadequate for this specific task. When residents or fellows are taught to perform RP in a stepwise fashion, PLND is often the first portion of the procedure taught during open technique, but it is usually the last part taught during robotic training, due to the potentially life-threatening situation caused by an inadvertent vascular injury.

Who Should Receive a PLND?

Omitting a PLND avoids potential complications, decreases the length of surgery, and saves $900–$3,000 in costs associated with the procedure [54]. But omission fails to provide important staging information and potential therapeutic value. Because the incidence of lymph node metastasis in most published surgical series is relatively low (usually below 10 %), various predictive tools such as nomograms have been proposed in order to maximize the benefit and minimize overtreatment. These nomograms have been created to determine the probability of lymph node involvement at the time of RP based on PSA, clinical stage, and Gleason score. Various guidelines suggest different cutoffs (Table 4.3). For example, the National Comprehensive Cancer Network (NCCN) guidelines recommend that PLND be performed in all patients undergoing RP who are estimated to have a ≥2 % risk of lymph node involvement, since this avoids 48 % of PLNDs at a cost of missing 12 % of positive lymph nodes [55]. The European Association of Urology (EAU) guidelines use a 5 % cutoff, in which the estimated risk of nodal involvement is between 15 and 40 % [56]. An important limitation of most nomograms is that they are based on cohorts of patients who underwent limited PLND and may therefore underestimate the true risk of nodal metastasis [57, 58]. A more complete evaluation of all existing nomograms is published elsewhere [15]; however, only two nomograms have been created and validated in sets of patients that have undergone extended PLND [59, 60]. Because both the American Urological Association (AUA) and EAU guidelines recommend extended PLND, these two nomograms likely more accurately predict true rates of nodal metastasis.

Table 4.3 Guidelines for pelvic lymph node dissection

Group	Recommendation	Limitations
AUA [61]	PLND is generally reserved for patients with higher risk of lymph node involvement	Fails to define "higher risk" and does not specify the extent of PLND
NCCN [55]	Extended PLND is recommended for all patients with a ≥2 % risk of lymph node involvement	Does not specify which nomogram to use to determine risk
EAU [56]	Extended PLND is recommended for all patients with a ≥5 % risk of lymph node involvement	Does not specify which nomogram to use to determine risk
MSKCC	PLND that includes external, internal, and obturator lymph nodes is recommended for all patients with a nomogram-estimated ≥2 % risk of lymph node involvement and for some patients with a <2 % risk, at the discretion of the surgeon	Unclear what factors should influence the surgeon's decision to perform PLND for patients with <2 % risk

PLND pelvic lymph node dissection

The AUA recommendations are the vaguest of the major guidelines regarding indications for and extent of PLND [61]. These state that PLND is "generally reserved for patients with higher risk of lymph node involvement," but fail to give specific cutoffs or definitions of "higher risk" disease.

In general, we recommend guiding patients with lower risk cancer toward active surveillance and reserving definitive treatment for patients with higher risk disease. As active surveillance becomes a more common recommendation for men with low-risk prostate cancer, the remaining pool of patients who undergo surgery will likely have more aggressive disease. Consequently, a higher percentage of the patients who receive an RP are likely to also benefit from a PLND [62]. Furthermore, if a PLND is performed, we recommend removal of all fibrofatty tissue surrounding the external, obturator, and internal vessels, from the node of Cloquet to the bifurcation of the internal/external iliac vessels. For patients at particularly high risk or with radiographic suspicion of nodal metastasis beyond these boundaries, the template may be expanded further.

Therapeutic Benefit of PLND

PLND provides staging information that can help to determine the extent of the patient's disease for both prognostic and treatment planning purposes. Removal of pelvic lymph node tissue—especially in the setting of minimal regional spread—can also provide therapeutic benefit. Multiple studies have demonstrated that a significant portion of patients with limited nodal involvement and favorable histopathologic features will not experience recurrence or progression following surgery, even without adjuvant treatment. Catalona et al. first demonstrated a 75 % recurrence-free survival rate at 6 years for patients who had undergone RP and had node-positive disease [63]. In the PSA era, Bader et al. demonstrated that the number of positive nodes correlated with the risk of biochemical recurrence following RP; for example, 42 % of patients with only one positive node remained free from biochemical recurrence at a median follow-up of 45 months [10]. More recently, Von Bodman et al. performed a retrospective review of 162 patients with lymph node metastases who received no adjuvant treatment. They found that patients with one positive node and a Gleason score of seven or lower had a recurrence-free probability of 79 % 2 years after RP, and those with greater numbers of positive nodes had greater rates of biochemical recurrence [9].

Detecting nodal positivity may direct subsequent adjuvant treatments with resulting therapeutic benefit. For example, adjuvant hormonal therapy in patients with positive lymph nodes may produce a long-term survival benefit compared with observation, as demonstrated by Messing et al. In a prospective randomized trial of 98 patients with prostate cancer, immediate long-term androgen deprivation therapy was associated with improved overall survival advantage, with a hazard ratio of 1.84 (95 % confidence interval 1.01–3.35, $p=0.04$) at a median follow-up

of 11.9 years [64]. This highly provocative study has received much criticism for its small size, lack of standardized PLND template, and the multiplicity of surgeons and centers involved. Additionally, it was conducted early in the era of widespread PSA screening, and the disease extent (i.e., disease stage at time of initial diagnosis) of these patients may not reflect current practice. Therefore, despite the overall, progression-free, and disease-specific survival advantages demonstrated in this study, we do not advocate adjuvant therapy for all patients. Men with minimal nodal disease found with thorough dissection can be carefully watched, receiving adjuvant treatment only after biochemical or clinical recurrence.

Interestingly, population-based studies have demonstrated that even in the absence of any pathologically positive lymph nodes, PLND may provide therapeutic benefit. Joslyn and Konety reviewed the SEER database and, after controlling for multiple patient- and disease-related factors, noted in a multivariate analysis that, even when restricting analysis to node-negative patients, there was a decreased risk of prostate cancer death when ten or more nodes were removed [65]. This benefit may be due in part to micrometastatic disease that is present in the nodal tissue but falsely determined to be negative on histopathologic observation [66]. Several authors have noted that reverse transcriptase polymerase chain reaction may identify such nodal metastases [67, 68]. While these tools are intriguing, they are currently most commonly reserved for the research setting.

Surgical Technique of Robot-Assisted Pelvic Lymph Node Dissection

The majority of RPs performed in the USA today is done via a robotic approach [34]. A successful robotic PLND requires not only a meticulous dissection but also a high degree of comfort and skill on the part of the surgeon in the use of the robotic platform. One of the fundamental keys to successful surgery, whether done by an open or minimal access approach, is learning how to achieve and maintain the exposure necessary to accomplish the task at hand. This necessitates a detailed knowledge of the anatomy of the region and an understanding of the most efficient use of traction and countertraction to facilitate dissection. Robotic surgery has an enormous, but often neglected, advantage in this regard. The robot allows the operator to become a three-handed surgeon, and with the help of a single assistant, a five-handed one. At any moment the surgeon can engage two of the robotic arms to provide traction and countertraction, while at the same time positioning and directing the bedside assistant to do the same through two assistant ports. Simultaneously the surgeon uses the remaining, or "fifth," hand for the primary task of cutting and dissecting. Patient position, bedside assistant utilization, and port placement become critical components in this process of efficient and successful robotic surgery.

When utilizing an intraperitoneal approach for robotic RP with PLND, port placement is modified only slightly, in that a slightly more cranial port placement is favored. The camera is inserted via a supraumbilical semi-circumferential incision and all additional ports are placed at or above the level of the umbilicus, or higher if the dissection is to be carried up to the inferior mesenteric artery as in a cystectomy. Surgeon preference varies as to the number and position of ports. For a right-handed surgeon, placing two robotic arms on the patient's right and one on the left is our preferred approach. This setup allows for opposing graspers, one on the left and one on the right, to provide traction and countertraction while keeping the dominant hand free to manipulate the scissors. When set up this way, instrumentation typically includes Maryland or fenestrated bipolar forceps in the left hand and ProGrasp forceps or similar device in the third arm on the far right. Scissors are placed on the right side in the number-one robotic port. Having grasping abilities in opposing hands facilitates achieving and maintaining exposure on either side of the pelvis. With this setup, the assistant will be on the patient's left side and work through two accessory ports—a 5 mm between the camera and left robotic port, and a 12 mm on the far left.

While an accessory 12 mm port is not absolutely necessary, it allows for a reusable specimen bag to be placed multiple times in order to retrieve the nodes in as many packets as the surgeon desires, and then it is available for prostate removal at the end of the procedure. Another advantage to an accessory 12 mm port is that the robotic camera can be placed through this port to look at the umbilical port if midline adhesions are encountered (Fig. 4.1).

Either a 30° down lens or a 0° lens is utilized for the PLND. The 30° down lens facilitates the removal of nodes underneath the iliac vessels proximally, but it is possible to perform an equivalent dissection using the 0° lens with a bit more effort. In terms of efficiency, in order to avoid scope changing, cleaning, and defogging, it is often best to use the same lens that is used for the RP portion of the operation. This also has the very real advantage of maintaining the same visual perspective for the entire case, as changing the camera angle requires the surgical team to shift their visual perception of the surgical anatomy.

Typical instruments used in the dissection of the nodes are a monopolar scissor in the dominant hand, a bipolar cautery (Maryland or fenestrated) in the opposite hand, and a grasper (ProGrasp™) in the third arm (Fig. 4.2). The Maryland bipolar, because of its pointed end, allows for finer dissection, while the fenestrated bipolar is much better at grasping the nodes, especially when they are encased in abundant adipose tissue. Medium-large (5 mm) Hem-o-Lok clips can be applied to large lymphatic channels by the assistant or by the surgeon. Placement by the surgeon is less efficient as it requires swapping out one of the instruments each time a clip is placed, but it has the advantage of affording the surgeon complete control of the process and allows for more accurate clip placement because of the wristed action of the robotic medium sized clip applier (Fig. 4.3). The robotic vessel sealer can also be used, but its large tip and higher cost make it a less attractive option.

The timing of PLND is also a matter of surgeon preference, but our inclination is to perform the dissection prior to removal of the prostate. Before an RP, the pelvic anatomy is in

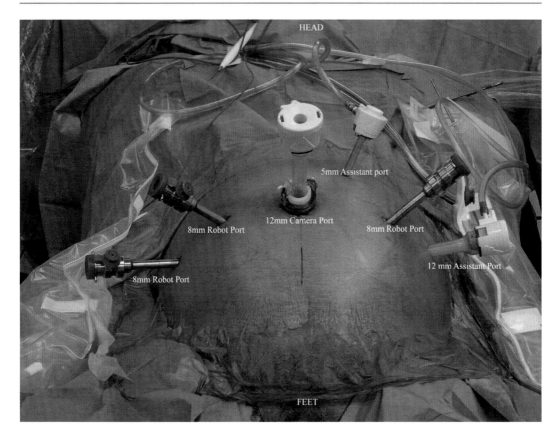

Fig. 4.1 External view of port placement. Port placement. (1) 12 mm assistant, (2) 8 mm robot, (3) 5 mm assistant, (4) 12 mm camera (midline, at umbilicus), (5) 8 mm robot, and (6) 8 mm robot

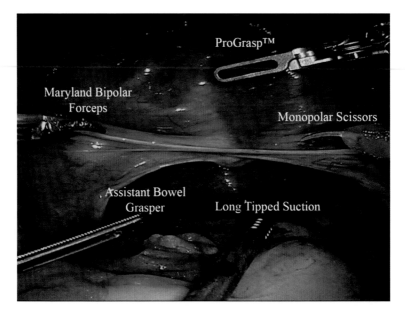

Fig. 4.2 Camera view of instrument position. Instruments: Clockwise: (1) ProGrasp™, (2) monopolar scissors, (3) Long tipped suction, (4) assistant bowel grasper, and (5) Maryland bipolar forceps

an undisturbed state, allowing for accurate and easy identification of all important landmarks. Additionally, a meticulous dissection requires patience and concentration, both of which are often in greater supply at the onset, rather than the later stages, of the case. The time required for a three-packet (iliac, obturator, and hypogastric) dissection is variable, dependent upon individual patient anatomy and surgeon skill. In a recent audit of 50 consecutive cases at MSKCC, the median time for the PLND was 26 min (range, 14–54; unpublished data, MSKCC).

The operation is begun by incising the peritoneum just lateral to the median umbilical ligament, starting above the vas deferens and continuing proximally to the mid common iliac artery (Fig. 4.4). The ligament is retracted medially, opening up the space between the bladder and the pelvic sidewall structures. On the left side, this proximal extent of the incision in the peritoneum mobilizes the sigmoid and distal left colon, which can then also be held medially by the assistant or the third arm. This maneuver should result in exposure of the important landmarks and boundaries of the dissection, which include the median umbilical ligament, common iliac artery, external iliac artery and vein, ureter, and hypogastric artery (Fig. 4.5). Further blunt dissection between the bladder and the vessels

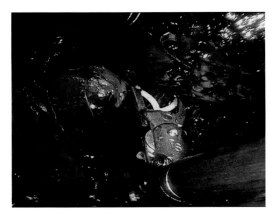

Fig. 4.3 Robotic clip applier. The wristed motion of robotic clip applier allows surgeon clip placement at any angle

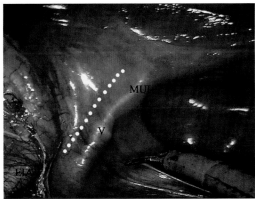

Fig. 4.4 Peritoneal incision. The initial peritoneal incision (*dotted line*) is made just lateral to the medial umbilical ligament above the vas and extended proximally along the ligament, over the vas, exposing the iliac vessels and ureter

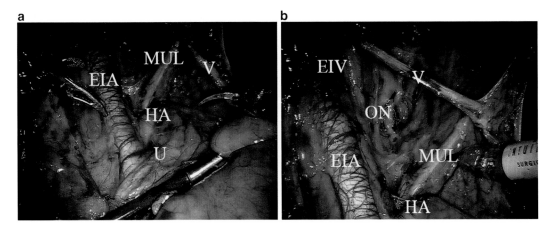

Fig. 4.5 Left pelvic anatomy. (**a**) wide view: *EIA* external iliac artery, *HA* hypogastric artery, *U* ureter, *MUL* medial umbilical ligament, *V* vas deferens. (**b**) closer view: *EIA* external iliac artery, *EIV* external iliac vein, *HA* hypogastric artery, *MUL* medial umbilical ligament, *V* vas deferens, *ON* obturator nerve

a

b

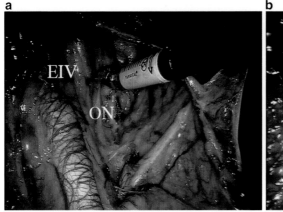
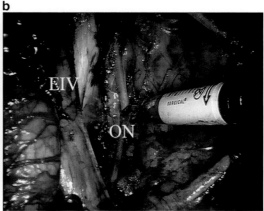

Fig. 4.6 Left iliac nodes. (**a**) Scissor pointing to the lymph node tissue between the external iliac vein (EIV) and the obturator nerve (ON), prior to removal. (**b**) Space between the external iliac vein (EIV) and obturator nerve (ON) following lymph node removal

a

b

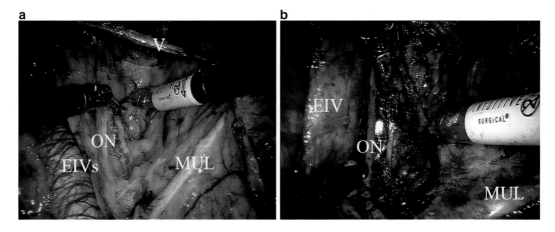

Fig. 4.7 Left obturator nodes. (**a**) Instruments point to the nodal tissue below the obturator nerve (ON) extending down to the peri-rectal fat. Vas deference (V), External Iliac vessels (EIVs), and the medial umbilical ligament (MUL) frame the dissection. (**b**) Obturator nodes removed. Obturator Nerve (ON), External Iliac vein (EIV), and the medial umbilical ligament (MUL)

will open up the anatomy and reveal the obturator nerve and vessels laterally as well as the peri-rectal fat posteriorly. Actually seeing the ureter as it courses over the common iliac artery medial to the umbilical ligament not only defines the upper extent of the dissection but goes a long way toward preventing inadvertent injury to this key structure. The vas deferens can be clipped and transected—which will get it out of the way—but the dissection can also be done with it intact, which may have the advantage of preserving the vasal artery to the testicle, thereby reducing the frequency or severity of postoperative orchalgia.

As a general guide, a standard PLND can be understood to involve three basic groups of nodes: those from the external iliac vein to the obturator nerve (Fig. 4.6), those below the obturator nerve to the peri-rectal space (Fig. 4.7), and those on the lateral aspect of the bladder along the anterior branches of the hypogastric artery (Fig. 4.8). While these nodes can be removed as three separate packets, the anatomic divisions are

a

b

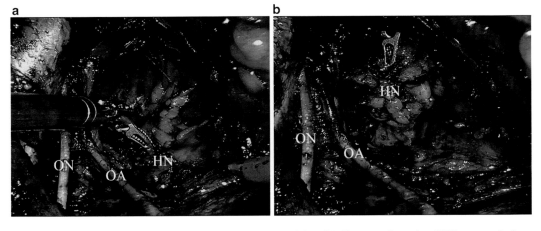

Fig. 4.8 Left hypogastric Nodes. (**a**) Instruments point to the hypogastric nodes (HN) located medial to the obturator nerve (ON) and artery (OA) on the side of the bladder. (**b**) Hypogastric nodes (HN) removed along bladder, medial to the obturator artery (OA) and obturator nerve (ON)

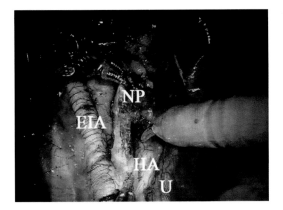

Fig. 4.9 Start of left side lymph node dissection. Dissection of the nodal packet (NP) begins at the bifurcation of the external iliac artery (EIA) and hypogastric artery (HA), lateral to the ureter (U)

somewhat nonspecific and the actual dissection can often be facilitated by dissecting the nodes en bloc, or at least nearly so. The standard PLND is started at the bifurcation of the external and hypogastric artery just lateral to the ureter (Fig. 4.9). The primary lymphatic channel in this location is clipped and the dissection proceeds distally, rolling all the tissue overlying the iliac vein medially to be included with the nodal tissue below the vein and the obturator nodes. The distal limit of the dissection is Cloquet's node, which is included if it facilitates termination of dissection in this area. While removal of

this node is typical, it is not required, since it is functionally related more to the superficial inguinal nodes than to the pelvic nodes. The literature is conflicting, but some suggest that Cloquet's node may actually be the sentinel or gateway node for inguinal-to-pelvic spread [69–71].

Of note, an accessory obturator artery and/or vein coursing toward the obturator fossa (defined as arising from the external iliac vessel or its branches instead of its more common hypogastric origin) can be encountered during the dissection of Cloquet's node (Fig. 4.10) [72]. Any dissection that includes Cloquet's node should seek to identify these vessels when present in order to avoid unnecessary bleeding. The artery should be spared in these circumstances, and it provides a visible landmark for the terminal edge of the distal dissection. Accessory veins often arise more proximally than their arterial counterparts and can be clipped and transected as needed to facilitate node removal.

Dissection proceeds beneath the iliac vein, stripping all the fibrofatty nodal tissue off the obturator internus fascia of the pelvic sidewall. Bipolar cautery is used to control the perforating muscular vessels. Identifying the obturator nerve very early in the dissection below the vein is particularly important in avoiding nerve injury. The most difficult part of the dissection to visualize from the angle of view of the robotic surgeon is

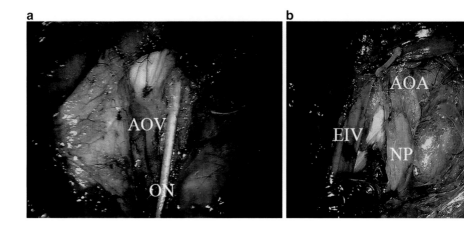

Fig. 4.10 Accessory obturator vessels. Frequently an accessory obturator vein (OV) and/or obturator artery (OA) is present surrounding Cloquet's node. (**a**) Accessory

obturator vein. (**b**). Accessory obturator artery and nodal packet (NP)

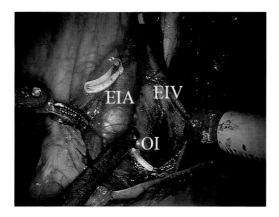

Fig. 4.11 Going behind the vein. It is sometimes necessary to dissect behind the iliac vessels in order to completely clear the nodal tissue along the pelvic wall. *EIA* external iliac artery, *EIV* external iliac vein, *OI* obturator internus

proximal and deep, at the convergence of the iliac vessel bifurcation and the nerve origin. The open surgeon can more easily work in this space because they can look up into this area and reach the tissue tucked under the vessels at the bifurcation and around the nerve proximally. The robotic surgeon, because of the midline and cephalad camera position, is forced to try to look down and back under at this same tissue. A 30° down lens can be very helpful in dissecting this region. Occasionally it is necessary to actually go behind (lateral) to the iliac vessels and then down along the obturator internus muscle in order to completely clean out this area (Fig. 4.11).

Medial dissection in the region of the iliac bifurcation exposes the takeoff of the medial umbilical ligament and the proximal aspect of the obturator artery and vein. These vessels can course either above or (more commonly) below the obturator nerve. All of the nodal tissue around and below these structures is removed. The posterior or deep limit of the dissection is the peri-rectal fat overlying the sciatic nerve, which can often be seen in very thin individuals. Small vascular branches from the obturator vessels often supply the nodes and are controlled with bipolar cautery. Occasionally the nodal tissue is quite adherent to the vessels, necessitating clipping the vessels proximally and distally and removing them en bloc. Concern has been raised regarding the potential effects on potency from the interruption of the obturator blood supply because approximately 80 % of accessory internal pudendal arteries arise from the obturator vasculature [73], and in rare circumstances the primary penile blood supply is based entirely off of the obturator artery rather than the internal pudendal system [74]. Given this, the obturator vessels should be preserved in most circumstances as long as this does not compromise the thoroughness of the node dissection.

The final part of a standard node dissection is designed to remove the nodes medial to the obturator nerve. These nodes are associated with the first branches of the hypogastric artery as it courses alongside the lateral aspect of the bladder.

They are interspersed between the medial umbilical ligament and the vesical arteries. These nodes are the ones most often neglected during many dissections, but they can be positive in over 48 % of patients with lymph node involvement and are the only site of node positivity in 26 % of patients [6].

Extension of the dissection beyond the standard three-packet template described above can be accomplished by further mobilization of the colon on the left and by continuing the incision in the posterior peritoneum on the right in a direction that frees the root of the small bowel mesentery. This will allow access to the common iliac nodes medial to the ureters, the presacral nodes on the sacral promontory, and the paraaortic and aortic nodes on top of and above the bifurcation up to the level of the inferior mesenteric artery. The number of nodes that can be removed with an extended dissection for prostate cancer depends in part on the time committed to the dissection. Node counts above 80 are not uncommon, as are lymphadenectomy times in excess of 90 min. Patients with very thick mesenteries or highly redundant sigmoid colons make for difficult extended dissections. In these cases, placement of additional 5 mm assistant ports along with the use of umbilical tape may facilitate retraction of interfering intestinal segments.

Even a meticulous extended PLND cannot be expected to remove all potentially involved nodes. For example, the sacral nodes that were described by Rouvière in 1938 [75] as draining the capsular lymphatics of the posterior prostate are located medially, below the sacral promontory, in an area that is more difficult to access and not commonly dissected. Individual lymphatic cancer cells "in transit" to nodes may be left behind during any surgical dissection. For these and other reasons, a PLND can only be viewed as one step in the management of the patient with high-risk prostate cancer. There is, however, ample reason to believe that a thorough dissection will provide significant prognostic information, can cure some patients with lymph node invasion, and may alter the pace of disease progression for others. Ultimately, this will allow for the more effective implementation and use of existing and developing adjuvant therapies.

References

1. Fowler Jr JE, Torgerson L, McLeod DG, Stutzman RE. Radical prostatectomy with pelvic lymphadenectomy: observations on the accuracy of staging with lymph node frozen sections. J Urol. 1981;126(5): 618–9.
2. Thomas R, Steele R, Smith R, Brannan W. One-stage laparoscopic pelvic lymphadenectomy and radical perineal prostatectomy. J Urol. 1994;152(4):1174–7.
3. Middleton RG. Value of and indications for pelvic lymph node dissection in the staging of prostate cancer. NCI Monogr. 1988;7:41–3.
4. Allaf ME, Palapattu GS, Trock BJ, Carter HB, Walsh PC. Anatomical extent of lymph node dissection: impact on men with clinically localized prostate cancer. J Urol. 2004;172(5 Pt 1):1840–4.
5. Bader P, Burkhard FC, Markwalder R, Studer UE. Is a limited lymph node dissection an adequate staging procedure for prostate cancer? J Urol. 2002;168(2): 514–8. discussion 518.
6. Godoy G, von Bodman C, Chade DC, Dillioglugil O, Eastham JA, Fine SW, Scardino PT, Laudone VP. Pelvic lymph node dissection for prostate cancer: frequency and distribution of nodal metastases in a contemporary radical prostatectomy series. J Urol. 2012; 187(6):2082–6.
7. Heidenreich A, Varga Z, Von Knobloch R. Extended pelvic lymphadenectomy in patients undergoing radical prostatectomy: high incidence of lymph node metastasis. J Urol. 2002;167(4):1681–6.
8. Smith Jr JA, Haynes TH, Middleton RG. Impact of external irradiation on local symptoms and survival free of disease in patients with pelvic lymph node metastasis from adenocarcinoma of the prostate. J Urol. 1984;131(4):705–7.
9. von Bodman C, Godoy G, Chade DC, Cronin A, Tafe LJ, Fine SW, Laudone V, Scardino PT, Eastham JA. Predicting biochemical recurrence-free survival for patients with positive pelvic lymph nodes at radical prostatectomy. J Urol. 2010;184(1):143–8. PMCID: PMC2927114.
10. Bader P, Burkhard FC, Markwalder R, Studer UE. Disease progression and survival of patients with positive lymph nodes after radical prostatectomy. Is there a chance of cure? J Urol. 2003;169(3):849–54.
11. Feifer AH, Elkin EB, Lowrance WT, Denton B, Jacks L, Yee DS, Coleman JA, Laudone VP, Scardino PT, Eastham JA. Temporal trends and predictors of pelvic lymph node dissection in open or minimally invasive radical prostatectomy. Cancer. 2011;117(17):3933–42. PMCID: PMC3136649.
12. Kawakami J, Meng MV, Sadetsky N, Latini DM, Duchane J, Carroll PR. Changing patterns of pelvic lymphadenectomy for prostate cancer: results from CaPSURE. J Urol. 2006;176(4 Pt 1):1382–6.
13. Abdollah F, Sun M, Thuret R, Budaus L, Jeldres C, Graefen M, Briganti A, Perrotte P, Rigatti P, Montorsi F, Karakiewicz PI. Decreasing rate and extent of lymph node staging in patients undergoing radical

prostatectomy may undermine the rate of diagnosis of lymph node metastases in prostate cancer. Eur Urol. 2010;58(6):882–92.

14. Brossner C, Ringhofer H, Hernady T, Kuber W, Madersbacher S, Pycha A. Lymphatic drainage of prostatic transition and peripheral zones visualized on a three-dimensional workstation. Urology. 2001; 57(2):389–93.

15. Briganti A, Blute ML, Eastham JH, Graefen M, Heidenreich A, Karnes JR, Montorsi F, Studer UE. Pelvic lymph node dissection in prostate cancer. Eur Urol. 2009;55(6):1251–65.

16. Whitmore 3rd WF, Blute Jr RD, Kaplan WD, Gittes RF. Radiocolloid scintigraphic mapping of the lymphatic drainage of the prostate. J Urol. 1980; 124(1):62–7.

17. Nepple KG, Rosevear HM, Stolpen AH, Brown JA, Williams RD. Concordance of preoperative prostate endorectal MRI with subsequent prostatectomy specimen in high-risk prostate cancer patients. Urol Oncol. 2013;31(5):601–6.

18. Meinhardt W, Valdes Olmos RA, van der Poel HG, Bex A, Horenblas S. Laparoscopic sentinel node dissection for prostate carcinoma: technical and anatomical observations. BJU Int. 2008;102(6):714–7.

19. van der Poel HG, Buckle T, Brouwer OR, Valdes Olmos RA, van Leeuwen FW. Intraoperative laparoscopic fluorescence guidance to the sentinel lymph node in prostate cancer patients: clinical proof of concept of an integrated functional imaging approach using a multimodal tracer. Eur Urol. 2011;60(4): 826–33.

20. Weissleder R, Elizondo G, Wittenberg J, Lee AS, Josephson L, Brady TJ. Ultrasmall superparamagnetic iron oxide: an intravenous contrast agent for assessing lymph nodes with MR imaging. Radiology. 1990;175(2):494–8.

21. Harisinghani MG, Barentsz J, Hahn PF, Deserno WM, Tabatabaei S, van de Kaa CH, de la Rosette J, Weissleder R. Noninvasive detection of clinically occult lymph-node metastases in prostate cancer. N Engl J Med. 2003;348(25):2491–9.

22. Triantafyllou M, Studer UE, Birkhauser FD, Fleischmann A, Bains LJ, Petralia G, Christe A, Froehlich JM, Thoeny HC. Ultrasmall superparamagnetic particles of iron oxide allow for the detection of metastases in normal sized pelvic lymph nodes of patients with bladder and/or prostate cancer. Eur J Cancer. 2013;49(3):616–24.

23. Briganti A, Chun FK, Salonia A, Suardi N, Gallina A, Da Pozzo LF, Roscigno M, Zanni G, Valiquette L, Rigatti P, Montorsi F, Karakiewicz PI. Complications and other surgical outcomes associated with extended pelvic lymphadenectomy in men with localized prostate cancer. Eur Urol. 2006;50(5):1006–13.

24. Clark T, Parekh DJ, Cookson MS, Chang SS, Smith Jr ER, Wells N, Smith Jr J. Randomized prospective evaluation of extended versus limited lymph node dissection in patients with clinically localized prostate cancer. J Urol. 2003;169(1):145–7. discussion 147–148.

25. Ji J, Yuan H, Wang L, Hou J. Is the impact of the extent of lymphadenectomy in radical prostatectomy related to the disease risk? A single center prospective study. J Surg Res. 2012;178(2):779–84.

26. Briganti A, Chun FK, Salonia A, Gallina A, Zanni G, Scattoni V, Valiquette L, Rigatti P, Montorsi F, Karakiewicz PI. Critical assessment of ideal nodal yield at pelvic lymphadenectomy to accurately diagnose prostate cancer nodal metastasis in patients undergoing radical retropubic prostatectomy. Urology. 2007;69(1):147–51.

27. Mazzola C, Savage C, Ahallal Y, Reuter VE, Eastham JA, Scardino PT, Guillonneau B, Touijer KA. Nodal counts during pelvic lymph node dissection for prostate cancer: an objective indicator of quality under the influence of very subjective factors. BJU Int. 2012;109(9):1323–8.

28. Bochner BH, Herr HW, Reuter VE. Impact of separate versus en bloc pelvic lymph node dissection on the number of lymph nodes retrieved in cystectomy specimens. J Urol. 2001;166(6):2295–6.

29. Joniau S, Van den Bergh L, Lerut E, Deroose CM, Haustermans K, Oyen R, Budiharto T, Ameye F, Bogaerts K, Van Poppel H. Mapping of pelvic lymph node metastases in prostate cancer. Eur Urol. 2013;63(3):450–8.

30. Yee DS, Katz DJ, Godoy G, Nogueira L, Chong KT, Kaag M, Coleman JA. Extended pelvic lymph node dissection in robotic-assisted radical prostatectomy: surgical technique and initial experience. Urology. 2010;75(5):1199–204.

31. Mattei A, Fuechsel FG, Bhatta Dhar N, Warncke SH, Thalmann GN, Krause T, Studer UE. The template of the primary lymphatic landing sites of the prostate should be revisited: results of a multimodality mapping study. Eur Urol. 2008;53(1):118–25.

32. Briganti A, Suardi N, Capogrosso P, Passoni N, Freschi M, di Trapani E, Gallina A, Capitanio U, Abdollah F, Tutolo M, Bianchi M, Salonia A, Da Pozzo LF, Montorsi F, Rigatti P. Lymphatic spread of nodal metastases in high-risk prostate cancer: the ascending pathway from the pelvis to the retroperitoneum. Prostate. 2012;72(2):186–92.

33. Intuitive Surgical, Inc. Investor faq [Internet]. http://investor.intuitivesurgical.com. Accessed 11 Mar 2013

34. Lowrance WT, Eastham JA, Savage C, Maschino AC, Laudone VP, Dechet CB, Stephenson RA, Scardino PT, Sandhu JS. Contemporary open and robotic radical prostatectomy practice patterns among urologists in the United States. J Urol. 2012;187(6):2087–92. PMCID: PMC3407038.

35. Silberstein JL, Derweesh IH, Kane CJ. Lymph node dissection during robot-assisted radical prostatectomy: where do we stand? Prostate Cancer Prostatic Dis. 2009;12(3):227–32.

36. Silberstein JL, Vickers AJ, Power NE, Parra RO, Coleman JA, Pinochet R, Touijer KA, Scardino PT,

Eastham JA, Laudone VP. Pelvic lymph node dissection for patients with elevated risk of lymph node invasion during radical prostatectomy: comparison of open, laparoscopic and robot-assisted procedures. J Endourol. 2012;26(6):748–53. PMCID: PMC3357075.

37. Silberstein JL, Su D, Glickman L, Kent M, Keren-Paz G, Vickers AJ, Coleman JA, Eastham JA, Scardino PT, Laudone VP. A case-mix-adjusted comparison of early oncological outcomes of open and robotic prostatectomy performed by experienced high volume surgeons. BJU Int. 2013;111(2):206–12.

38. Vickers AJ, Bianco FJ, Serio AM, Eastham JA, Schrag D, Klein EA, Reuther AM, Kattan MW, Pontes JE, Scardino PT. The surgical learning curve for prostate cancer control after radical prostatectomy. J Natl Cancer Inst. 2007;99(15):1171–7.

39. Zorn KC, Katz MH, Bernstein A, Shikanov SA, Brendler CB, Zagaja GP, Shalhav AL. Pelvic lymphadenectomy during robot-assisted radical prostatectomy: assessing nodal yield, perioperative outcomes, and complications. Urology. 2009;74(2):296–302.

40. Cooperberg MR, Kane CJ, Cowan JE, Carroll PR. Adequacy of lymphadenectomy among men undergoing robot-assisted laparoscopic radical prostatectomy. BJU Int. 2010;105(1):88–92.

41. Truesdale MD, Lee DJ, Cheetham PJ, Hruby GW, Turk AT, Badani KK. Assessment of lymph node yield after pelvic lymph node dissection in men with prostate cancer: a comparison between robot-assisted radical prostatectomy and open radical prostatectomy in the modern era. J Endourol. 2010;24(7):1055–60.

42. Sogani PC, Watson RC, Whitmore Jr WF. Lymphocele after pelvic lymphadenectomy for urologic cancer. Urology. 1981;17(1):39–43.

43. Paul DB, Loening SA, Narayana AS, Culp DA. Morbidity from pelvic lymphadenectomy in staging carcinoma of the prostate. J Urol. 1983;129(6):1141–4.

44. Khoder WY, Trottmann M, Buchner A, Stuber A, Hoffmann S, Stief CG, Becker AJ. Risk factors for pelvic lymphoceles post-radical prostatectomy. Int J Urol. 2011;18(9):638–43.

45. Orvieto MA, Coelho RF, Chauhan S, Palmer KJ, Rocco B, Patel VR. Incidence of lymphoceles after robot-assisted pelvic lymph node dissection. BJU Int. 2011;108(7):1185–90.

46. Musch M, Klevecka V, Roggenbuck U, Kroepfl D. Complications of pelvic lymphadenectomy in 1,380 patients undergoing radical retropubic prostatectomy between 1993 and 2006. J Urol. 2008;179(3):923–8. discussion 928–929.

47. Catalona WJ, Kadmon D, Crane DB. Effect of mini-dose heparin on lymphocele formation following extraperitoneal pelvic lymphadenectomy. J Urol. 1980;123(6):890–2.

48. Kropfl D, Krause R, Hartung R, Pfeiffer R, Behrendt H. Subcutaneous heparin injection in the upper arm as a method of avoiding lymphoceles after lymphadenectomies in the lower part of the body. Urol Int. 1987;42(6):416–23.

49. Waldert M, Remzi M, Klatte T, Klingler HC. FloSeal reduces the incidence of lymphoceles after lymphadenectomies in laparoscopic and robot-assisted extraperitoneal radical prostatectomy. J Endourol. 2011;25(6):969–73.

50. Simonato A, Varca V, Esposito M, Venzano F, Carmignani G. The use of a surgical patch in the prevention of lymphoceles after extraperitoneal pelvic lymphadenectomy for prostate cancer: a randomized prospective pilot study. J Urol. 2009;182(5):2285–90.

51. Pepper RJ, Pati J, Kaisary AV. The incidence and treatment of lymphoceles after radical retropubic prostatectomy. BJU Int. 2005;95(6):772–5.

52. Keegan KA, Cookson MS. Complications of pelvic lymph node dissection for prostate cancer. Curr Urol Rep. 2011;12(3):203–8.

53. Secin FP, Jiborn T, Bjartell AS, Fournier G, Salomon L, Abbou CC, Haber GP, Gill IS, Crocitto LE, Nelson RA, Cansino Alcaide JR, Martinez-Pineiro L, Cohen MS, Tuerk I, Schulman C, Gianduzzo T, Eden C, Baumgartner R, Smith JA, Entezari K, van Velthoven R, Janetschek G, Serio AM, Vickers AJ, Touijer K, Guillonneau B. Multi-institutional study of symptomatic deep venous thrombosis and pulmonary embolism in prostate cancer patients undergoing laparoscopic or robot-assisted laparoscopic radical prostatectomy. Eur Urol. 2008;53(1):134–45.

54. Loeb S, Partin AW, Schaeffer EM. Complications of pelvic lymphadenectomy: do the risks outweigh the benefits? Rev Urol. 2010;12(1):20–4. PMCID: PMC2859138.

55. Mohler JL, Armstrong AJ, Bahnson RR, Boston B, Busby JE, D'Amico AV, Eastham JA, Enke CA, Farrington T, Higano CS, Horwitz EM, Kantoff PW, Kawachi MH, Kuettel M, Lee RJ, MacVicar GR, Malcolm AW, Miller D, Plimack ER, Pow-Sang JM, Roach 3rd M, Rohren E, Rosenfeld S, Srinivas S, Strope SA, Tward J, Twardowski P, Walsh PC, Ho M, Shead DA. Prostate cancer, Version 3.2012: featured updates to the NCCN guidelines. J Natl Compr Canc Netw. 2012;10(9):1081–7.

56. Heidenreich A, Bellmunt J, Bolla M, Joniau S, Mason M, Matveev V, Mottet N, Schmid HP, van der Kwast T, Wiegel T, Zattoni F. EAU guidelines on prostate cancer. Part 1: screening, diagnosis, and treatment of clinically localised disease. Eur Urol. 2011;59(1):61–71.

57. Cagiannos I, Karakiewicz P, Eastham JA, Ohori M, Rabbani F, Gerigk C, Reuter V, Graefen M, Hammerer PG, Erbersdobler A, Huland H, Kupelian P, Klein E, Quinn DI, Henshall SM, Grygiel JJ, Sutherland RL, Stricker PD, Morash CG, Scardino PT, Kattan MW. A preoperative nomogram identifying decreased risk of positive pelvic lymph nodes in patients with prostate cancer. J Urol. 2003;170(5):1798–803.

58. Abdollah F, Sun M, Suardi N, Gallina A, Capitanio U, Bianchi M, Tutolo M, Passoni N, Karakiewicz PI, Rigatti P, Montorsi F, Briganti A. National Comprehensive Cancer Network practice guidelines

2011: need for more accurate recommendations for pelvic lymph node dissection in prostate cancer. J Urol. 2012;188(2):423–8.

59. Briganti A, Karakiewicz PI, Chun FK, Gallina A, Salonia A, Zanni G, Valiquette L, Graefen M, Huland H, Rigatti P, Montorsi F. Percentage of positive biopsy cores can improve the ability to predict lymph node invasion in patients undergoing radical prostatectomy and extended pelvic lymph node dissection. Eur Urol. 2007;51(6):1573–81.

60. Briganti A, Chun FK, Salonia A, Zanni G, Scattoni V, Valiquette L, Rigatti P, Montorsi F, Karakiewicz PI. Validation of a nomogram predicting the probability of lymph node invasion among patients undergoing radical prostatectomy and an extended pelvic lymphadenectomy. Eur Urol. 2006;49(6):1019–26. discussion 1026–1027.

61. Thompson I, Thrasher JB, Aus G, Burnett AL, Canby-Hagino ED, Cookson MS, D'Amico AV, Dmochowski RR, Eton DT, Forman JD, Goldenberg SL, Hernandez J, Higano CS, Kraus SR, Moul JW, Tangen CM. Guideline for the management of clinically localized prostate cancer: 2007 update. J Urol. 2007;177(6): 2106–31.

62. Silberstein JL, Vickers AJ, Power NE, Fine SW, Scardino PT, Eastham JA, Laudone VP. Reverse stage shift at a tertiary care center: escalating risk in men undergoing radical prostatectomy. Cancer. 2011;117(21):4855–60. PMCID: PMC3181272.

63. Catalona WJ, Miller DR, Kavoussi LR. Intermediate-term survival results in clinically understaged prostate cancer patients following radical prostatectomy. J Urol. 1988;140(3):540–3.

64. Messing EM, Manola J, Yao J, Kiernan M, Crawford D, Wilding G, di'SantAgnese PA, Trump D. Immediate versus deferred androgen deprivation treatment in patients with node-positive prostate cancer after radical prostatectomy and pelvic lymphadenectomy. Lancet Oncol. 2006;7(6):472–9.

65. Joslyn SA, Konety BR. Impact of extent of lymphadenectomy on survival after radical prostatectomy for prostate cancer. Urology. 2006;68(1):121–5.

66. Theodorescu D, Frierson Jr HF. When is a negative lymph node really negative? Molecular tools for the detection of lymph node metastasis from urological cancer. Urol Oncol. 2004;22(3):256–9.

67. Okegawa T, Nutahara K, Higashihara E. Detection of micrometastatic prostate cancer cells in the lymph nodes by reverse transcriptase polymerase chain reaction is predictive of biochemical recurrence in pathological stage T2 prostate cancer. J Urol. 2000;163(4): 1183–8.

68. Martinez-Pineiro L, Rios E, Martinez-Gomariz M, Pastor T, de Cabo M, Picazo ML, Palacios J, Perona R. Molecular staging of prostatic cancer with RT-PCR assay for prostate-specific antigen in peripheral blood and lymph nodes: comparison with standard histological staging and immunohistochemical assessment of occult regional lymph node metastases. Eur Urol. 2003;43(4):342–50.

69. Shen P, Conforti AM, Essner R, Cochran AJ, Turner RR, Morton DL. Is the node of Cloquet the sentinel node for the iliac/obturator node group? Cancer J. 2000;6(2):93–7.

70. Heyns CF, Fleshner N, Sangar V, Schlenker B, Yuvaraja TB, van Poppel H. Management of the lymph nodes in penile cancer. Urology. 2010;76(2 Suppl 1):S43–57.

71. Chu CK, Zager JS, Marzban SS, Gimbel MI, Murray DR, Hestley AC, Messina JL, Sondak VK, Carlson GW, Delman KA. Routine biopsy of Cloquet's node is of limited value in sentinel node positive melanoma patients. J Surg Oncol. 2010;102(4):315–20.

72. Pai MM, Krishnamurthy A, Prabhu LV, Pai MV, Kumar SA, Hadin GA. Variability in the origin of the obturator artery. Clinics. 2009;64(9):897–901.

73. Park BJ, Sung DJ, Kim MJ, Cho SB, Kim YH, Chung KB, Kang SH, Cheon J. The incidence and anatomy of accessory pudendal arteries as depicted on multidetector-row CT angiography: clinical implications of preoperative evaluation for laparoscopic and robot-assisted radical prostatectomy. Korean J Radiol. 2009;10(6):587–95. PMCID: PMC2770828.

74. Kawanishi Y, Muguruma H, Sugiyama H, Kagawa J, Tanimoto S, Yamanaka M, Kojima K, Numata A, Kishimoto T, Nakanishi R, Kanayama HO. Variations of the internal pudendal artery as a congenital contributing factor to age at onset of erectile dysfunction in Japanese. BJU Int. 2008;101(5):581–7.

75. Rouvière H. Anatomy of the human lymphatic system: a compendium. Ann Arbor, Mich: Edwards Bros; 1938.

The Transperitoneal Robotic-Assisted Radical Prostatectomy

5

Aaron A. Laviana, Stacey C. Carter, and Jim C. Hu

Preoperative Considerations

We consider all men who are candidates for open radical prostatectomy to be candidates for robotic-assisted radical prostatectomy: men with clinically organ-confined disease who meet the National Comprehensive Cancer Network (NCCN) guidelines based on risk of recurrence [1]. Previous abdominal surgeries, obesity, and a significantly enlarged prostate may add to the challenge of the robotic approach, particularly early in the learning curve. However, we have performed transperitoneal robotic-assisted radical prostatectomy following aborted open radical prostatectomy due to poor exposure secondary to obesity and a narrow pelvis [2]. In men with more advanced disease, such as higher volume and/or higher-grade disease, we obtain magnetic resonance imaging to determine the degree of nerve sparing that may be safely performed without compromising cancer control. Additionally,

S.C. Carter, M.D.
Urology Department, UCLA Medical Center,
STE 1000, 924 Westwood Blvd, Los Angeles,
CA 90024, USA
e-mail: JCHu@mednet.ucla.edu

A.A. Laviana • J.C. Hu, M.D., M.P.H. (✉)
Director and Henry E. Singleton Chair of Robotic
and Minimally Invasive Surgery, Associate Professor
Department of Urology, David Geffen School
of Medicine at UCLA, STE 1000, 924 Westwood
Blvd, Los Angeles, CA 90024, USA

for men with high-risk disease, including PSA greater than 20 ng/mL, a Gleason score of 8–10, clinical stage T3a or higher, or clinical symptoms, we obtain bone scan and cross-sectional imaging to rule out metastatic disease [1].

Men are placed on a clear liquid diet the day prior to surgery. They are given a laxative, usually 300 cc of magnesium citrate, with nothing by mouth after midnight. While we prefer the stoppage of aspirin and anti-platelet therapy at least 7 days prior to surgery, we perform robotic-assisted radical prostatectomy for those unable to come off of aspirin or clopidogrel, due to coronary artery disease and/or cardiac stents, without changing our surgical technique. Similar to others, we have not found a difference in outcomes for those who continue or stop aspirin therapy prior to robotic-assisted radical prostatectomy [3, 4].

Before skin incision, parenteral antibiotics are administered and sequential compression devices are placed. For those at high risk, we administer 5,000 U of subcutaneous heparin prior to induction [5]. An eye mask is always used intraoperatively to prevent corneal abrasions that may result from being in the Trendelenberg position. This risk increases with longer operative times that typically occur early in learning curve. Another rare but known risk of prolonged Trendelenberg position is posterior ischemic neuropathy. To date there are two documented cases, the latter leading to complete blindness [6]. We limit intravenous fluids intraoperatively to less than 2 L of crystalloid, which minimizes the degree of facial edema and the amount of urine that accumulates

J.A. Eastham and E.M. Schaeffer (eds.), *Radical Prostatectomy: Surgical Perspectives*,
DOI 10.1007/978-1-4614-8693-0_5, © Springer Science+Business Media New York 2014

in the operative field, since the bladder neck is divided early during the procedure. Finally, we find an oro-gastric tube unnecessary.

We prefer split legs to the lithotomy position, due to greater efficiency in manipulating the legs into and out of stirrups. After placement of an arterial line at the anesthesiologist's discretion and adequate intravenous access is established, the patient's arms are appropriately padded and tucked using the operating room sheets. The arm boards are removed and 4-in. tape is used to secure the sternum to the operating table over a surgical towel, allowing a fingerbreadth width for adequate chest wall expansion. Securing the patient to the table is critical in minimizing slippage in steep Trendelenberg position. The assistant surgeon stands to the right of the patient, simultaneously controlling two laparoscopic ports for retraction and suctioning.

Transperitoneal Versus Extraperitoneal Approach

With the advent of the minimally invasive radical prostatectomy, the transperitoneal approach has been more popular than the extraperitoneal approach and is our preferred technique. In men with prior open/laparoscopic appendectomy, cholecystectomy, or inguinal hernia repair, we prefer the transperitoneal approach due to the larger working space and minimal lysis of adhesions that may be required. However, in men with extensive abdominal surgery, such as bowel resection, gastric bypass, or exploratory laparotomy, we prefer the extraperitoneal approach to avoid extensive adhesions. During the extraperitoneal approach, all ports are shifted 1–2 cm caudad. This approach is more costly due to the use of the OMS-XB2 Extra View™ balloon dilator (Covidien, Norwalk CT) and the processing of an additional 10 mm laparoscope. Additionally, there is greater CO_2 absorption via the extraperitoneal approach, requiring anesthesia to correct hypercarbia and acidosis, particularly during longer cases [7]. However, because bowel is avoided with the extraperitoneal approach, it does not require the steeper Trendelenberg position critical to the transperitoneal approach. Finally, because the urachus and medial umbilical liga-

ments are not divided during the extraperitoneal approach, there is greater tension during the anastomosis. This is overcome by lowering the pneumoperitoneum to 5 mmHg during this step.

Instrumentation for Transperitoneal Robotic-Assisted Radical Prostatectomy

Robotic Instruments

- Curved monopolar scissors set to 25 W (robotic arm number 1)
- Maryland bipolar dissector set to 25 W (robotic arm number 2)
- ProGrasp™ (robotic arm number 3)
- Zero degree/straight lens
- Large needle driver
- Large suture-cut needle driver

Surgical Assistant Laparoscopic Instruments

- Laparoscopic scissors
- Laparoscopic needle driver
- Laparoscopic grasper (blunt tip)
- Suction irrigator with long bariatric tip
- 10 mm laparoscopic specimen entrapment bag
- Purple (medium) and Green (small) Hem-o-lok clip applier and clips
- 16-French Foley working catheter and 20-French Foley end catheter

Trocars

- 12 mm trocar x2
- 8 mm robotic trocar x3
- 5 mm trocar x1
- Veress needle

Sutures

- *Vesicourethral anastomosis*: Two 3–0 Vicryl CT-3 needles with sutures cut to 7 and 10 in. (Ethicon, Inc., Cincinnati, OH)

- *Fascial closure of extraction site*: 0-Vicryl UR-6 needle (Ethicon, Inc., Cincinnati, OH)
- *Skin closure*: 4–0 monocryl (poliglecaprone 25) for extraction site and DERMABOND for other port sites (Ethicon, Inc., Cincinnati, OH)

Access and Trocar Configuration (Fig. 5.1)

After abdominal wall hair is clipped in the right upper quadrant and the lower abdomen, the Veress needle is inserted 1–2 cm supraumbilically in the midline. The peritoneum is then insufflated to 15 mm of mercury, the Veress needle removed, and the scalpel used to make a 12 mm vertical skin incision at the site of the Veress needle. Electrocautery is used to dissect through the dermis. We then place a 12 mm port by feel, with a "give" indicating the tip of the port is through the posterior rectus sheath. In men with prior abdominal surgery, the Hassan technique is used to place the initial 12 mm port. The zero degree robotic lens and camera are then inserted through this supraumbilical 12 mm port to guide placement of the remaining trocars. Another 12 mm port is placed 1–2 cm medial to the right anterior iliac spine for the assistant laparoscopic graspers and placement of the Hem-o-Lok® (Medline Industries, Inc. Mundelein, Illinois). Care is taken to ensure that this 12 mm port is not placed lateral to the anterior axillary line, as this will force the assistant to come in at an upward trajectory before dropping down into the surgical field. Additionally, insufflation tubing is placed on this 12 mm port. Next, a 5 mm trocar is placed in the right upper quadrant, medial to the lateral rectus margin. This serves as the point of access for the assistant surgeon's bariatric tip suction irrigator. Care is taken to place this port at least 2 cm below the costal margin, as placement closer to the costal margin may inhibit the fulcrum of the suction irrigator into the pelvis.

Next, the 8 mm robotic trocars are placed in the same horizontal plane as the assistant 12 mm port site. These three robotic trocars are placed at the right (number 1 robotic arm) and left rectus margin (number 2 robotic arm), and 1–2 cm medial to the left anterior iliac spine (number 3 robotic arm). For men with prior appendectomy, it is often necessary to place the left lower quadrant robotic trocars initially. Laparoscopic scissors are then inserted through these ports to a perform lysis of adhesions, in order to safely place the right lower quadrant trocars.

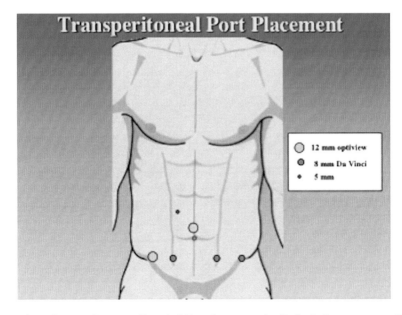

Fig. 5.1 Transperitoneal trocar placement. From Lei Y., et al. Athermal Division and Selective Suture Ligation of the Dorsal Vein Complex During Robot-Assisted Laparoscopic Radical Prostatectomy: Description of Technique and Outcomes. *Eur Urol 2011*;59: 235–243. Reprinted with permission from Elsevier Limited

Dropping the Bladder, Entry into the Space of Retzius

While we initially conformed to the traditional Montsouris approach of performing a posterior dissection of the peritoneal cul-de-sac to dissect out the seminal vesicles and ligate the vas deferens before dropping the bladder, we converted to the anterior approach for several reasons [8]. First, in men with extensive prior abdominal surgery, the posterior approach is incompatible with an extraperitoneal approach. Second, the posterior approach ties up robotic arm number 3 to retract the sigmoid colon as well as an assistant's instrument to hold up the anterior leaflet of the cut peritoneal edge. Therefore exposure may be more challenging, necessitating more "one-handed" dissection and greater use of monopolar cautery. Finally, incision of the peritoneal cul-de-sac, while not time consuming, is an additional step that is not required with the anterior approach.

With the curved monopolar scissors in robotic arm number 1, the Maryland bipolar dissector in robotic arm number 2, and the ProGrasp™ in robotic arm number 3, we incise the medial umbilical ligaments and the urachus as cephalad as possible. Care must be taken to fully cauterize these structures, as patent vessels may traverse the medial umbilical ligaments. We then downwardly retract the cut edge, and dissect beneath the preperitoneal fat in the midline of the fibro-areolar plane until we encounter the symphysis pubis. Next, the peritoneal incision is extended posterolaterally from the incised medial umbilical ligament to the vas deferens at its intersection with the iliac vessels. This is repeated on the contralateral side. We deliberately incise the peritoneum medial to the internal ring to avoid weakening the abdominal wall and increasing the susceptibility to an inguinal hernia. The bladder is retracted medially, away from the iliac vessels and pelvic sidewall, and this firm traction facilitates identification of the fibroareolar, anatomic plane lateral to the bladder. The final maneuver to mobilize the bladder away from the sidewall is accomplished by turning the ipsilateral robotic instrument tip at a right angle toward the symphysis pubis. The rounded, hinged part of the endowrist is used to sweep between the bladder and the pelvic sidewall toward the ipsilateral shoulder, stopping where the common iliac artery bifurcates. After fully mobilizing the bladder, the area over the mid-prostate is then de-fatted using bipolar cautery. We do not defat over the apex of the prostate, as this is unnecessary with our antegrade approach. If anything, this maneuver increases the risk of venous bleeding, which requires additional time to control.

Bladder Neck Sparing Dissection

In contrast to our initial description [9, 10], we no longer suture ligate the mid-prostate or anterior bladder prior to bladder neck dissection. The ProGrasp™ (in robotic arm number 3 arm) grasps and tents the bladder wall anteriorly and cephald to identify the detrusor apron's intersection with the vesico-prostatic junction (Fig. 5.2). Staying midline, sharp dissection is used through the

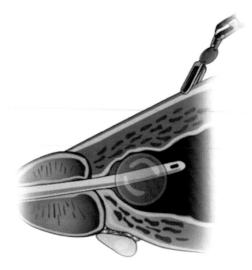

Fig. 5.2 Robotic arm number 3 provides upward tension on the prostate base while the assistant grasps the posterior lip of the bladder neck to provide countertension. From Freire MP., et al. Anatomic Bladder Neck Preservation During Robotic-assisted Laparoscopic Radical Prostatectomy: Description of Technique and Outcomes. *Eur Urol. 2009*;56(6):972–80. Reprinted with permission from Elsevier Limited

connective tissue of the detrusor apron until bladder fibers are seen. We prefer sharp dissection, since monopolar cautery may obliterate or obscure these fibers. Bipolar electrocautery is used in short bursts for hemostasis. After reaching the bladder fibers, the prostatic contour in the sagittal plane is followed proximally to the bladder neck. This incision is extended lateral in an arced fashion to avoid vessels that traverse the prostate from the lateral pedicle to the dorsal vascular complex.

Next, blunt dissection is performed in a caudal direction over the anterior bladder neck, identifying the vertical fibers of the prostatic urethra. We then perform blunt dissection lateral to the bladder neck by opening the Maryland dissector and manipulating the scissors caudally, resulting in a triangular spread on the lateral lobes of the prostate. This also defines the funneled shape of the bladder neck and its junction with the prostatic urethra. The bladder neck is opened anteriorly, and the urethral catheter is withdrawn after deflating the balloon. The posterior bladder mucosa is then incised using monopolar electrocautery, while the ProGrasp™ is used to elevate the prostatic base, avoiding the need for catheter manipulation during this step. The surgical assistant then provides countertraction on the bladder neck to allow the dissection to continue posteriorly to the detrusor apron. Dissecting laterally before identification of the detrusor apron may result in inadvertent cystotomy or ureteral injury.

After identification of the posterior longitudinal detrusor layer, we turn the dissection laterally until adipose tissue is encountered. The adipose tissue is lateral to the bladder neck and found at the cephalad portion of the endopelvic fascia. This landmark was originally named the fat pad of Whitmore, and it defines the posterolateral bladder neck dissection boundary, as the neurovascular bundle is in very close proximity to the lateral prostatic pedicle [9, 10]. Complete division of the bladder neck to the fat pad of Whitmore allows for better exposure during the seminal vesicle dissection. The posterior detrusor layer is then opened as posteriorly as possible, close to the seminal vesicle tips, and the vasa deferentia are identified behind a layer of adipose tissue. This layer is thicker in obese men and almost nonexistent in very thin individuals.

Seminal Vesicle and Posterior Dissection

After identification of the vasa, the ProGrasp™ lifts them anteriorly, while the Maryland bipolar dissects around them to create space for a purple Hem-o-lok clip. Care must be taken to avoid closing the clip on the seminal vesicle located behind the vasa. After clipping each vas but prior to transection, assistant grasper countertraction is provided below the clip and the vas pulled toward the assistant trocar. This exposes the tip of the seminal vesicle, allowing for safe transection of the vas to proceed. The artery of the vas usually courses between the vas and medial aspect of the seminal vesicle. Hemostasis is controlled by either the aforementioned clip or with bipolar cautery prior to division. After dividing each vas, the ProGrasp™ grasps the proximal aspect of the seminal vesicle and lifts it anteriorly. Blunt dissection is used to define the medial and typically avascular border of the seminal vesicle [11]. The arterial blood supply of the seminal vesicle originates inferolaterally, and bipolar cautery is used sparingly away from the seminal vesicle tips to control arterioles (Fig. 5.3).

Particularly for larger seminal vesicles, the ProGrasp™ must be continuously repositioned as progress is made toward the seminal vesicle tip. The temptation to dissect the lateral proximal border of the seminal vesicle to its origin must be avoided, as this may result in capsular incision and/or bleeding from the lateral pedicle vessels. The dissection is ultimately finished when the lateral pedicles are ligated and divided in a subsequent step [11].

Attention is then turned posteriorly. The ProGrasp™ again grasps the seminal vesicles and lifts them anteriorly. Denonvilliers' fascia is incised in the midline and blunt dissection is used to define the posterior prostate contour (Fig. 5.4). The nerve-sparing dissection plane is recognized by a layer of glistening Denonvilliers' fascia coursing above the pre-rectal fat [12]. This plane of dissection is continued distally toward the apex of the prostate and then laterally until the medial border of the neurovascular bundle is encountered. The neurovascular bundle

a

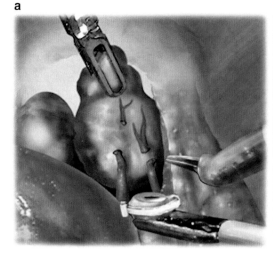

b

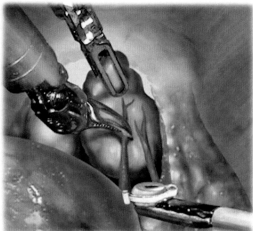

Fig. 5.3 (a) Fourth-arm ProGrasp™ anterior traction and assistant laparoscopic grasper countertraction facilitate the high isolation of arterioles proximal to the seminal vesicle tip. From Kowalczyk KJ., et al. Stepwise Approach for Nerve Sparing Without Countertraction During Robot-assisted Radical Prostatectomy: Technique and Outcomes. *Eur Urol. 2011*;60(3):536–47. Reprinted with permission from Elsevier Limited.

(**b**) Bipolar 25-W current fulguration of arterioles prior to cut-and-peel technique to divide and bluntly sweep arterioles beyond the seminal vesicle tip. From Kowalczyk KJ., et al. Stepwise Approach for Nerve Sparing Without Countertraction During Robot-assisted Radical Prostatectomy: Technique and Outcomes. *Eur Urol. 2011*;60(3):536–47. Reprinted with permission from Elsevier Limited

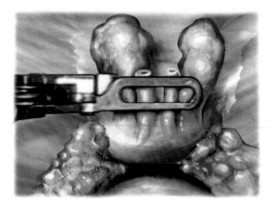

Fig. 5.4 After seminal vesicle dissection and prior to defining the anterior prostatic contour (endopelvic fascia intact), the posterior dissection is performed. Denonvilliers' fascia is separated posteriorly from the prostatic fascia in the midline, and the posterior contour is defined. This dissection is carried out lateral to the lateral pedicle fat pad proximally. Distally, veins that provide the landmark of the medial border of the neurovascular bundle are commonly encountered at the mid- and apical prostate and serve as the lateral border of the dissection. From Lei Y., et al. Athermal Division and Selective Suture Ligation of the Dorsal Vein Complex During Robot-Assisted Laparoscopic Radical Prostatectomy: Description of Technique and Outcomes. *Eur Urol 2011*;59: 235–243. Reprinted with permission from Elsevier Limited

may be landmarked by veins coursing longitudinally along the prostate. Alternatively, for men with high volume, high Gleason grade disease for whom interfascial or extrafascial nerve sparing is preferable, this dissection plane is carried out beneath Denonvilliers' fascia onto the prerectal fat. Greater prostatic volume impedes visualization and limits the extent of the posterior dissection distally. This requires subsequent rotation of the prostate after antegrade neurovascular bundle release to complete the apical dissection posteriorly [13].

Lateral Pelvic Fascia Separation and Development of the Anterior Prostatic Contour

At our institution, we prefer to perform right versus left nerve sparing first because of the better working angles with the robotic scissors already entering to the right of midline. The left-sided nerve sparing is technically easier after increased prostate mobility from releasing the right-sided attachments. Beginning at the right mid-prostate,

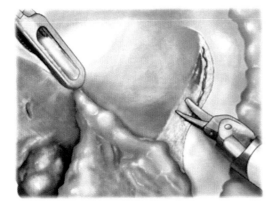

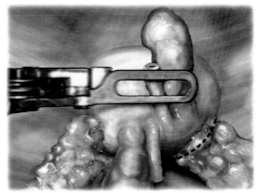

Fig. 5.5 Prostatic rub used for periprostatic fascia separation. Nerve bundle components are encountered on the medial aspect of the levator fascia and pushed laterally. The outer prostatic fascia remains medically on the prostate distal to the lateral pedicle and the fat pad located posterolaterally between the bladder and the prostate. In thinner men with finer or more translucent prostatic fascia, fibroadipose tissue may be seen underlying the outer prostatic fascia. From Lei Y., et al. Athermal Division and Selective Suture Ligation of the Dorsal Vein Complex During Robot-Assisted Laparoscopic Radical Prostatectomy: Description of Technique and Outcomes. *Eur Urol 2011*;59: 235–243. Reprinted with permission from Elsevier Limited

Fig. 5.6 After division of the lateral pedicle fat pad, the confluence of the right anterior and posterior contours, serves as a landmark for lateral pedicle ligation and division before antegrade nerve sparing. In addition, the medial neurovascular bundle edge is visible after incision of the outer prostatic fascia. From Lei Y., et al. Athermal Division and Selective Suture Ligation of the Dorsal Vein Complex During Robot-Assisted Laparoscopic Radical Prostatectomy: Description of Technique and Outcomes. *Eur Urol 2011*;59: 235–243. Reprinted with permission from Elsevier Limited

Lateral Vascular Pedicle Ligation

The intersection of the anterior and posterior prostate contours and distal fold of the lateral pedicle comprise the landmarks for the lateral vascular pedicle ligation (Fig. 5.6). The prostatic pedicles are placed on gentle 45° supra-medial tension. Hem-o-lock clips are placed on both the stay and specimen side to avoid back bleeding, since the dorsal vascular complex has not been ligated. The vascular pedicles are then sharply divided between the stay and specimen clips with cold scissor division, and antegrade intrafascial versus interfascial nerve sparing is then executed (Fig. 5.7) [12].

a "prostatic rub" is used medial to the fascial tendinous arch to split the pelvic fascia, leaving the levator fascia laterally and the prostatic fascia with the prostate (Fig. 5.5) [12]. "Rubbing" proximally toward the base helps define the distal fold of the lateral pedicle. The thickness of the prostatic fascia is not uniform and in men with more translucent prostatic fascia, fibro-adipose tissue is seen underlying this fascia. The junction between the medial aspect of the fibro-adipose tissue and prostate capsule defines the intrafascial dissection plane. Incision of the outer prostatic fascia allows the medial edge of the neurovascular bundle to be identified. We do not routinely perform this move, however, especially when prominent capsular veins course below the outer prostatic fascia. While pneumoperitoneum typically results in thrombosis and hemostasis if inadvertent venotomies occur, avoiding these veins is prudent to prevent venous oozing that impedes visualization and takes time to control [11]. After completing the lateral pelvic fascia separation on the right, we then proceed in a similar manner on the left.

Athermal, Antegrade Neurovascular Bundle Release

In developing the intrafascial nerve-sparing plane, which is largely avascular distal to the already clipped lateral pedicle, the medial leaf of the prostatic fascia is entered to identify the neurovascular bundle components. This bundle courses between the inner and outer prostatic fascia [14]. In dissecting this plane, the venous components are

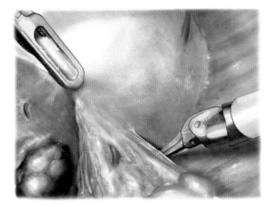

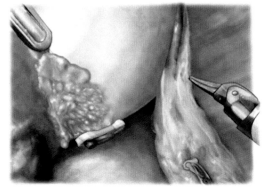

Fig. 5.7 The robotic scissors are inserted at the confluence of contours and the distal fold of the lateral pedicle to create space for clip placement and ligation prior to division. The medial edge of fibroadipose neurovascular bundle tissue is identified just lateral to the vein coursing on the prostate. From Lei Y., et al. Athermal Division and Selective Suture Ligation of the Dorsal Vein Complex During Robot-Assisted Laparoscopic Radical Prostatectomy: Description of Technique and Outcomes. *Eur Urol 2011*;59: 235–243. Reprinted with permission from Elsevier Limited

Fig. 5.8 Denonvilliers' fascia dissected away from the prostate capsule posteriorly. After lateral pedicle division, intrafascial nerve sparing is performed by dissecting the prostate capsule away from the inner prostatic fascia, covering the medial neurovascular bundle border. Neurovascular bundle veins lateral to the prostatic fascia also serve as a landmark for the medial aspect of the neurovascular bundle during intrafascial nerve sparing. From Lei Y., et al. Athermal Division and Selective Suture Ligation of the Dorsal Vein Complex During Robot-Assisted Laparoscopic Radical Prostatectomy: Description of Technique and Outcomes. *Eur Urol 2011*;59: 235–243. Reprinted with permission from Elsevier Limited

often the most medial component of the neurovascular bundle, as they are often found just lateral to the inner prostatic fascia during intrafascial nerve sparing (Fig. 5.8). During interfascial nerve sparing, in contrast, a layer of the periprostatic fibroadipose tissue is purposely left overlying the inner prostatic fascia. The veins of the neurovascular bundle may be intentionally split, leaving a portion of the vein and inner prostatic fascia with the prostate during this latter approach (Fig. 5.9). Arterioles are often found in this plane as well, and these are controlled with 5-mm Hem-o-lock clips. Finally, in those with high-volume, high-risk disease, non-nerve sparing may be performed via an extrafascial dissection, leaving the neurovascular bundle with the prostate.

During our initial experience, we relied on continuous countertraction to facilitate dissection of the nerve-sparing plane, with the assistant laparoscopic suction tip on the right and the robotic Maryland dissector on the left (Fig. 5.10) [11, 13]. Moreover, we were over-reliant on pealing the neurovascular bundle away from the prostate. Both of these maneuvers exacerbate neurapraxia, and over the course of several hundred cases, we modified our technique. We now use more sharp dissection and spread along, rather than against,

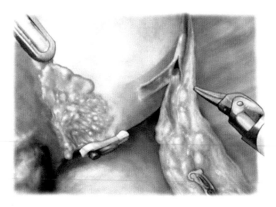

Fig. 5.9 Following interfascial nerve-sparing venotomy, the neurovascular bundle is split, leaving the medial edge of the venous wall, inner prostatic fascia, and fibroadipose components of the neurovascular bundle with the prostate. Fibroadipose tissue is also noted on the medial border of the neurovascular bundle. From Lei Y., et al. Athermal Division and Selective Suture Ligation of the Dorsal Vein Complex During Robot-Assisted Laparoscopic Radical Prostatectomy: Description of Technique and Outcomes. *Eur Urol 2011*;59: 235–243. Reprinted with permission from Elsevier Limited

the neurovascular bundle (Fig. 5.11) [15, 16]. These modifications have resulted in earlier and better recovery of sexual function.

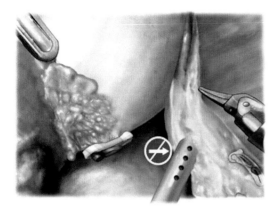

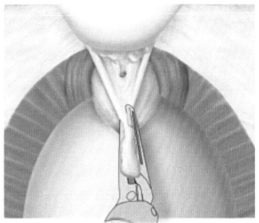

Fig. 5.10 Demonstration of the prior technique of nerve sparing with assistant suction (or robotic instrument) neurovascular bundle countertraction to facilitate nerve-sparing dissection that leads to neuropraxia. From Lei Y., et al. Athermal Division and Selective Suture Ligation of the Dorsal Vein Complex During Robot-Assisted Laparoscopic Radical Prostatectomy: Description of Technique and Outcomes. *Eur Urol 2011*;59: 235–243. Reprinted with permission from Elsevier Limited

Fig. 5.12 With elective suture ligation of the dorsal vein complex, the prostate is rotated medially to release the neurovascular bundle from the prostatic apex. The ProGrasp™ then bunches the detrusor apron while creating slight cephalad tension to allow visualization of the anterolateral prostatic contour. From Lei Y., et al. Athermal Division and Selective Suture Ligation of the Dorsal Vein Complex During Robot-Assisted Laparoscopic Radical Prostatectomy: Description of Technique and Outcomes. *Eur Urol 2011*;59: 235–243. Reprinted with permission from Elsevier Limited

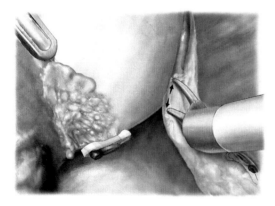

Fig. 5.11 As opposed to our previous dependence on countertraction, we now use sharp dissection and spread along, rather than against, the neurovascular bundle. This has attenuated neuropraxia and resulted in better sexual function recovery. From Lei Y., et al. Athermal Division and Selective Suture Ligation of the Dorsal Vein Complex During Robot-Assisted Laparoscopic Radical Prostatectomy: Description of Technique and Outcomes. *Eur Urol 2011*;59: 235–243. Reprinted with permission from Elsevier Limited

Apical Dissection and Selective Suture Ligation of the Dorsal Vein Complex

After bilateral neurovascular bundle release is achieved up to or past the midprostate, we rotate the prostate medially to allow release of

the neurovascular bundle away from the prostate apex. The ProGrasp™ forceps in robotic arm number 3 then bunches the detrusor apron while creating slight cephalad tension (Fig. 5.12) [17]. This also allows for visualization of the anterolateral prostatic contour. After pushing levator fibers away from the prostatic apex, vascular structures between the detrusor apron and the apical prostate are divided sharply. Pinpoint bipolar cautery is used to control the arterioles comprising the dorsal vascular complex. Critical to adequate visualization is maintenance of pneumoperitoneum to minimize venous bleeding. This may be accomplished with the use of the AirSeal® (SurgiQuest, Milford, CT) [18]. Additionally, the bedside assistant uses the suction sparingly, primarily with the sucker tip submerged within a puddle of blood to prevent lowering of the pneumoperitoneum [19].

An anatomic plane extends sagittally from the detrusor apron's attachment on the pubic bone to the prostatic-urethral junction, lying anterior to the urethra and medial to the ischio-prostatic

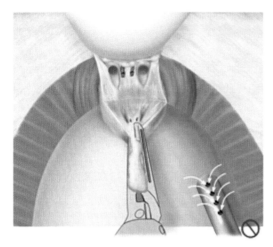

Fig. 5.13 Vascular structure residing within the detrusor apron are sharply divided until blunt dissection is used to identify the avascular plane anterior to the urethra and the pillars of Walsh laterally. Arterioles are controlled with pinpoint bipolar energy set to 25 W. Maintenance of pneumoperitoneum and avoidance of assistant suction allows visualization for dissection. From Lei Y., et al. Athermal Division and Selective Suture Ligation of the Dorsal Vein Complex During Robot-Assisted Laparoscopic Radical Prostatectomy: Description of Technique and Outcomes. *Eur Urol 2011*;59: 235–243. Reprinted with permission from Elsevier Limited

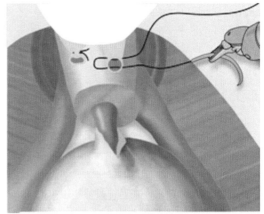

Fig. 5.14 Selective horizontal mattress suture ligation of the dorsal vein complex components prior to anastomosis with a 22 cm 3–0 vicryl suture cut to 22 cm that is used for selective suturing and 50 % of the anastomosis. From Lei Y., et al. Athermal Division and Selective Suture Ligation of the Dorsal Vein Complex During Robot-Assisted Laparoscopic Radical Prostatectomy: Description of Technique and Outcomes. *Eur Urol 2011*;59: 235–243. Reprinted with permission from Elsevier Limited

ligaments (Walsh's pillars). Identification of this avascular plane is achieved with blunt dissection after the vascular structures have been sharply divided. Once this cleavage plane is established, Walsh's pillars are sharply divided (Fig. 5.13) [20]. The ProGrasp™ then grasps the prostatic base and rotates it to exposure the remaining posterior rhabdosphincter attachments which are divided.

Next, the anterior urethra is sharply transected. The robotic Maryland and the curved scissors are removed, and replaced with robotic needle drivers. Selective suturing of the dorsal vein sinuses is accomplished with a 3–0 Vicryl cut to 10 in. on a CT-3 needle (Ethicon, Somerville, NJ) in a horizontal mattress fashion (Fig. 5.14). Identification of the venotomies is facilitated by lowering the pneumoperitoneum, either by assistant suctioning of the pneumoperitoneum, or setting the insufflator to

<5 mmHg. The bleeding venotomies are repaired with a mattress suture, using the same suture used for selective suturing of the dorsal venous complex. It is critical to take thin bites of the venotomies, avoiding wider needle trajectories that may ensnare the anterior rhabdosphincter. Approximately two to three venotomies are typically encountered.

For efficiency, the remaining suture following selective suture ligation of the dorsal vascular complex is used for 50 % of the urethral anastomosis [21]. The first stitch is preplaced as a posterior anastomotic suture prior to division of the posterior urethra (Fig. 5.15). The assistant then divides the posterior urethra using laparoscopic scissors (Fig. 5.16). This sequence prevents retraction of the urethral stump and avoids another instrument change back to robotic scissors. The prostate is then placed in the 10 mm specimen entrapment bag and the neurovascular bundles are inspected for arterial bleeding after irrigating. This bleeding is controlled via suture ligation or by delicate placement of 5 mm hemo-lok clips.

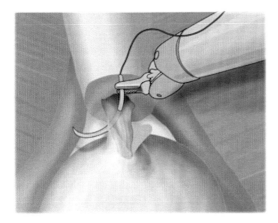

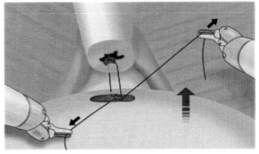

Fig. 5.17 A surgeon's knot on the bladder mucosa is used to parachute down the bladder. Tying the knot on the inside versus the outside of the anastomosis allows the surgeon to directly visualize the suture and ensure that the knot is down. From Williams SB., et al. Randomized Controlled Trial of Barbed Polyglyconate Versus Polyglactin Suture for Robot-assisted Laparoscopic Prostatectomy Anastomosis: Technique and Outcomes. *Eur Urol. 2010*;58(8):875–81. Reprinted with permission from Elsevier Limited

Fig. 5.15 Six o'clock anastomotic suture placed inside-out of the urethral mucosa prior to transection of the posterior urethra to avoid retraction of the urethral stump. From Williams SB., et al. Randomized Controlled Trial of Barbed Polyglyconate Versus Polyglactin Suture for Robot-Assisted Laparoscopic Prostatectomy Anastomosis: Technique and Outcomes. *Eur Urol. 2010*;58(8):875–81. Reprinted with permission from Elsevier Limited

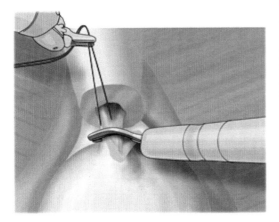

Fig. 5.16 An assistant divides the posterior urethra with laparoscopic scissors to avoid additional robotic instrument change, and the specimen is placed into a laparoscopic bag. From Williams SB., et al. Randomized Controlled Trial of Barbed Polyglyconate Versus Polyglactin Suture for Robot-assisted Laparoscopic Prostatectomy Anastomosis: Technique and Outcomes. *Eur Urol. 2010*;58(8):875–81. Reprinted with permission from Elsevier Limited

Anastomosis

The 3–0 vicryl suture placed in the urethral stump prior to division of the posterior urethra is then placed outside-in at the six o'clock (posterior)

position on the bladder neck. A surgeon's knot is used to bring this down to the urethral stump. Advancement of the bladder to the urethra is facilitated by placing the needle drivers in a "water-skier" position: pulling in a 45° anterior-cephalad direction (Fig. 5.17) [22]. Often lowering the pneumoperitoneum to 3–5 mmHg is helpful. Next, two lateral posterior sutures are placed with the knots tied on the bladder mucosa and the needles left on the suture. The reinforcement of the posterior aspect of the anastomosis minimizes the likelihood of false catheter passage and creates watertight mucosal apposition. This is confirmed by passage of a working catheter under direct camera vision. The needles are then placed through the urethra in an inside-out fashion, preparing for two continuous sutures. Using the contralateral needle driver, the next posterior lateral anastomotic bite is placed, taking full-thickness bites outside-in the bladder neck and inside-out the urethra (Fig. 5.18). Use of the contralateral versus ipsilateral robotic needle driver allows an optimal working angle for the running suture line component of the anastomosis. Alternative bites are taken until both suture lines comprising the sides of the anastomosis reach the 12 o'clock (anterior) position on the urethra. At this point, the left suture is placed inside-out the bladder to allow tying of the

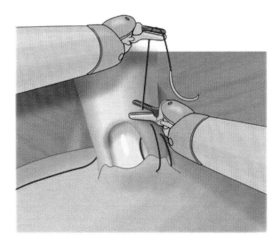

Fig. 5.18 To remove slack from the suture line during the running component of the anastomosis, the suture is pulled through perpendicular to the urethral stump versus pulling it back toward the camera. Simultaneously, the other needle driver forms a "V" where the suture exits the urethra and buttresses as slack is removed from the suture line. However, this maneuver must be avoided with barbed polyglyconate sutures to avoid overtightening and potential tissue strangulation. From Williams SB., et al. Randomized Controlled Trial of Barbed Polyglyconate Versus Polyglactin Suture for Robot-assisted Laparoscopic Prostatectomy Anastomosis: Technique and Outcomes. *Eur Urol. 2010*; 58(6):875–81. Reprinted with permission from Elsevier Limited

to spread under the external iliac vein to the pelvic sidewall. The plane between the medial edge of the external iliac vein and the lateral aspect of the lymph node packet is developed predominantly by blunt dissection. This plane extends distally to Cooper's ligament and proximally until becoming obscured by the confluence of the lateral proximal bladder wall with the iliac vessels. Posteriorly, the obturator nerve is identified prior to placement of a large (purple) hem-o-lock clip onto the distal aspect of the lymph node packet. The packet is then teased away from the proximal aspect of the pelvic sidewall underneath the external iliac vein. No clips are required proximally, and the packet is gently plucked out. Care is taken to avoid injury to the obturator artery and vein, which run alongside the nerve. Occasionally, the lymph nodes are matted down to these vessels, and they are taken after placement of hem-o-lok clips. After completion of the dissection, the left lymph node packet is tagged with a clip and both are placed into a 10 mm laparoscopic bag separate from the one for the prostate. The prostate and lymph node specimen bags are then removed together just prior to abdominal wall closure.

two sutures across the anterior anastomosis. Integrity of the anastomosis is tested by filling the bladder with 120 cc of saline. The working catheter is exchanged for a final 20-French catheter and the return of irrigant confirms its correct positioning [22].

Lymph Node Dissection

Consistent with current guidelines, we perform pelvic lymph node dissection for men with intermediate or high-risk disease [1]. The lymph node dissection is typically performed prior to the apical dissection and after the bilateral antegrade nerve sparing. Division of the bladder neck allows greater medial mobilization of the bladder by the robotic arm number 3 ProGrasp™ to create better exposure during lymph node dissection. The first step involves identification of the external iliac vein. The robotic Maryland dissector is then used

Wound Closure

Although the likelihood of urine leak and postoperative bleeding is very uncommon at this point in our experience, we continue to place a 15-French round Blake drain (Ethicon Inc., Somerville NJ) through the robotic arm number 3 trocar. This is typically removed the following day.

The specimen bag is retrieved by enlarging the supra-umbilical camera port vertically. Under guidance, the surgeon grasps the end of the string on the entrapment bag in his right hand with a needle driver and lines this up directly with the camera trocar. The string is then brought out through the camera port and all the trocars are removed. Two 0-polyglactin sutures on UR-6 needles are used to close the anterior rectus sheath fascia in a figure-of-eight interrupted fashion. The skin of the extraction site is closed with a 4–0 monocryl (poliglecaprone 25) suture in a subcuticular fashion. We do not close the fascia of the other port sites. After infiltration with local analgesics, DERMABOND™ is used to re-approximate the skin of the trocar sites including reinforcement of the subcuticular closure at the extraction site.

References

1. Guidelines. N. Prostate cancer version 3.2012. www.nccn.org. Clinical practice guidelines in oncology

2. Kowalczyk KJ, Huang AC, Williams SB, Yu H, Hu JC. Robotic-assisted laparoscopic radical prostatec-tomy after aborted retropubic radical prostatectomy. J Robotic Surg. 2013;7(3):301–304.

3. Parikh A, Toepfer N, Baylor K, Henry Y, Berger P, Rukstalis D. Preoperative aspirin is safe in patients undergoing urologic robot-assisted surgery. J Endourol. 2012;26(7):852–6.

4. Eberli D, Chassot PG, Sulser T, et al. Urological surgery and antiplatelet drugs after cardiac and cerebrovascular accidents. J Urol. 2010;183(6):2128–36.

5. Forrest JB, Clemens JQ, Finamore P, Leveillee R, Lippert M, Pisters L, Touijer K, Whitmore K. AUA Best Practice Statement for the prevention of deep vein thrombosis in patients undergoing urologic sur-gery. American Urological Association Education and Research, Inc. 2009;181(3):1170–7.

6. Weber ED, Colyer MH, Lesser RL, Subramanian PS. Posterior ischemic optic neuropathy after minimally invasive prostatectomy. J Neuroophthalmol. 2007;27(4):285–7.

7. Meininger D, Byhahn C, Wolfram M, Mierdl S, Kessler P, Westphal K. Prolonged intraperitoneal ver-sus extraperitoneal insufflation of carbon dioxide in patients undergoing totally endoscopic robot-assisted radical prostatectomy. Surg Endosc. 2004;18(5):829–33.

8. Guillonneau D, Vallancien G. Laparoscopic radical prostatectomy: the Montsouris technique. J Urol. 2000;163:1643–9.

9. Friedlander DF, Alemozaffar M, Hevelone ND, Lipsitz SR, Hu JC. Stepwise description and out-comes of bladder neck sparing during robot-assisted laparoscopic radical prostatectomy. J Urol. 2012;188(5):1754–60.

10. Freire MP, Weinberg AC, Lei Y, et al. Anatomic bladder neck preservation during robotic-assisted laparoscopic

11. Kowalczyk KJ, Huang AC, Hevelone ND, et al. Stepwise approach for nerve sparing without countertraction during robot-assisted radical prosta-tectomy: technique and outcomes. Eur Urol. 2011;60(3):536–47.

12. Berry A, Korkes F, Hu JC. Landmarks for consistent nerve sparing during robotic-assisted laparoscopic rad-ical prostatectomy. J Endourol. 2008;22(8):1565–7.

13. Alemozaffar M, Duclos A, Hevelone ND, et al. Technical refinement and learning curve for attenuat-ing neurapraxia during robotic-assisted radical prostatectomy to improve sexual function. Eur Urol. 2012;61(6):1222–8.

14. Menon M, Shrivastava A, Kaul S, et al. Vattikuti Institute prostatectomy: contemporary technique and analysis of results. Eur Urol. 2007;51(3):648–57. discussion 657–48.

15. Carter SC, Le JD, Hu JC. Anatomic and technical considerations for optimizing recovery of sexual function during robotic-assisted radical prostatec-tomy. Curr Opin Urol. 2013;23(1):88–94.

16. Kowalczyk KJ, Huang AC, Hevelone ND, et al. Effect of minimizing tension during robotic-assisted laparo-scopic radical prostatectomy on urinary function recovery. World J Urol. 2012;31:515–21.

17. Carter SC, Konijeti R, Hu J. Selective suture ligation of the dorsal vein complex during robot-assisted lapa-roscopic radical prostatectomy. J Endourol. 2012;26(12):1576–7.

18. Lepor H. Status of radical prostatectomy in 2009: is there medical evidence to justify the robotic approach? Rev Urol. 2009;11(2):61–70.

19. Lei Y, Alemozaffar M, Williams SB, et al. Athermal division and selective suture ligation of the dorsal vein complex during robot-assisted laparoscopic radical prostatectomy: description of technique and out-comes. Eur Urol. 2011;59(2):235–43.

20. Walsh PC. Urologic surgery: radical retropubic pros-tatectomy—an anatomic approach with preservation of sexual function. New York: Bristol Laboratories S; 1986.

21. Williams SB, Alemozaffar M, Lei Y, et al. Randomized controlled trial of barbed polyglyconate versus poly-glactin suture for robot-assisted laparoscopic prosta-tectomy anastomosis: technique and outcomes. Eur Urol. 2010;58(8):875–81.

22. Berry AM, Korkes F, Ferreira M, Hu JC. Robotic ure-throvesical anastomosis: combining running and interrupted sutures. J Endourol. 2008;22(9):2127–9.

Robotic-Assisted Radical Prostatectomy: A Surgical Guide to the Extraperitoneal Approach

6

Christian P. Pavlovich and Adam C. Reese

Background

Laparoscopic urologic oncology essentially started when the first laparoscopic radical nephrectomy was reported in 1991 [1]. Until then, although laparoscopic cholecystectomy had become accepted, removing solid organs was considered impractical. Within a few years the first laparoscopic radical prostatectomy was performed by some of the same urologists, and this initial series was finally reported in 1997 [2]. For a variety of reasons, this procedure did not immediately catch on, but instead was re-pioneered by several European groups over the coming years, resulting in a reproducible technique by 2001 [3]. This approach became popular in Europe, but caught on at only a few centers in the USA until the advent of robot-assisted surgery. Few would have imagined however, that within 10 years, robot-assisted laparoscopic radical prostatectomy would become the most common approach to radical prostatectomy in the USA.

C.P. Pavlovich, M.D. (✉)
Brady Urological Institute, Johns Hopkins Bayview
Medical Center, Johns Hopkins University School of
Medicine, 301 Building, Suite 3100, 4940 Eastern
Ave., Baltimore, MD 21224, USA
e-mail: cpavlov2@jhmi.edu

A.C. Reese, M.D.
Brady Urological Institute, Johns Hopkins University
School of Medicine, Baltimore, MD 21287, USA

The first-generation laparoscopic assist robot that saw widespread adoption was Aesop™ (Computer Motion, USA), a camera-holding device that could be remotely manipulated with voice control. This device was important to the development of streamlined laparoscopic radical prostatectomy, providing stable and reproducible camera focusing and movement controlled by the primary surgeon. The same company then worked towards creating a more versatile robotic platform that could assist with other instruments, while in parallel another company (Intuitive Surgical, USA) was developing its own robotic system. These companies eventually merged, and Intuitive's da Vinci™ became the sole platform for contemporary robotic surgery. This proved to be a boon for minimally invasive radical prostatectomists, as the laparoscopic radical prostatectomy was considered by a consensus panel of expert urologic laparoscopists to be "extremely difficult", the highest level of laparoscopic surgical complexity [4].

As the transperitoneal approach to laparoscopic radical prostatectomy was perfected, some surgeons turned back to the space of Retzius and developed a totally extraperitoneal approach to laparoscopic radical prostatectomy [5, 6]. It was just a matter of time until robot-assisted radical prostatectomy was performed extraperitoneally [7, 8], a development facilitated by the smaller next-generation robotic platform, the da Vinci S™. The smaller arms allow for less clashing in the relatively more confining space of Retzius,

J.A. Eastham and E.M. Schaeffer (eds.), *Radical Prostatectomy: Surgical Perspectives*,
DOI 10.1007/978-1-4614-8693-0_6, © Springer Science+Business Media New York 2014

and the robot decreases the physical demands of the laparoscopic approach.

How-to-Guide

The concept is both to mimic open radical retropubic prostatectomy as far as possible, and to use the advantages of robotic instrumentation and pneumoperitoneum to minimize blood loss and facilitate careful dissection. Compared to open radical retropubic prostatectomy, extraperitoneal robotic radical prostatectomy utilizes essentially the same steps, albeit in a slightly different order. After all, both procedures are performed in the retropubic or extraperitoneal space of Retzius and with the same goal: complete prostate extirpation and, in many cases, bilateral pelvic lymphadenectomy.

Patient Positioning and Port Placement

The patient is placed supine on a butterfly beanbag specifically made for robotic pelvic surgery that is secured to the operating table. Legs are placed in Allen stirrups and spread apart and then lowered slightly with flexion at the hip joints. Arms are carefully tucked and secured at the sides and held in place by the beanbag. The beanbag is molded to cradle both the arms and the shoulders to prevent cranial migration of the patient during Trendelenburg positioning, and air is aspirated out of the beanbag when the patient is in final position for surgery. All pressure points are double-checked and reinforced with padding and/or tape as necessary to avoid positional injuries. The abdomen is then prepped and draped up to the tenth rib/costal margin and lateral to the mid-axillary lines. The scrotum and perineum are included in the prep of the abdomen. After draping, a Foley catheter is placed sterilely in order to decompress the bladder.

Rather than using Veress needle insufflation, the retropubic space is entered through a 12 mm infra-umbilical skin incision that is either vertical or smile-shaped, in a similar fashion as total extraperitoneal inguinal hernia repair. Through this

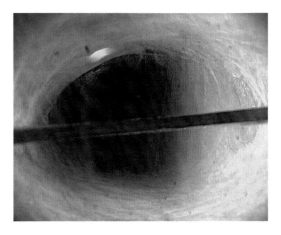

Fig. 6.1 View through the Visiport as anterior rectus fascia is incised *horizontally*. Left rectus m. belly is the *red* structure visible through incised fascia, midline is the *yellow* area to the right

incision the anterior rectus fascia is identified and incised (Fig. 6.1). Our preference is to incise directly with a Visiport angled 80° to the vertical aiming slightly caudally (Fig. 6.2a), though others prefer the open cut-down Hasson technique (note that the Visiport does not accommodate the standard 12 mm robotic camera, but only a laparoscopic 10 mm or robotic 8 mm camera). The Visiport allows for excellent visualization without making the incision any larger than 12 mm. At this point the Visiport is gently advanced between the rectus muscle bellies, generally to the left of the linea alba and is then slid over the posterior sheath toward the arcuate line at a far more acute angle (30° to the skin) aiming caudally and into the space of Retzius (Fig. 6.2b). The arcuate line is passed over as the horizontal fibers of the posterior sheath give way to transversalis fascia, and then the Visiport is pushed left and right in a fan-shaped manner to gently open up the retropubic potential space for subsequent balloon dilatation. The Visiport is removed and a kidney-shaped laparoscopic balloon (PDBS2 AutoSuture™, Covidien, Mansfield, MA) is blindly inserted into the infraumbilical incision just past the incised anterior rectus fascia and angled Southward into the space of Retzius in front of the bladder and behind the pubis. At this point the balloon is manually insufflated and the expanding balloon is visualized through the port with the laparoscopic 0° lens (Fig. 6.3). The inferior epigastric arteries

a   b

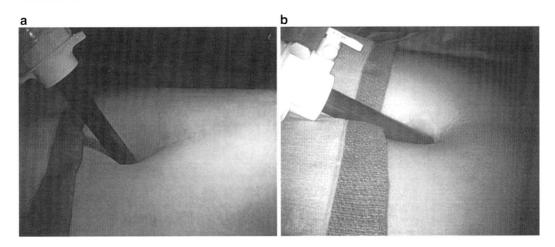

Fig. 6.2 Angles shown during initial incision of anterior rectus fascia (**a**) and then as space of Retzius is entered (**b**)

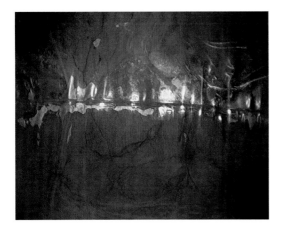

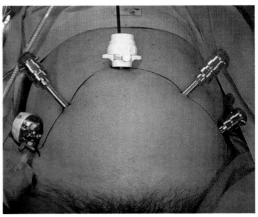

Fig. 6.3 View of the pelvis from within the just-deployed balloon that is creating the potential space in which the operation will take place

Fig. 6.4 Port configuration for extraperitoneal robotic-assisted radical prostatectomy. The four robotic ports (the metal ports plus the midline camera port must each be at least 8 cm from each other

and veins are easily identified superolaterally through the clear developing balloon as it pushes the parietal peritoneum away superiorly. Finally, the balloon is deflated and removed, and the Visiport trocar is reinserted into the space and insufflation is started. The whole case can be performed with pressures ranging from 12 to 20 mm Hg; it is always safest to use the lowest possible insufflation pressure to maintain the space. If the space is intact it should appear concave, football-shaped, and have flimsy areolar tissue within it overlying the structures of the deep pelvis.

At this point the remaining ports are placed, all with blunt trocars, and essentially in a fan-shaped position around the pubic midline. 3 mm × 8 mm Reusable metal robotic ports are used, as well as a 12 mm disposable assistant port (Ethicon Xcel for example). The configuration is as in (Fig. 6.4), with ports *angled caudally* about 45–70° from the vertical and generally placed along the line from the anterior superior iliac spine (ASIS) to the umbilical incision, with a minimum of 8 cm between robotic ports. The first port is 8–9 cm left lateral to the umbilical port along the line to the left ASIS; then that is

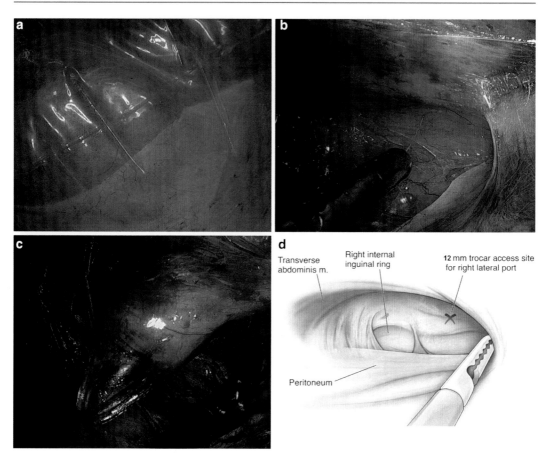

Fig. 6.5 (**a**) The peritoneal reflection is noted in the *right lower* aspect of the figure, appearing as a pale line going across the image from *lower left* to *upper right*. The balloon is pushing it inferiorly as it is being inflated. (**b**) Here the balloon has been removed and an alligator grasper is being used to push the peritoneum more inferiorly and superiorly such that the sidewall can be identified over the spermatic cord. (**c**) The spermatic cord is being held down as the assistant port is being placed caudal and superior to the peritoneal lining in the *right lower* quadrant. (**d**) A graphic depiction of (**b**)

used to insert a blunt alligator grasper which can facilitate dissection of the peritoneum cranially and posteriorly for right lateral-most port placement 2 cm superior and 2 cm medial to the right ASIS. This port gets *tunneled subcutaneously* until it reaches the line between the right ASIS and the umbilical port. It then gets pushed in deeper and into the true pelvis gliding over the spermatic cord and lateral to the peritoneal reflection which is often noted here (Fig. 6.5). Finally, the right medial 8 mm robotic trocar is placed 8–9 cm to the right of the umbilical port along the line toward the right ASIS, and then the left-most 8 mm robotic port for the fourth robotic arm is placed near the left ASIS but again some 2 cm superior and medial to it, then tunneled subcuta-neously toward the left ASIS–umbilical port line, before passing into the pelvis and over the spermatic cord. It is crucial to angle all of the ports approximately 45–70° caudally on insertion (e.g., toward the legs) in order to avoid the perito-neal space, which is often visible at the time of port placement, and to watch the trocars go in under direct vision.

The patient is then placed in modest Trendelenburg (full Trendelenburg is rarely needed) and the space is analyzed. A peritoneot-omy would be noticed at this point as the space would appear small and its supero-posterior wall (peritoneum) would be billowing into the field. This relatively rare occurrence (about 1/20 cases in experienced hands) need not change one's operative plan. A small/microscopic peritoneotomy which lets gas into the peritoneal cavity can be managed by inserting a Veress needle into the abdomen for continuous venting of this space during the operation. Alternately, since the bladder has been "taken down" already, a small inadvertent peritoneotomy can purposely be enlarged on one or both sides side to render the extra- and trans-peritoneal spaces contiguous but still without losing some of the advantages of extraperitoneal surgery, such as the fact that the bladder is already taken down, and the veil of tissue composed of the urachus and medial umbilical ligaments maintain separation between the patient's bowels and the pelvic space.

The Da Vinci robot is then moved into place between the legs. If the legs need to be spread a bit more or lowered to avoid clashing with the robot, this is easily accomplished by adjusting the Allen stirrups. Docking is done carefully and remembering to keep the ports angled even while docking to avoid inadvertent peritoneotomy. The fourth robotic arm (robot arm "3") comes in left lateral-most and must be docked such that it does not clash with the stirrup, left knee, left foot or pelvis. Then, under direct vision, the robotic instruments should be advanced into the retropubic space. Our preference is for a ProGrasp forceps in the arm at far left, a bipolar Maryland grasper in the left arm, a monopolar scissor in the right robotic port, and a 0° lens in the camera port. The 12 mm assistant port is used for a right-sided assistant and allows for retraction, suction, clip placement, and also specimen (lymph node packet(s)) extraction.

The Extraperitoneal Space

The extraperitoneal space at this point only needs to be expanded a bit in order to appear identical to the standard open retropubic space that surgeons have grown accustomed to over the last decades. It is worthwhile to spend several minutes dissecting through areolar tissue until the entire pubis and midline symphysis are clearly identified (Fig. 6.6a, b show the area first as it looks on removal of the balloon and subsequent insufflation, then after the areolar tissue has been cleared away). It then helps to defat the area as well until the endopelvic fasciae are visible (Fig. 6.6c). The superficial dorsal vein is usually apparent as fat gets dissected off of the anterior prostate and it should be taken with electrocautery. The fat overlying it generally ramifies along with its proximal branching to the right, left, and center over the prostate toward the bladder, but with bipolar diathermy these branches can easily be taken and the fat and superficial dorsal venous complex removed to better expose the prostate. We have in recent years been sending this fatty tissue for pathologic analysis as a minority of patients (5–15 %) will have periprostatic lymph node(s) contained within.

Flimsy tissues overlying the external iliac vessels and spermatic cords should then be incised to facilitate easy access to the pelvis for the assistant and fourth robotic arm. Any inguinal hernias or herniated fat that are in the way should be reduced. Finally, identification of important landmarks should ensue, the puboprostatic ligaments and endopelvic fasciae for the prostatectomy, and the external iliac veins (EIV) and obturator nerves for men who will be receiving pelvic lymph node dissection (PLND). It is particularly important to make sure to assess the position of the right EIV in comparison to the right assistant port, and ideally to advance that port *past* the vein such that instruments that are placed through the port do not risk traumatizing it.

Pelvic Lymph Node Dissection

We prefer to perform the PLND prior to the prostatectomy, though it certainly can be accomplished subsequent to the mobilization of the prostate. In either case, preparation for PLND involves identifying the EIV and obturator nerves. The former can usually be found, even if there is much fat overlying them, by looking for venous waveforms just above the pelvic brim. Once found, the fascia overlying the EIVs must be incised and the sidewall accessed under the veins. The assistant's suction device can be placed in this space while the operator dissects the nodes off the EIV and looks for the obturator nerve. If not obviously under the EIV it can often

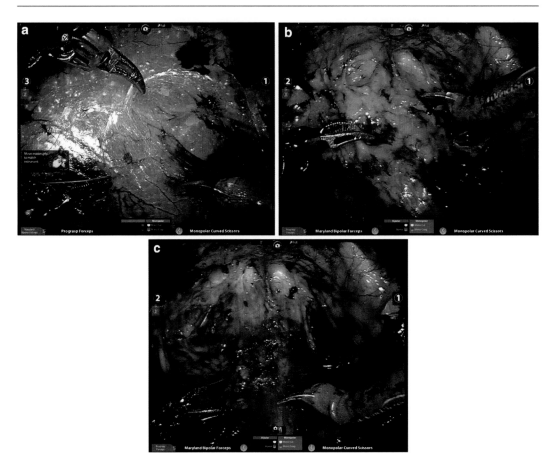

Fig. 6.6 (**a**) The space of Retzius after the balloon has been removed and all ports have been placed and instruments loaded. (**b**) The same space (and patient) after the areolar tissue has been cleared away, leaving residual periprostatic fat. (**c**) After the fat has been cleared away the endopelvic fascia and puboprostatic ligaments are more identifiable

be found by looking for the obturator foramen which often has a fat plug in it. The nerve courses through the foramen and out of the pelvis by hugging the foramen superolaterally; once it is found the nodal packet under the EIV and above the obturator nerve should be clipped distally and handled with the ProGrasp for dissection as proximally as indicated. A standard PLND can certainly be performed in this space, taking all level I and II nodes, as the bifurcation of the iliac vessels is reachable (as in open radical prostatectomy which, as mentioned, is performed in the same space and with the same limitations). With the ProGrasp holding the nodes anteriorly, two arms remain for dissection, cautery, and retraction (Fig. 6.7). In addition, the wrist of the arm on the side of the PLND can be used to hold back

pre-peritoneal fat if it gets in the way, while still allowing the instrument to be used as a grasper/dissector. Extended PLND depending on the definition may or may not be able to be performed, as presacral nodes are not reachable without mobilizing the bladder more than can be done extraperitoneally; a 30° lens may be used to facilitate deeper and more medial dissections at the internal iliac artery(ies) and vein(s). In any case, we favor using Hem-o-lok™ clips (Weck, Teleflex, Limerick, PA) to secure lymphatic pedicles, rather than bipolar cautery or suction whenever possible. A harmonic scalpel is also a great tool for PLND and for sealing small lymphatics, but is certainly not necessary. The nodes are typically extracted after the dissection, through the 12 mm assistant port (Fig. 6.8), though they can also be

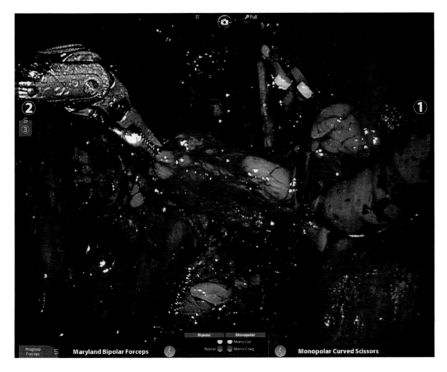

Fig. 6.7 The ProGrasp is an excellent tool for atraumatically grasping lymph node packets and leaving the other robotic arms free for dissection. The right obturator nerve and right external iliac vein are in plain view

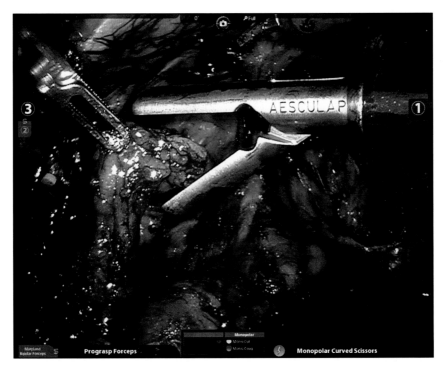

Fig. 6.8 The freed right pelvic lymph node packet is being given to the assistant for extraction through the assistant 12 mm port with a spoon forceps. An alligator grasper often does the trick as well if the specimen is too bulky. Remember to open the port for specimen extraction

left in their location for later extraction with the prostate specimen. A drain should be placed at the conclusion of the case whenever PLND is performed, particularly when confined to the extraperitoneal space.

Radical Prostatectomy

The subsequent steps can be performed in much the same manner as a radical prostatectomy would be done in open retropubic fashion or in transperitoneal laparoscopic/robotic fashion. The order of the steps and the tools used may differ, but fundamentally the retropubic potential space, once expanded, allows for a comparable retropubic view of the cancerous prostate. An advantage to remaining extraperitoneal, or preperitoneal, as in open radical retropubic radical prostatectomy, is that steep Trendelenburg is not necessary prior to docking the robot, although some minor Trendelenburg is helpful. The reason is that the bladder and peritoneum form a natural superior and posterior floor to the operation until Denonvilliers' fascia is reached, preventing small and large bowel and any prior intra-abdominal adhesions from complicating access to the prostate. The critical aspect of the case that differs from most other approaches and that must be mastered in order to perform successful extraperitoneal radical prostatectomy is identification, dissection and taking of the posterior genital structures the vasa deferentia and seminal vesicles. These are taken after bladder neck transection and not accessed transperitoneally nor retrograde as in open retropubic radical prostatectomy. Nerve sparing on the other hand, may be accomplished antegrade, retrograde, or in a combined manner regardless of the approach to the prostate and is performed as per the preferences of the operating surgeon.

- Step 1: *Incising the endopelvic fasciae and puboprostatic ligaments*

  The surgeon should search for the relatively avascular plane between the prostate and its lateral attachments. The optimal place to start is at the proximal shoulder of the prostate on either side, just distal to the vasculature of the bladder at the lateral prostate–bladder interface. The endopelvic fascia at its proximal origin is easily identifiable and can be swept toward the apex until at one point it needs to be incised and will no longer sweep away. This incision line, made by scissor or with monopolar cautery (Fig. 6.9), should be continued to the puboprostatic ligaments, which are then carefully taken at their midpoint in order to allow for better ligation of the deep dorsal vein beneath them. The more distal and inferior aspects of the puboprostatics should not be taken as they lend support to the urethra as it exits the prostate apically. Ideally, after incision of the endopelvic fascia, the lateral prostatic fascia is kept on the prostate, the levator ani fascia is left on the levator ani muscle, and a plane between them develops with venous channels (often quite prominent) notable on the prostate side and just covered by lateral prostatic fascia. For intrafascial dissections, if desired, these veins can be left lateral to the plane of dissection and contiguous with the levator fascia, allowing the surgeon to get right onto the prostate capsule. This dissection is however more difficult, associated with more bleeding, and should ideally only be undertaken in low–intermediate risk patients with minimal to no apparent disease on that side. As an additional note, accessory pudendal arteries are sometimes identified during dissection through the endopelvic fasciae and are spared when possible to assist in preservation of erectile function. Electrocautery is kept to a minimum to prevent damage to the neurovascular bundles and external urethral sphincter.

- Step 2: *The dorsal vein*
- Once the endopelvic fasciae and puboprostatic ligaments have been incised, the prostatic apex becomes readily apparent. Most of what is seen is deep dorsal vein and supporting connective tissue over the prostate, and the urethra and its Foley catheter are surprisingly deep yet. Tugging on the Foley by the assistant can help demonstrate the level of the urethra, but with experience and with meticulous dissection deep and lateral to the puboprostatics the sides of the deep dorsal vein of the penis become apparent and its posterior extent is usually visible. Once the surgeon is content with both sides of the apical dissection

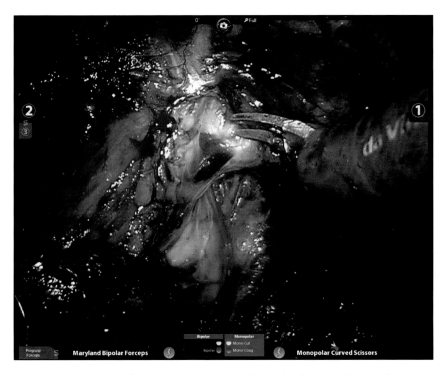

Fig. 6.9 Incision of the endopelvic fasciae starts proximally for the most avascular result. Here the right endopelvic fascia is being incised—note the vessel in the fascia that has been found and not traumatized due to carefully incising from base to apex lateral to the gland

a prudent move is to simulate where a dorsal vein stitch would be thrown from one side to the other, and place an instrument there such as a Maryland or PK dissector and gently spread its jaws to prepare the area and move the vein away from it. Then the assistant switches to the Large Needle Drivers and a stitch is thrown. The ligation is performed as distally as possible to ensure that the prostatic apex is not inadvertently entered during subsequent division of the DVC. We prefer to use a 2–0 braided suture (e.g., Polysorb) on a large needle (GS-21) for most dorsal venous complexes and throw the needle right-to-left and horizontally under the dorsal vein but above the urethra, then again throw it horizontally in figure-of-eight and locking fashion just anterior to the dorsal vein and through the remaining anterior portion of the incised puboprostatic ligaments (Fig. 6.10). The placement of these throws and the locking of

the suture promotes upward traction on the final knot, and the braided nature of the suture as well as an initial surgeon's knot facilitates the knot holding fast. After three throws the stitch is cut short so that it does not interfere with the anastomosis later in the course of the case. Most surgeons prefer not to actually divide the dorsal venous complex until later in the operation, at the time of the apical prostatic dissection.

- Step 3: *The bladder neck transection*
- Attention is then turned to the bladder neck. Several different maneuvers can aid in identification of the interface between the prostate and bladder neck. First, with the assistant gently pulling on the urethral catheter, the surgeon can visually identify the junction between these two structures. This junction can often be further delineated as the point where the perivesical fat gives way to the prostatic contour. Finally, the two robotic arms can be used

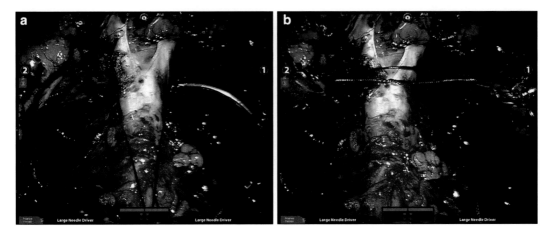

Fig. 6.10 (**a**) The dorsal vein stitch (2–0 Polysorb) has been thrown from right to left under the deep dorsal vein. A second throw is about to be made superior to the vein and through the more anteriorly placed remnant puboprostatic ligaments. (**b**) Having completed the second throw a figure-of-eight knot is made and tied

in a pinching maneuver to confirm the interface between prostate and bladder neck. Once this junction is identified, the anterior bladder neck is divided using electrocautery. The bladder is retracted cranially and posteriorly during this maneuver to facilitate dissection.

- Once the lumen of the bladder is entered, the urethral catheter is identified and the balloon is deflated. The catheter is grasped with the fourth robotic arm and tented anteriorly over the pubic symphysis to suspend the prostate. At this point, as the assistant retracts the anterior neck inferiorly, the surgeon should attempt to check for the presence of a median lobe, identify the trigone, and judge the position of or actually see the ureteral orifices. The mucosa of the posterior bladder neck is then divided in an upward smile shape under and proximal to the prostatic urethra (Fig. 6.11). When a median lobe is present, this dissection can be more challenging, and necessitates division of the posterior bladder neck more cranially and posteriorly to ensure that the median lobe remains en bloc with the prostate specimen. The detrusor muscle of the posterior bladder neck is then divided, taking care not to enter the prostate but also ensuring that this layer is sufficiently thick to later hold anastomotic stitches.

- Step 4: *The posterior genital structures*
- After division of the posterior bladder neck, the vasa deferentia are identified deep and near the midline (Fig. 6.12). Once reasonably well-exposed, these are grasped with the ProGrasp as it is no longer needed in order to suspend the prostate anteriorly by the urethral catheter; the vasa are retracted anteriorly one at a time and carefully dissected free from surrounding structures as they head laterally towards the deep inguinal rings. The vasa are then clipped and divided. This exposes the seminal vesicles, and the more proximally the vasa are taken the closer to the tips of the seminal vesicles the surgeon will find themselves. One at a time, each seminal vesicle is then grasped and dissected free from surrounding tissues. It is easier to identify the medial border first and sweep Denonvilliers' fascia posteriorly off of the seminal vesicle, and then work toward the proximal tip and lateral border (Fig. 6.13). A neurovascular pedicle is typically present at the tip of each seminal vesicle; this structure is clipped and divided without cautery to prevent damage to the neurovascular bundle. Once both seminal vesicles are dissected free, they are retracted anteriorly, exposing more of Denonvilliers' fascia and the lateral pedicles to the prostate.

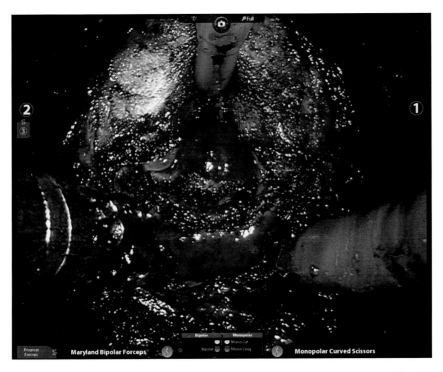

Fig. 6.11 The bladder neck has been transected anteriorly and the posterior bladder mucosa has been scored for subsequent transection just under a small median lobe. The instruments are in the bladder, holding down the anterior bladder neck for purposes of the photo

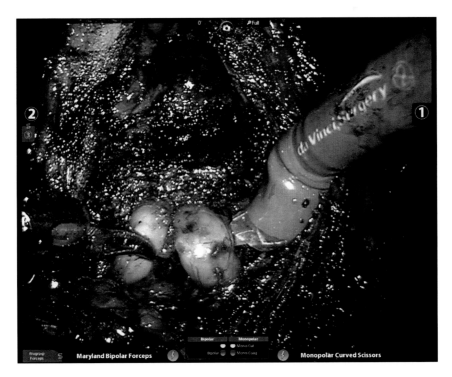

Fig. 6.12 The bladder has been transected from the prostate, a layer of fascia anterior to the posterior genital structures has been incised, and the midline vasa deferentia have come into view

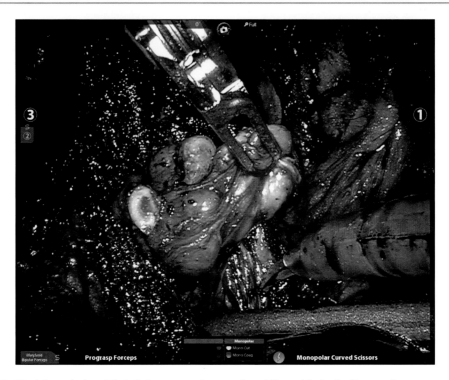

Fig. 6.13 The left seminal vesicle is being retracted across the midline with the ProGrasp to better access the left pedicle. The cut ends of the vasa deferentia can be seen flanking the seminal vesicle

Denonvilliers' is then divided horizontally in the midline, a few millimeter from the junction of the posterior prostate and seminal vesicle insertion, in order to leave a healthy posterior margin on the prostate. Division of Denonvilliers' fascia exposes the underlying prerectal fat (Fig. 6.14). The plane between the prostate and rectum can then be gently developed in the midline using a combination of sharp and blunt dissection, proceeding towards the apex of the prostate. Care is taken not to proceed too far laterally with this dissection, as this can result in troublesome bleeding from the vascular pedicles which have not yet been ligated.

- Step 5: *The pedicles and nerve-sparing*
- At this point, the tip of a seminal vesicle is grasped with the fourth arm ProGrasp and retracted cranially and medially. This exposes the ipsilateral neurovascular pedicle. Depending on preoperative disease characteristics, the surgeon can then choose to perform nerve-sparing or to take a wider soft-tissue margin. In a nerve-sparing procedure, the prostatic fascia is identified at the level of the mid prostate and incised. This identifies the plane between the prostate and the prostatic fascia and its posterolateral attachments which include branches from the neurovascular bundle of Walsh. This neurovascular pedicle is identified, clipped with on more Hem-o-lok clips close to its junction with the prostate, and divided. This dissection is carried from the base of the prostate toward the apex. By minimizing the use of cautery, clipping and cutting the main pedicle and any remaining neuro-vasculature as it enters the prostate, and staying as close to the gland as possible, less damage is done to the posterolateral neurovascular bundles. Such a dissection has been termed intrafascial and gets a surgeon as close to the prostate as is oncologically permissible (Fig. 6.15). Working toward the apex is challenging in that one must stay aware of the

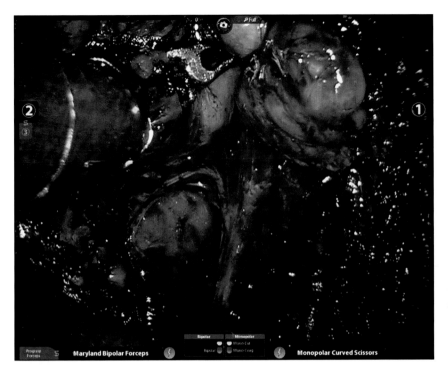

Fig. 6.14 The left seminal vesicle pedicle has now been taken and Denonvilliers' fascia has been incised. Note the prerectal fat (*yellow*) evident in the deep pelvis. The dissection will continue to the left and toward the apex with clips and careful use of cautery

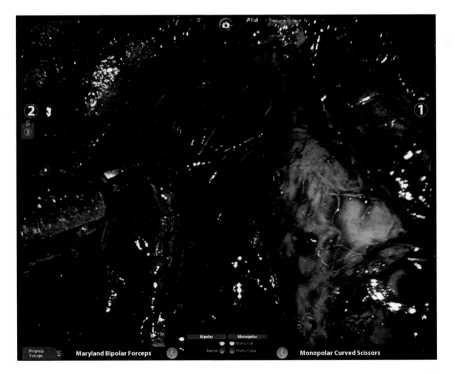

Fig. 6.15 An intrafascial dissection from prostate base to apex has been performed. The healthy veil of tissue overlying the left neurovascular bundle that was spared is being shown by the Maryland bipolar. Note the smooth left side of the prostate on the *right side* of the figure

changing countour of the ellipsoid prostate gland as it courses apically, and use clips and cutting between the bundle and the prostate to sever their neurovascular attachments.

In a more conventional but less prostate-hugging nerve-sparing procedure, an interfascial dissection is performed. The prostatic fascia is left intact in such cases, and the neurovascular pedicle is divided a little further from its junction with the prostate to allow for a slightly wider soft-tissue margin. Dissection towards the apex is done leaving this fascia overlying the posterolateral prostate and clips are again used to secure the pedicles and other smaller branches emanating toward the prostate. Degrees of partial nerve sparing can also be accomplished during such dissections by taking wider margins and clipping in general all around the prostatic fascia and some associated tissue, at all points staying a few mm away from the prostatic fascia. In a non-nerve-sparing approach, the neurovascular bundle is clipped and severed at the base of the gland and then dissection is performed more widely all the way to the apex, with care to avoid rectal injury. In a non-nerve-sparing case, or when rectal injury is suspected, it is prudent to check for such an occurrence by inserting a Foley catheter in the rectum, inflating its balloon to 20 cc, and then instilling 60–120 cc of air into the catheter with a Toomey syringe as the prostatectomy bed is filled with sterile water. Any bubbles noted should elicit a search for a rectal laceration.

Finally, the surgeon must remain vigilant in all cases about leaving any permanent foreign bodies (e.g., Hem-o-lok clips) near proximal urethra and upcoming anastomosis. To prevent subsequent erosion into the neo-bladder neck and proximal urethra, clips and similar nonabsorbables should never be left within a few centimeter of this area. Options to control bleeding more distally are to use gentle bipolar cautery to specific arterial bleeders, and to use fine absorbable suture ligation, bipolar cautery, and/or topical hemostatic agents for any open venous channels that may remain atop the neurovascular bundles after they have been separated from the prostate. Later, it is important also to reassess the bladder neck as it is brought down for re-anastomosis, to

remove any clips from it that would find themselves in proximity to the new anastomosis.
- Step 6: *The apical dissection*
- Prior to moving onto the apex, it is a good idea to grasp the posterior structures (both vasa, both SVs, or a combination as necessary to elevate them and see posteriorly) and retract them anteriorly. The anterior rectal wall and cut Denonvilliers' fascia are seen posteriorly, and the neurovascular bundles laterally. Inspection for any remaining posterior attachments, particularly in the midline allows for these to be taken sharply and prevents them anchoring the prostate once a decision has been made to go to the apex. Once the posterior is all freed up, the prostate is allowed to fall back into the pelvis, and attention is turned toward the apical dissection.
- The deep dorsal venous complex, which was previously ligated, is now divided, leaving a ½ cm cuff of tissue between the cut and the stitch. If troublesome bleeding occurs at this point, it is best managed initially by simply finishing the transection of the complex such that the cut distal end retracts up into the suture and under the pubis. If bleeding continues, particularly if arterial (rare) or venous (through large open sinuses that are not compressed by the stitch) the placement of an additional hemostatic suture may be necessary. One easy way of dealing with this is to re-ligate the complex, this time with a 2–0 absorbable braided suture on a GU needle passed horizontally from one side to the other in figure-of-eight fashion.
- Following division of the DVC, the urethra is visible and is divided in a location that maximizes urethral length but leaves sufficient tissue coverage on the prostate to avoid a positive margin. Division of the urethra frees up most if not all of the specimen, which is then grasped with the fourth arm at its right and then left shoulders (or seminal vesicles) and retracted medially such that the posterior urethral plate or striated sphincter can be accessed. Any remaining fibers here between the transected urethra anteriorly and the previously freed up posterior overlying the rectum

are carefully divided, thus freeing up the specimen completely. The specimen is then retracted out of the operative field by grasping it with the fourth arm and retracting it cranially and just lateral to the camera on the left. Placing the prostate specimen in an EndoCatch bag at this point actually hinders construction of the anastomosis—it is far better to just retract and hold onto the specimen with the fourth arm's ProGrasp until the anastomosis is complete and the EndoCatch bag can be deployed for specimen extraction.

- Step 7: *Assessment of the specimen and prostatectomy bed*
- The field is then inspected for bleeding, which can be facilitated with irrigation of sterile water by the assistant, and the lowering of insufflation pressure to 10–12 mm Hg. Arterial bleeders should be clipped or managed with pinpoint electrocautery. Venous bleeders can be oversewn, although this is rarely necessary. Clips or bipolar cautery can be judiciously used, but if the venous oozers are distal and large caliber it is often best to proceed with the anastomosis and then undermine it with a hemostatic agent once it is half complete. Reinspection at this point makes sense but rarely will venous bleeding not have stopped by now.
- The specimen itself is inspected prior to re-anastomosis of bladder and urethra and any areas suspicious for capsular incision should elicit consideration of resecting a portion of matching tissue from the prostatectomy bed, for frozen or permanent section. Similarly, areas in the bed suspicious for prostate or cancer tissue should be resected and sent for analysis. At this point, a barbed suture can optionally be run in order to approximate the cut edges of Denonvilliers' fascia near the urethral stump and proximally near the bladder neck. The aim is to reduce tension on the upcoming anastomosis, and reinforce the posterior plate.
- Step 8: *The anastomosis*
- The vesicourethral anastomosis is then performed. We prefer to perform the anastomosis with two 9″ V-Loc-90™ (Covidien) barbed

sutures tied together at 7″, such that there are barbs throughout the anastomosis and no areas of unbarbed suture remain. The anastomosis is performed in running fashion as per van Velthoven [9], beginning at the bladder neck at the 6 o'clock position. One suture is run clockwise and the other counterclockwise, meeting at the 12 o'clock position, where the sutures are tied together. It is our preference to tie *across* the anastomosis rather than on one side of it, so the suture on one side is thrown in an outside-in, inside-out fashion bridging the 12 o'clock position on the bladder neck, exiting at either 11 or 1 o'clock and tied to the matching suture from the contralateral side which is exiting the urethra at pretty much the same position. An 18 French silicone urethral catheter is placed just prior to tying the anastomosis. The bladder is then irrigated with 120 cc of normal saline to check for an anastomotic leak, and then the catheter balloon is inflated to 15 cc.

- Often the caliber of the bladder neck opening will be significantly larger than that of the urethra. In this setting, we prefer to "parachute" the bladder down, spacing neighboring sutures further apart on the bladder neck than on the urethra. In some cases it is helpful to narrow the bladder neck at each side with a barbed suture until it more closely approximates the caliber of the urethral stump. If a cystotomy persists at the completion of the anastomosis, an anterior reconstruction can be performed to close the defect in the bladder onto itself, often with a simple figure-of-eight suture at 12 o'clock. The anastomosis is checked for leakage by instilling up to 180 cc through the Foley, then the Foley balloon is inflated to 15 cc and gently pulled to make sure that it settles in the appropriate place at the bladder neck.
- Step 9: *Closure*
- After completing the anastomosis, the specimen is placed into a laparoscopic entrapment sack and the robot is undocked. A closed suction drain is placed through the left-lateral robotic port and sewn to the skin. The medial robotic ports are then removed, taking care to

inspect for inferior epigastric plexus injury, and then the 12 mm assistant port is removed, all under direct vision through the infraumbilical port. Finally, the specimen is extracted through the infraumbilical incision, which is opened up at the skin level in a smile configuration under the umbilicus, and at the level of the anterior rectus fascia in the midline superiorly and inferiorly. The anterior rectus fascia is closed with interrupted #1 Maxon suture with two or three figure-of-eight throws, making sure to capture at least 1 cm of fascia on either side with each bite. Skin incisions are closed with absorbable suture and/or skin glue and all specimen(s) are sent for histopathologic analysis.

Special Considerations

The extraperitoneal approach is rather ideal for men with a variety of factors which make them more challenging surgical patients:

- *Obese men*: These patients are typically challenging to operate on, but more so when they have central obesity. The distances traveled in order to reach the prostate are greater and therefore the use of bariatric length ports is recommended. The extraperitoneal approach is helpful in these men because no intraabdominal fat is encountered, and the bowels are kept out of the way by the peritoneum which acts as a retractor would. The safety of the extraperitoneal approach in obese men has been demonstrated [10]. It helps to use more Trendelenburg in obese men than one would otherwise use in order to keep the trocar/instrument angles more standard and not excessively angled due to a protuberant abdomen.
- *Men with prior abdominal surgery*: Men with prior surgery, particularly low abdominal operations including appendectomy for perforated appendix, low anterior resection for colon cancer or diverticulitis, or umbilical/ventral hernia repair, are at greater risk for enterotomy during port placement and lysis of adhesions than are men without a prior similar surgical history. Angling the ports into the extraperitoneal space and performing

robot-assisted radical prostatectomy extraperitoneally is simply ideal for such patients, and has resulted in 0 enterotomies in over 1,000 cases at our institution, even without a Hasson-type access approach. By gliding infraumbilically with the camera port, and then carefully placing subsequent ports under direct vision and at least 2 cm away from any prior incisions, access for extraperitoneal robot-assisted radical prostatectomy can be achieved in almost every patient. Small peritoneotomies are more commonly encountered in patients with prior surgery, but are usually of little consequence if they are enlarged somewhat and/or vented transperitoneally with a Veress needle for the duration of the case.

- *Men with concomitant inguinal hernia(s)*: Relative contraindications to extraperitoneal robot-assisted radical prostatectomy are men with prior bilateral mesh inguinal hernia repairs, especially if performed laparoscopically and even more so if performed totally extraperitoneally. Not only the pieces of mesh occasionally meet in the midline, they also result in significant reaction and adhesion in the exact space in which the radical prostatectomy is supposed to be performed. In such men a transperitoneal robot-assisted approach would be wiser. On the other hand, men with unilateral or bilateral reducible inguinal hernias pose only minor inconvenience, and can have their hernia defects repaired during the prostatectomy prior to conclusion of the case. We have performed many mesh inguinal hernia repairs in the same setting as the extraperitoneal robot-assisted radical prostatectomy, but often undock the robot and perform the repair laparoscopically (and in difficult cases with a general surgery colleague). No recurrences have been noted to date, and the incidence of incisional (port site hernia) is also very low (0.3 %) despite the fact that we only formally close fascia at the infraumbilical specimen extraction site [11]. The angled extraperitoneal nature of the ports and the blunt trocars used are likely explanations for why we see virtually no port-related hernias with this approach.

References

1. Clayman RV, Kavoussi LR, Soper NJ, et al. Laparoscopic nephrectomy. N Engl J Med. 1991;324(19):1370–1.
2. Schuessler WW, Schulam PG, Clayman RV, Kavoussi LR. Laparoscopic radical prostatectomy: initial short-term experience. Urology. 1997;50(6):854–7.
3. Guillonneau B, Vallancien G. Laparoscopic radical prostatectomy: the montsouris technique. J Urol. 2000;163(6):1643–9.
4. Guillonneau B, Abbou CC, Doublet JD, et al. Proposal for a "European Scoring System for laparoscopic operations in urology". Eur Urol. 2001;40(1):2–6. discussion.
5. Stolzenburg JU, Do M, Pfeiffer H, et al. The endoscopic extraperitoneal radical prostatectomy (EERPE): technique and initial experience. World J Urol. 2002;20(1):48–55.
6. Gettman MT, Hoznek A, Abbou CC, et al. Laparoscopic radical prostatectomy: description of the extraperitoneal approach using the Da Vinci robotic system. J Urol. 2003;170:416–9.
7. Esposito M, Dakwar G, Ahmed M, et al. Extraperitoneal robotic prostatectomy: comparison of technique and results at one institution. J Endourol. 2004;18:691–706.
8. Joseph JV, Rosenbaum R, Madeb R, et al. Robotic extraperitoneal radical prostatectomy: an alternative approach. J Urol. 2006;175:945–50.
9. Van Velthoven RF, Ahlering TE, Peltier A, et al. Technique for laparoscopic running urethrovesical anastomosis: the single knot method. Urology. 2003;61(4):699–702.
10. Boczko J, Madeb R, Golijanin D, et al. Robot-assisted radical prostatectomy in obese patients. Can J Urol. 2006;13(4):33169–73.
11. Lin BM, Hyndman ME, Steele KE, et al. Incidence and risk factors for inguinal and incisional hernia after laparoscopic radical prostatectomy. Urology. 2011; 77(4):957–62.

Open Radical Retropubic Prostatectomy

Stephen A. Poon and Peter T. Scardino

Abbreviations

RP   Radical prostatectomy
PSA   Prostate-specific antigen
DRE   Digital rectal examination
PLND   Pelvic lymph node dissection
NVB   Neurovascular bundle
BCR   Biochemical recurrence
PCSM   Prostate cancer specific mortality

Introduction

Patients with clinically localized prostate cancer are faced with an ever-growing list of treatment options, including conservative management with active surveillance or "watchful waiting," external beam radiation and/or brachytherapy, cryotherapy, high-intensity focused ultrasound (HIFU), and focal therapies, as well as surgical resection. Physicians should support patients' decision-making by providing fair, unbiased, comprehensive information about treatment effectiveness and morbidity, considering each individual's life expectancy and his concerns about quality of life.

S.A. Poon, M.D.
Southern California Permanente Medical Group,
Fontana, CA, USA

P.T. Scardino, M.D. (✉)
Department of Surgery, Urology Service, Memorial
Sloan-Kettering Cancer Center, New York, NY, USA
e-mail: scardinp@mskcc.org

Radical prostatectomy (RP) is a highly effective treatment for potentially lethal prostate cancers, but most patients with low-risk cancers are best suited for active surveillance. RP has undergone a number of refinements since its introduction by Millin in 1948 [1], most notably the modifications introduced by Walsh [2]. However, it remains one of the most technically complex operations performed by urologists. The surgeon must navigate a difficult balancing act to remove the cancer completely, while minimizing blood loss and preserving urinary and sexual functions.

Modern outcomes research has documented the outcomes of RP in great detail. We now understand periprostatic anatomy much more clearly, and, as a result, a number of refinements in surgical technique that decrease blood loss and improve urinary and sexual function outcomes have occurred. Hospital stays have been reduced to 1–2 days, and rates of positive margins are lower. But the most powerful factor affecting outcomes is the skill and experience of the surgeon, regardless of the surgical approach—traditional, laparoscopic, or robot-assisted [3, 4].

The prostate surgeon should be well versed in periprostatic anatomy (Fig. 7.1) and in the principles of surgery for prostate cancer. This chapter will provide surgeons with a detailed description of our approach to this operation, with an emphasis on surgical techniques to minimize treatment morbidity. Other successful approaches have been described, but we emphasize these key steps in the operation that have stood the test of time and led to progressively better outcomes.

J.A. Eastham and E.M. Schaeffer (eds.), *Radical Prostatectomy: Surgical Perspectives*,
DOI 10.1007/978-1-4614-8693-0_7, © Springer Science+Business Media New York 2014

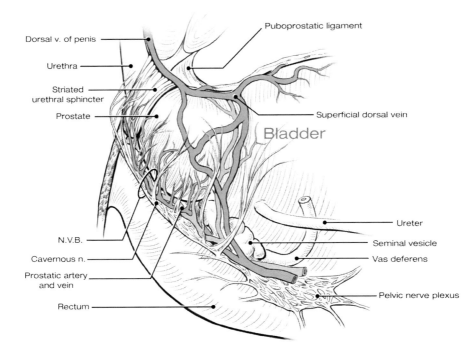

Fig. 7.1 Periprostatic anatomy. The nerves (NVB) run along the posterolateral aspect of the prostate, surrounded by the periprostatic (lateral pelvic) fascia. Until the nerves are fully released from the prostate, traction on the prostate should be kept to a minimum to avoid damaging these delicate structures. Courtesy of Memorial Sloan-Kettering Cancer Center © 2013. Used with permission

Preoperative Assessment

A successful operation begins with proper patient selection and careful surgical planning, so that the operation best suited to the patient's anatomy and the characteristics of his cancer can be performed. Before entering the operating theater, the surgeon must have a detailed understanding of the size, grade, and location of the patient's cancer, as well as the tumor's relationship to critical periprostatic structures. The patient's serum prostate-specific antigen (PSA) levels; digital rectal examination (DRE) results; the grade, the location and extent of cancer in each biopsy core; and the presence of perineural and lymphovascular invasion and extraprostatic extension (EPE) can help to define the location and extent of the cancer. This information can also be incorporated into preoperative nomograms to estimate the probable pathologic stage of the cancer, the site of EPE, and the chances of long-term cancer control [5].

Magnetic resonance imaging (MRI) can be helpful in delineating the anatomic details to assist in tailoring the operation, particularly with regard to dissection of the neurovascular bundles [6], the apical dissection and vesicourethral anastomosis, and the extent of bladder neck excision [7]. Most tumors are grossly localized to the prostate, but areas of microscopic EPE may be present. Knowledge of the presence and location of EPE allows the surgeon to perform wider excision in the involved areas to decrease the risk of positive margins and cancer recurrence. Measurement of the length of the membranous urethra on MRI helps to predict the risk of postoperative urinary incontinence, and it allows the surgeon to avoid over-dissection of the urethra beyond the apex and to take small bites of the urethra with the anastomotic sutures. In a study of 211 consecutive patients treated with RP by a single surgeon from 1999 to 2001, 120 of the 134 patients (89 %) with preoperative urethral length greater than 12 mm were continent at 1 year, versus only 35 of the 46 patients (77 %) with a length of 12 mm or less [7]. After controlling for age and surgical technique, a multivariate analysis found membranous urethral length to be associated with a shorter time to stable postoperative continence ($p = 0.02$). Thus, in a patient with a long urethra, variations in surgical technique may not be significant, but in a patient with a short urethra, imprecise surgical technique may substantially reduce recovery of continence.

Patients with newly diagnosed clinically localized prostate cancer (T1–T2) have a low probability of occult metastases. "Extent-of-disease" imaging, or a metastatic work-up, is unnecessary unless the patient's PSA levels or Gleason grade are high. Bone scans are rarely positive if the PSA is less than 20 ng/mL [8, 9]. However, patients with an aggressive cancer (PSA > 20 ng/mL or Gleason sum > 7), advanced local lesions (T3–T4), or symptoms suggestive of metastases should undergo axial skeletal imaging with bone scan or body MRI before a final treatment decision is made. An MRI of the prostate is adequate to assess the pelvic lymph nodes, but in high-risk patients an abdominal pelvic CT should be obtained if an MRI is not performed.

Pelvic Lymph Node Dissection

Pelvic lymph node dissection (PLND) has not been shown to improve survival in patients with localized prostate cancer, but long-term observational studies consistently show freedom from biochemical and clinical recurrence in 10–30 % of patients with nodal metastases, suggesting a therapeutic benefit of PLND [10–12]. In a recent article by Schumacher et al., 122 patients with limited lymph node metastases at RP had 60 % 10-year cancer-specific survival without the use of immediate adjuvant androgen deprivation therapy [13]. Because PLND may delay or prevent biochemical recurrence and the need for additional therapy, we recommend PLND if the risk of nodal metastases predicted by nomogram is ≥2 %. Few patients whose risk is <2 % are appropriate candidates for RP; most are managed expectantly by active surveillance [14–16].

No prospective studies have delineated the appropriate anatomic limits of PLND, and much controversy exists over appropriate templates. Some surgeons remove only the few nodes near the inguinal ligament (node of Cloquet); others take only the external iliac lymph nodes above the obturator nerve, while others routinely perform a more extensive dissection that includes the obturator and hypogastric areas. Extended lymph node dissections not only remove a greater number of lymph nodes, they also are more likely to detect positive lymph nodes. In a study by Heidenreich et al., lymph node metastases were diagnosed in 27 % of patients with extended PLND, compared with only 12 % of patients who underwent standard PLND [17]. We confirmed Studer's finding that 60 % of all positive nodes lie beneath the obturator nerve. Thus, performing a full, extended PLND in intermediate- and high-risk patients is important, both for its increased staging accuracy and for its potential therapeutic benefit. (See Chap. 4 for further details on pelvic lymphadenectomy.)

Surgical Technique for RP

The patient is positioned flat on the operating room table in the supine position, with the pubis over the break in the table. As the operation proceeds, the table can be flexed to improve exposure (Fig. 7.2). Excessive flexion should be avoided and the duration of flexion minimized, particularly in patients with a history of lower back pain or sciatica, to decrease the risk of spinal flexion injuries. Prophylactic antibiotics should be given *before* the incision is made. The patient is prepped with antiseptic solution (chlorhexidine), and an 18 Fr Foley catheter is placed in the bladder. An 8–10-cm midline skin incision is carried down through subcutaneous tissues. The fascia is sharply incised along the linea alba in the midline, exposing both rectus muscles, which are freed from the posterior rectus sheath laterally, elevating the inferior epigastric vessels. The fascial dissection can be 4–6 cm longer than the skin incision, allowing sufficient exposure. A Turner Warwick retractor is placed

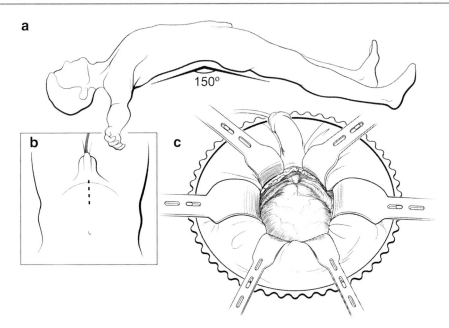

Fig. 7.2 Patient positioning. The patient is placed in the supine position with arms perpendicular to the body (**a**). The table is slightly flexed and placed in Trendelenburg to make the suprapubic area level. An 8- to 10-cm midline skin incision is made to expose the retropubic space (**b**). A Turner Warwick retractor is used to expose the operative field (**c**). Courtesy of Memorial Sloan-Kettering Cancer Center © 2013. Used with permission

superiorly to gain full exposure of the deep pelvic nodes. The vas is mobilized anteriorly but not transected, exposing the external iliac vessels to the hypogastric artery. The prevesical space is opened and the lymphadenectomy is performed at this time, if indicated. Care is taken to seal all large lymphatic vessels with clips or sutures to minimize lymphocele formation.

Dorsal Vascular Complex

The first step in mobilizing the prostate is to divide the endopelvic fascia and isolate and ligate the dorsal vascular complex (DVC). The fat anterior to and lateral to the prostate is teased away to expose the underlying anatomy, and the endopelvic fascia is incised laterally in the deep natural groove between the prostate and the levator ani muscles (Fig. 7.3). Only the fascia itself should be incised (a few millimeters thick); the remaining fibers of the levators attached to the prostate should be dissected bluntly to minimize bleeding.

Extensive cauterization of bleeding in the levators could damage the pudendal nerve, leading to incontinence. The fascial incision is extended anteriorly and the puboprostatic ligaments divided only if necessary. The surgeon should be able to pass his index and middle fingers around the apex of the prostate (Fig. 7.4). It is critical that this step be done using tactile and not visual feedback. The apex of the prostate need not be completely visualized, as this often results in over-dissection and possible damage to the external rhabdosphincter. The puboprostatic ligaments need not be divided if the apex of the prostate is adequately mobilized, but if necessary, these ligaments should be sharply incised at their attachment to the pubic bone, with care taken to not damage the DVC.

A figure-of-eight suture ligature is then placed approximately 1 cm cephalad to the anterior bladder neck, to ligate the *superficial* DVC roughly at the equator of the Foley balloon when placed on tension. This suture is also helpful in identifying the proper location for dividing

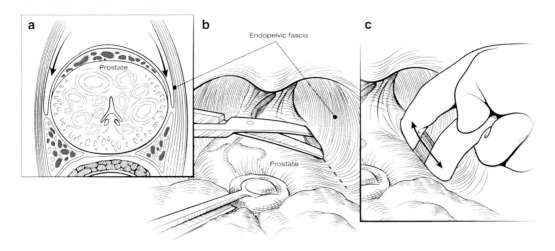

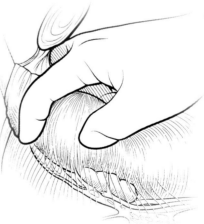

Fig. 7.3 Opening the endopelvic fascia. Adipose tissue overlying the apex of the prostate and endopelvic fascia is teased free and sent for pathology examination, because it may contain lymph nodes. The endopelvic fascia is incised within the natural groove between the prostate and levator ani muscles (**a**, **b**). Blunt digital dissection is used to accentuate the incision (**c**). Fibers of the levator ani muscle can be swept off the prostate bluntly. Care must be taken to avoid rupturing the venous plexus on the lateral aspect of the prostate. Courtesy of Memorial Sloan-Kettering Cancer Center © 2013. Used with permission

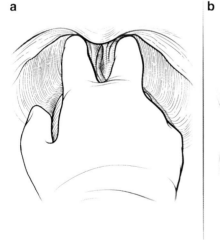

Fig. 7.4 Mobilizing the apex of the prostate. Once the endopelvic fascia has been opened bilaterally, blunt dissection is used to gently mobilize the apex before proceeding with ligation of the dorsal vascular complex (DVC). The surgeon should be able to pass his index and middle fingers around the apex and feel the urethra to ensure adequate mobilization. This step should be done only with tactile feedback. If the apex can be completely visualized, it has probably been over-dissected, potentially risking damage to the external rhabdosphincter. Any suspicious nodules at the apex, particularly with an anterior tumor, should be noted. The puboprostatic ligaments do not typically need to be divided to gain adequate exposure. However, in patients with a wide DVC or large gland, releasing the puboprostatic ligaments may assist with adequate mobilization. Scissors can be used to incise the ligaments at their attachment to the pubic bone to avoid lacerating the superficial dorsal veins. Courtesy of Memorial Sloan-Kettering Cancer Center © 2013. Used with permission

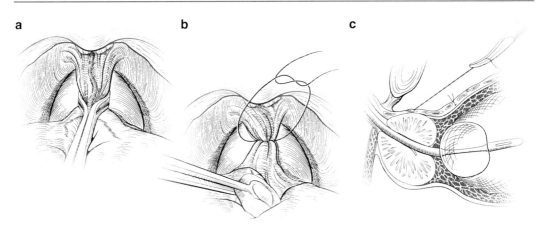

Fig. 7.5 Control of the deep dorsal vascular complex (DVC). The superficial branch of the dorsal vascular complex is ligated proximally (**a** and **b**) and distally (Fig. 7.7) before incising the DVC over the urethra. A second figure-of-eight suture is placed around the deep DVC at the mid-prostate. It may be helpful to gather up the DVC between the cut edges of the endopelvic fascia using a Babcock clamp (**a**) or a sponge stick (**b**). The suture should not be placed too laterally, to avoid tethering the neurovascular bundles. This stitch is kept long and tagged for later use in the apical dissection (**c**). Courtesy of Memorial Sloan-Kettering Cancer Center © 2013. Used with permission

the bladder neck later in the operation and to minimize bleeding. The first deep figure-of-eight suture is placed around the superficial and deep DVC at the mid-prostate, encompassing both cut edges of the endopelvic fascia. A Babcock clamp can facilitate the placement of this suture by cinching the fascial edges (Fig. 7.5a), or, alternatively, a sponge stick can be used to retract the fascial edges (Fig. 7.5b) as the suture is placed.

The deep DVC is ligated distally after the DVC is isolated from the urethra just beyond the apex of the prostate. The fascial layer surrounding the DVC and urethra is bluntly ruptured (Fig. 7.6) with the index finger, allowing the surgeon to appreciate an indentation between the urethra, filled with the Foley catheter, and the DVC. Gentle traction on the Foley catheter can help identify the urethra. A long, blunt-tipped right-angle clamp is passed between the DVC and the urethra and is used to grasp a 26-gauge stainless steel wire (Fig. 7.7). The wire is pulled through, and the ends are grasped with a heavy clamp. The wire loop will be used as a guide to transect the DVC after the distal suture ligature is placed through the DVC a few millimeters dorsal and caudal to the wire. The suture is anchored through the posterior periosteum of the pubis and tied securely, controlling bleeding from the DVC when it is divided. Care is taken to not encompass the levator muscles or the urethra. This maneuver reduces blood loss by several hundred cubic centimeters (cc).

Holding the steel wire vertically as a template, the DVC is transected sharply with a fresh No. 15 surgical blade (Fig. 7.8). The surgeon can adjust the amount of upward tension on the wire and downward traction on the prostate with a sponge stick to divide the DVC sufficiently distal to the apex, minimizing the chance of a positive anterior surgical margin. Transection too distally, however, risks incontinence by damaging the anterior supporting structures of the distal sphincter mechanism. Any residual DVC bleeding can be controlled by sewing the incised edges of the lateral pelvic fascia over the DVC with a running vertical suture. Again, this suture is anchored

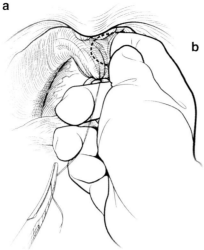

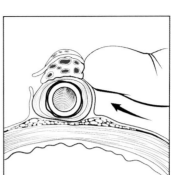

Fig. 7.6 Disruption of the lateral pelvic fascia over the dorsal vascular complex (DVC) and urethra. Tension is maintained on the tagged suture to provide countertraction. The surgeon uses his pointer finger to feel the subtle indentation between the urethra and DVC (**a**). Manipulation of the Foley catheter can assist in properly identifying the limits of the urethra. The fascia is digitally disrupted on both sides (**b**). With one finger in the space as a guide, the surgeon passes a long-tipped right angle clamp beneath the DVC. The clamp must be placed as close to the apex as possible to avoid damaging the rhabdosphincter. Courtesy of Memorial Sloan-Kettering Cancer Center © 2013. Used with permission

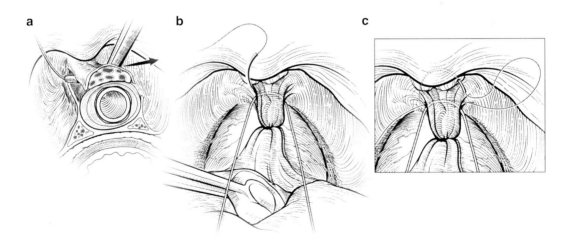

Fig. 7.7 Ligation of the dorsal vascular complex (DVC). A blunt-tipped (Mixter) right-angle clamp is used beneath the DVC to grasp a 26-gauge stainless steel wire, which is pulled through and clamped. This wire serves as a guide to delineate the DVC. A suture ligature is placed a few mm caudal and dorsal to the wire (**b**) and is then anchored through the periosteum of the symphysis pubis (**c**). The stitch is slowly tightened, cinching the DVC against the public bone to secure hemostasis. Courtesy of Memorial Sloan-Kettering Cancer Center © 2013. Used with permission

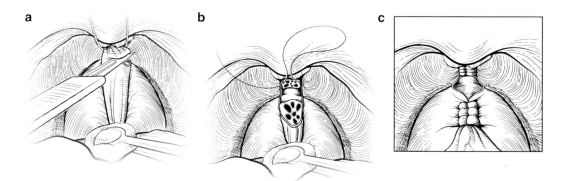

Fig. 7.8 Division of the dorsal vascular complex (DVC). The wire serves as a guide to allow a guillotine transection of the DVC. With the wire held vertically and a sponge stick on the prostate for countertraction, the surgeon uses a No. 15 blade scalpel to incise the DVC (**a**). Tension on the wire and sponge stick can be adjusted to ensure that the DVC is divided sufficiently distal to the apex to minimize the chance of a positive anterior surgical margin. The anterior urethra should be fully visible once the DVC is fully transected. If neces-

sary, a scalpel or scissors can be used to cut any remaining DVC tissue to fully expose the urethra. Bleeding is controlled, if necessary, by sewing the incised edges of the pelvic fascia lateral to the DVC with a running vertical suture (**b**), which is anchored through the periosteum. A running suture can be placed on the prostate side to minimize back-bleeding (**c**). Care must be taken to avoid medial displacement of the neurovascular bundles (NVBs). Courtesy of Memorial Sloan-Kettering Cancer Center © 2013. Used with permission

through the periosteum of the symphysis pubis to compress the vessels and reestablish the suspension provided by the puboprostatic ligaments. If necessary, back-bleeding from the prostate can be controlled with a hemostatic suture, clips, or bipolar cautery. Care should be taken to not draw the neurovascular bundles (NVB) medially if a suture is used.

Nerve Sparing

Once adequate hemostasis is achieved, the apex of the prostate and the urethra should be readily visible. The surgeon must now mobilize the prostate away from the NVBs while minimizing traction or cautery on these delicate nerves. Gentle dissection is essential at this stage of the operation. The surgeon should feel as if (s)he were operating on the sacral nerve roots of the spinal cord. The patient's recovery of erectile function is highly dependent on the care with which these fragile structures are handled. The following procedural steps are neither serial nor exclusive; they are often done concurrently, depending on the patient's anatomy.

Early Lateral Release of the NVB

The NVBs may be released using a lateral approach (Fig. 7.9) [18]. Early release of the NVB minimizes traction on the nerves during further manipulation of the prostate. A sponge stick is used to retract the prostate medially, and the fascia is incised medial to the NVBs using scissors or a scalpel. A Kittner ("peanut") dissector helps to gently widen the plane between the NVB and the prostate. The incision can be made more medial or lateral, based on the extent and location of the patient's cancer. At this point the surgeon must decide whether to dissect between Denonvilliers' fascia and the capsule of the prostate ("intrafascial dissection"), leaving the fascia covering the medial NVB, or to dissect more widely, outside the fascia, preserving the NVB but leaving Denonvilliers' fascia on the prostate ("interfascial dissection"). Small venous branches of the NVB are encountered that can be isolated and ligated with small hemoclips placed parallel to the NVB. The fasciotomy is extended from the apex to the level of the seminal vesicles. Once a sufficient plane has been developed, it can be extended dorsally and medially around the prostate in the same plane. Once the NVB is released,

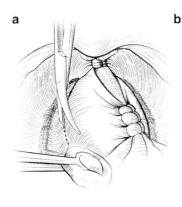

Fig. 7.9 Lateral release of the left neurovascular bundle (NVB). Early release of the NVB will minimize traction on the nerves while mobilizing the prostate. A sponge stick is used to rotate the prostate to the contralateral side. A small fasciotomy is made in the groove between the NVB and the prostate (**a**). Depending on the location of the tumor, the incision can be made more medial or lateral. The fasciotomy is then extended using a Kittner or sharp tipped right-angle clamp (**b**). Small vessels are controlled with small hemoclips or bipolar focused electrocautery. Once the NVB has been completely released anteriorly, Denonvilliers' fascia will be encountered posteriorly once the NVB is mobilized. This layer should be sharply incised so that the anterior rectal fat is visualized, allowing for complete lateral release. Courtesy of Memorial Sloan-Kettering Cancer Center © 2013. Used with permission

Denonvilliers' fascia must be sharply incised posteriorly, leaving Denonvilliers' fascia covering the posterior prostate to minimize the risk of a positive margin. The yellow anterior fat of the rectal wall should be clearly visualized, indicating a proper depth of the dissection. Throughout this dissection, the surgeon must follow the contour of the prostate to assure complete resection of the cancer and avoid injury to the NVB.

Retrograde Release of the NVB

In some patients, the lateral fascial planes may not develop easily, and release of the NVBs may be easier if the dissection starts at the apex of the prostate. The anterior two-thirds of the urethra is sharply divided at the apex of the prostate (Fig. 7.10), with care taken to maximize the length of the urethral stump. When the prostate is retracted cephalad, the plane between the urethra medially and the NVB laterally can be gently developed using a Kittner inserted just distal to the apex of the prostate. The Kittner is repeatedly inserted into the groove and rotated with gentle but persistent downward force toward the rectum, following the contour of the prostate. This manipulation will slowly push the NVB lateral, away from the urethra and expose the

digital apex. Further dissection with a Kittner, scissors, or a right-angle clamp can then be used to extend this plane around the apex, releasing the NVBs laterally.

Planes of Dissection of NVBs

Using a combination of these techniques, the NVBs can be spared routinely. Preservation of NVBs is generally not an all-or-nothing phenomenon. Often, all or most of each bundle can be spared, even in patients with a high risk of EPE. A more detailed description of periprostatic anatomy [19, 20] has further defined the alternative planes of dissection for releasing the NVBs (Fig. 7.11). The initial fasciotomy can be made directly adjacent to the prostatic capsule for an intrafascial plane of dissection (complete nerve sparing), which preserves the layer of Denonvilliers' fascia over the NVBs, protecting the nerve for optimal recovery of function. The fasciotomy can be made more laterally, leaving Denonvilliers' fascia on the prostate (interfascial plane; partial nerve sparing) to minimize the risk of a positive margin. A wide extrafascial dissection, with complete resection of a nerve, is rarely necessary except when the presence of gross extension of cancer into the NVB is readily

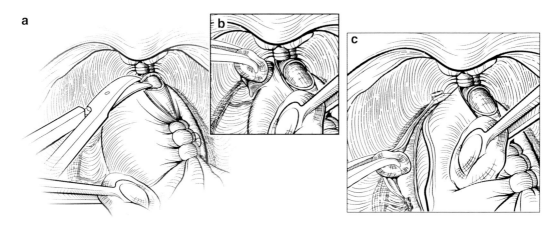

Fig. 7.10 Retrograde release of the neurovascular bundles (NVB). An alternate approach to the lateral release is to explore the plane between the NVBs and the urethra distal to the apex of the prostate. The anterior urethra is divided at the apex of the prostate (**a**). A Kittner dissector is gently inserted between the urethra medially and the NVBs laterally, developing a space between the urethral stump and apex of the prostate (**b**). This plane can then be extended laterally around the remainder of the prostate. Finally, Denonvilliers' fascia is incised to fully release the NVBs (**c**). Courtesy of Memorial Sloan-Kettering Cancer Center © 2013. Used with permission

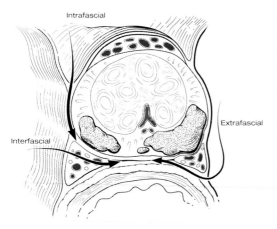

Fig. 7.11 Transverse section of the prostate depicting the planes for release of the neurovascular bundles (NVB). The type of nerve dissection performed must be tailored to the tumor location. The initial fasciotomy can be made directly adjacent to the prostatic capsule for an intrafascial plane dissection (complete nerve sparing), within the lateral prostatic fascia (interfascial plane; partial nerve sparing), or outside the lateral prostatic fascia (extrafascial plane; nerve resection). Courtesy of Memorial Sloan-Kettering Cancer Center © 2013. Used with permission

apparent. The proper plane for dissection should be chosen based on careful preoperative and intraoperative evaluation of the location, extent, and grade of the cancer. We find MRI particularly useful in this setting to help evaluate the anatomy of the prostate and of the cancer. During the operation, palpable indication or fixation of the layers of fascia can help identify areas of possible extracapsular extension.

In some high-risk patients, if an extrafascial dissection may be required to achieve negative margins, a CaverMap device (Uromed, Boston, MA) can be used to confirm the functionality of the remaining NVBs [21, 22]. If one or both NVBs are resected, a sural nerve graft is then considered. We believe that this step is best accomplished in collaboration with a plastic surgeon who has microsurgical expertise.

Apical Dissection and Urethral Division (Anastomotic Sutures)

Once the NVBs have been released laterally, the apex of the prostate can be mobilized. If not already completed, the anterior two-thirds of the urethra is sharply divided using scissors or a scalpel. The anterior and lateral anastomotic sutures are placed at 9, 11, 1, and 3 o'clock positions in the urethral stump with the Foley catheter in place (Fig. 7.12). We use a 2-0 monofilament

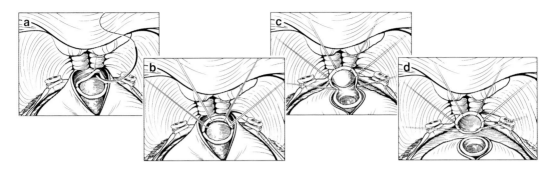

Fig. 7.12 Placement of urethral sutures. If not already done, the anterior urethra is incised over the Foley catheter. Care must be taken to maximize urethral length without creating a positive apical margin. The urethral sutures are then placed in an inside-to-outside fashion. Three-millimeter bites are taken with the urethra under slight trac-tion with a sponge stick. Once the 9, 11, 1, and 3 o'clock sutures are placed, the Foley is withdrawn. The final 5 and 7 o'clock sutures are placed outside-to-inside and should include the fascia posterior to the urethra. The remainder of the urethra is then incised (**d**). Courtesy of Memorial Sloan-Kettering Cancer Center © 2013. Used with permission

suture on a 5/8 circle needle (UR-6 Monocryl, Ethicon, Inc.). If the urethra is thin, 3-0 Monocryl can be substituted. With the urethra on mild trac-tion and the prostate retracted cephalad, the ure-thral sutures can be placed, including only 3–4 mm of urethral tissue. Larger bites will shorten the effective urethral length and compro-mise recovery of urinary continence. We prefer to place these urethral sutures from inside to out-side. The catheter is then removed, exposing the undivided posterior urethra. The posterior anas-tomotic sutures are placed from outside to inside at 5 and 7 o'clock positions so that the deep fibrous layers of Denonvilliers' fascia are included for added strength. The remaining pos-terior urethra is then divided, and the dissection continued, lifting the prostate off the rectum beneath Denonvilliers' fascia.

Posterior Dissection of Lateral Vascular Pedicle and Excision of Seminal Vesicles

As the prostate is mobilized off the rectum, upward retraction on the apex of the prostate allows sharp and blunt dissection all the way to the base of the prostate. If a large, high-grade cancer invades through this thick posterior fascia (rare), this plane can be further deepened to keep perirectal fat on the prostate. Once the prostate has been mobilized, a plastic Foley catheter can be inserted to assist with upward traction. While blunt digital dissection is potentially quicker, we discourage it because it creates traction on the NVBs and may leave some of Denonvilliers' fas-cia on the rectum, risking positive posterior margins.

At the base of the prostate the NVBs give off a vascular pedicle, which must be carefully identified, clipped, and divided, allowing the NVBs to separate from the prostate fully. Once the NVBs are completely freed, the thick lateral vascular pedicles of the prostate can be felt on each side as tight bands (Fig. 7.13) as the pros-tate is retracted ventrally and cephalad. The pedicles contain the large prostatic artery and must be isolated, securely clipped or ligated, to expose the seminal vesicles and fully mobilize the prostate. The pedicles can be isolated with a sharp right-angle clamp, clamped with a long tonsil clamp, or cut and ligated with 2-0 ties. All of the lateral vascular pedicle must be isolated, ligated, and divided to fully expose the seminal vesicles.

Blunt finger dissection between the seminal vesicles and bladder at the upper third of the sem-inal vesicles will separate the seminal vesicles (Fig. 7.14), exposing a large arterial pedicle between the bladder and seminal vesicles about

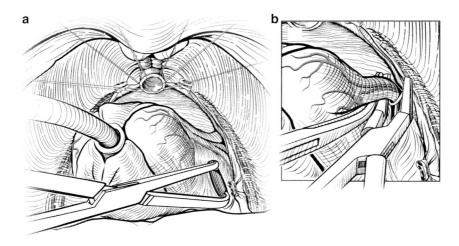

Fig. 7.13 Posterior dissection of the prostate. Once the urethra has been divided, the prostate is placed on upward traction and sharp dissection is used to develop the plane below Denonvilliers' fascia. A Foley catheter is placed into the bladder to assist with traction. The lateral vascular pedicles require sequential ligation with clips or ties from superficial to deep. Courtesy of Memorial Sloan-Kettering Cancer Center © 2013. Used with permission

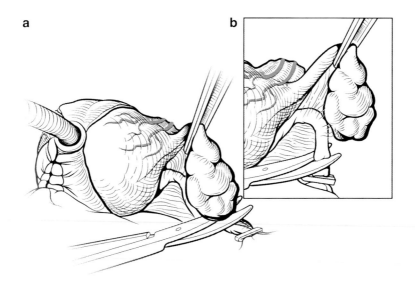

Fig. 7.14 Dissection of the seminal vesicles. A plane is created between the bladder and the seminal vesicles to expose the large vessels at the tips of the seminal vesicles (**a**). These are controlled with hemoclips and divided (**b**). Fibrovascular tissue surrounding the seminal vesicles is taken en bloc. The ampulla of the vas deferens is clipped to include the vasal arteries and divided. Courtesy of Memorial Sloan-Kettering Cancer Center © 2013. Used with permission

midway along the seminal vesicles. These vessels and the small arteries at the tip of the seminal vesicles must be carefully ligated or controlled with bipolar cautery. The vas deferens are also clipped and divided at the level of the tip of the seminal vesicles.

Once the seminal vesicles and vasa deferentia are free, the tips can be bluntly dissected off the base of the bladder all the way to the bladder neck. The remaining lateral vascular pedicles contain the prostatic artery and the major vessels from the bladder to the prostate [23]. This "beard"

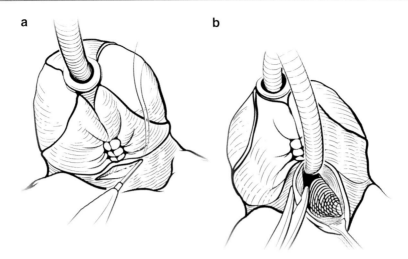

Fig. 7.15 Bladder neck incision. Cautery is used to incise the bladder neck anteriorly over the Foley catheter balloon (**a**). The balloon is deflated and the Foley is looped to provide traction. The bladder neck incision is carried circumferentially to free the specimen (**b**). Care is taken to avoid damage to the ureteral orifices. Courtesy of Memorial Sloan-Kettering Cancer Center © 2013. Used with permission

of tissue in the hilum of the prostate should be widely dissected to provide a margin of resection, comparable to the tissue in the hilum of the kidney during a radical nephrectomy.

Bladder Neck Division and Reconstruction

The prostate is divided from the bladder at the bladder neck, beginning anteriorly where the superficial dorsal vein was marked with a stitch. Electrocautery helps control bleeding (Fig. 7.15). Attempting to spare the bladder neck by tapering it into the prostatic urethra should be avoided to minimize the risk of a positive surgical margin [24]. Sparing the bladder neck has not been shown to improve long-term continence. Traction on the prostate facilitates the dissection. Care is taken to identify the ureteral orifices, which can be confirmed by inserting Number 5 Fr pediatric feeding tubes or simply administering indigo carmine or methylene blue to ensure that the ureters are patent, steps rarely necessary.

The Specimen

Once the specimen is freed, we carefully inspect the entire surface to ensure that there are no obvious positive surgical margins that might require more tissue to be removed (Fig. 7.16). Frozen sections can be used to confirm a positive margin but are of little value for routine detection of positive margins during the operation [23]. Next, the field is irrigated and meticulously inspected for bleeding. Postoperative bleeding after RP inevitably leads to a pelvic hematoma, which can disrupt the bladder anastomosis and lead to a bladder neck contracture or urinary incontinence [25]. In rare cases, patients with postoperative bleeding will need to be re-explored to evacuate the hematoma and control bleeding.

When adequate hemostasis has been achieved, the divided bladder neck is reconstructed. The bladder neck is closed posteriorly in a tennis-racquet fashion tight to a 32 Fr red rubber catheter (Fig. 7.17). The mucosa is everted with fine 4-0 polyglactin absorbable sutures. Sutures are placed at 10, 12, 2, and 4 o'clock, approximately

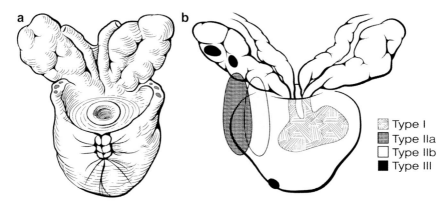

Fig. 7.16 Possible areas of seminal vesicle involvement [22]. The removed specimen should contain both entire seminal vesicles as well as the surrounding fibrovascular tissue at the seminal vesicle base (**a**). High-risk patients may have seminal vesicle involvement that is direct spread from the ejaculatory duct complex (Type 1); direct spread from the base of the prostate (Type IIa); retrograde spread from the tumor through periprostatic tissue into the seminal vesicles (Type IIb); or isolated skip metastases (Type III) (**b**). Courtesy of Memorial Sloan-Kettering Cancer Center © 2013. Used with permission

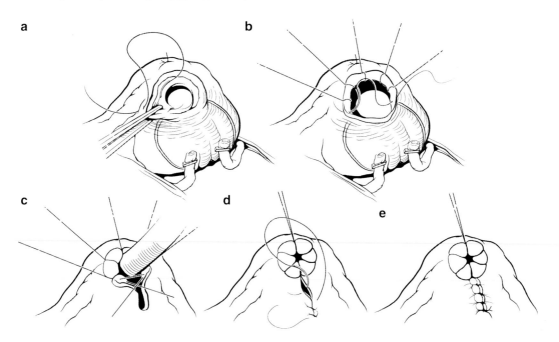

Fig. 7.17 Bladder neck reconstruction. The mucosa is everted anteriorly with interrupted sutures placed at 8, 10, 12, 2, and 4 o'clock approximately 5 mm apart (**b**). The 6 o'clock suture is placed through muscle on both sides to coapt the mucosal edges and sized to 32 Fr using a red rubber catheter (**c**). The remaining posterior bladder neck is closed with a running suture (**d**, **e**). Courtesy of Memorial Sloan-Kettering Cancer Center © 2013. Used with permission

8 mm apart. At 6 o'clock a suture is placed deep through bladder muscle on both sides to coapt the mucosal edges around the 32 Fr red rubber catheter, which should slide with some resistance through the newly created bladder neck. The placement of the 6 o'clock suture can be adjusted, if necessary, to ensure proper diameter of the bladder neck before this suture is tied. The mucosa should be fully everted 360° around the reconstructed bladder neck. The remaining

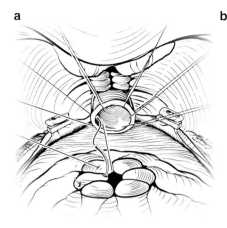 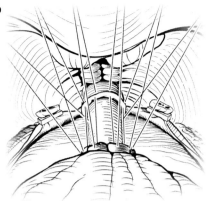

Fig. 7.18 Urethrovesical anastomosis. A Ferguson needle is loaded with the inner arm of each urethral anastomotic suture. The suture is placed inside-out on the corresponding aspect of the newly reconstructed bladder neck in a posterior-to-anterior fashion. Deep bites of bladder muscle should be included in these stitches (**a**). A new 18 Fr Foley is passed and inflated with 15 mL of sterile water, and is used to pull the bladder to the urethra as the sutures are securely tied (**b**). Courtesy of Memorial Sloan-Kettering Cancer Center © 2013. Used with permission

posterior bladder neck is closed with a running two-layer 3-0 polyglactin absorbable suture. Care must be taken to avoid the ureteral orifices near the trigone by incorporating large bites of detrusor muscle but very small bites of mucosa.

Once the bladder neck is reconstructed, the retractor is removed and the table leveled, releasing any flexion. An 18 Fr 5 cc Foley catheter is inserted through the urethra. The previously placed urethral sutures are now placed inside out through the newly reconstructed bladder neck using a Ferguson needle (Fig. 7.18). Mucosa and muscle should be included in each of these stitches. The Foley catheter is inflated with 15 mL of sterile water. The catheter is placed on traction to bring the bladder neck down to the urethra, slack is taken out of the sutures, and the bladder is gently retracted with the anastomotic sutures tied in an anterior-to-posterior fashion. The bladder is irrigated to remove clots and to test that the anastomosis is watertight to 180 cc. A proper anastomosis will be watertight with no traction on the catheter. A small self-suction drain is then placed through the anterior abdominal wall through a separate stab incision, and the incision is closed with a running suture. The skin is closed with a running 4-0 Monocryl stitch, and the catheter is secured.

Postoperative Care

We place all RP patients on a standardized postoperative care pathway. Ketorolac, acetaminophen, and intravenous narcotics are administered for pain control via a patient-controlled analgesia device. Patients are permitted to take a full liquid diet. Sequential compression devices are placed on the lower extremities during the operation to prevent deep venous thrombosis (DVT). Early ambulation within a few hours after surgery is strongly encouraged. We do not routinely use low molecular weight heparin, unless there are specific indications, because of the increased risk of bleeding and lymphocele. Hemoglobin is checked in the recovery room and the following morning. Patients are advanced to oral analgesics and regular diet on postoperative day 1 and are discharged on postoperative day 1 or 2. The drain is removed prior to discharge. If drain output exceeds 50 cc in 8 h, drain fluid can be sent for creatinine analysis to assess for a urine leak. The Foley catheter is removed in 7–10 days. A fluoroquinolone antibiotic is given, beginning on the day before catheter removal and continuing for a 3-day course.

The Surgeon

The surgeon's expertise is one of the most important factors influencing a patient's functional outcome and cancer control after RP; this has been demonstrated in studies of the surgical learning curve and achievement of the surgical "trifecta." Vickers et al. examined the association of increasing surgeon experience and biochemical recurrence-free survival rates [26]. In a cohort of 7,765 patients treated with RP alone by one of 72 surgeons at four major US academic medical centers, there was a strong, statistically significant relationship between surgical experience and biochemical recurrence rates (BCR) (Fig. 7.19). Optimal cancer control rates were not achieved, on average, until a surgeon had performed approximately 250 operations, suggesting a steep learning curve. Surgeons who had performed only 10 operations had a 17.9 % probability of BCR at 5 years versus 10.7 % BCR at 5 years for surgeons with at least 250 previous operations (difference = 7.2 %, 95 % CI 4.6–10.1 %; $p < 0.001$). In a separate study using the same patient cohort, fellowship training was found to

shorten the learning curve [27]. In addition to the beneficial effect of multiple years of surgical experience, having an operation performed by a high-volume surgeon at a high-volume hospital has also been shown to decrease postoperative and later urinary complications [3].

Several investigations have shown that the rate of positive margins is more closely related to surgical technique than to tumor biology [28]. Some have suggested that a tradeoff may exist between cancer control and functional outcomes, so that to ensure complete tumor removal surgeons would have to abandon nerve sparing or perform a wider resection, which may hamper return of urinary continence. However, in a study of 1,910 RP patients treated by 11 surgeons at Memorial Sloan-Kettering Cancer Center, there was substantial and statistically significant heterogeneity in rates of recovery of erectile and urinary function among surgeons, even when fully adjusting for case mix (age, PSA, pathologic stage and grade, and comorbidity) [29]. Several surgeons consistently had better outcomes (Fig. 7.20), and those with better cancer control rates also had better functional recovery rates. These findings suggest that specific surgical techniques performed

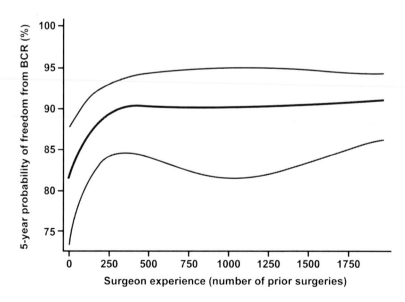

Fig. 7.19 The surgical learning curve for cancer control after radical prostatectomy [26]. The 5-year probability of freedom from biochemical recurrence (BCR) (*black curve*) and 95 % confidence intervals (*gray curves*) improve with each subsequent radical prostatectomy for

an individual surgeon during the first 250 operations. From Vickers et al. The surgical learning curve for prostate cancer control after radical prostatectomy. J Natl Cancer Inst 2007;99:1171–7, by permission of Oxford University Press

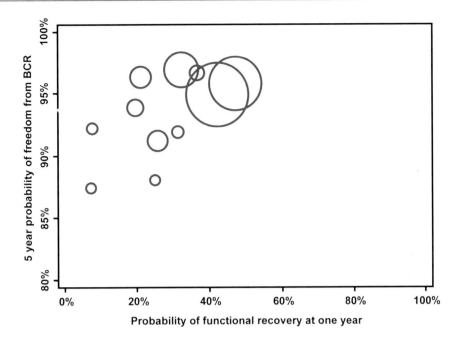

Fig. 7.20 Scatter plot of adjusted 5-year probability of freedom from biochemical recurrence (BCR) versus probability of recovery of urinary and sexual function at 12 months [29]. Each circle represents a single surgeon and the size of the circle represents the number of patients treated. Several high-volume surgeons have both favorable functional and oncologic outcomes, suggesting that these are not mutually exclusive goals. Reprinted from Vickers et al. Cancer control and functional outcomes after radical prostatectomy as markers of surgical quality: analysis of heterogeneity between surgeons at a single cancer center. Eur Urol 2011;59:317–22, with permission from Elsevier

by experienced surgeons are associated with overall improved outcomes.

In this chapter, we have outlined the steps of our method of performing RP, which has been refined over time. One of the primary benefits of experience is learning how to adapt the operation to the specific anatomy of each patient, his prostate, and his cancer.

Complications

Early perioperative complications reported in several surgical series are listed in Table 7.1 [5, 30–35]. Among the 7,220 men summarized in these studies, no intraoperative mortality was reported. One patient died at home from a myocardial infarction within the 30-day period after surgery [34]. Rectal injuries were uncommon (and should they occur, they can be repaired primarily). No colostomies were performed because of rectal injury in these series. Venous thromboembolic events and pulmonary embolism (VTE/PE)

were reported in less than 2 % of patients, consistent with a prior report [36]. Bladder neck contractures were not common. Several groups noted that these contractures occurred more frequently in their early experience [3, 5, 27], but they became rare with the adoption of the technical steps described in this chapter.

Cancer Control After Radical Prostatectomy

Localized prostate cancer is a heterogeneous disease, and progression rates depend on the clinical stage and Gleason grade of the tumor and on the patient's serum PSA level before surgery, as well as on pathologic findings in the prostatectomy specimen. After a patient has undergone RP, his serum PSA level should become undetectable. Due to the effectiveness of RP and thus the slow clinical progression of prostate cancer after RP [37], PSA recurrence has often been used as an endpoint in many studies. Several

Table 7.1 Perioperative complications and mortality in radical prostatectomy from large single-surgeon and -institution series

	Catalona [5, 32]		Lepor [33, 34]		Dorin et al. [31]		Lerner et al. [35]		Augustin et al. [30]	
	Single-surgeon		Single-surgeon		USC		Mayo clinic		University of Hamburg	
	1983–2003		1994–2002[a]		1988–2008		1989–1992		1999–2002	
	N=3,477		N=1,500		N=2,487		N=1,000		N=1,243	
Complications	N	%	N	%	N	%	N	%	N	%
Intra operative:	–	–	–	–	–	–	–	–	–	–
Obturator nerve injury	–	–	–	–	–	–	–	–	1	0.08
Rectal injury	1	0.03	5	0.33	1	0.04	6	0.6	3	0.24
Ureteral injury	1	0.03	2	0.13	1	0.04	–	–	4	0.32
Mortality (30 day)	0	0	1	0.07	–	–	–	–	0	–
Bladder neck contracture	95[b]	2.73	10	0.67	–	–	87	8.7	–	–
Hemorrhage/pelvic hematoma	–	–	8	0.53	9	0.36	–	–	14	1.13
Hernia	88	2.53	–	–	–	–	–	–	–	0
Ileus	–	–	6	0.4	14	0.56	–	–	4	0.32
Infection/sepsis	26	0.75	–	–	–	–	3	0.3	25	2.01
Lymphocele	7	0.2	1	0.07	–	–	1	0.1	37	2.98
Myocardial infarction	3	0.09	8	0.53	–	–	7	0.7	1	0.08
Neurological	5	0.14	2	0.13	–	–	–	–	13	1.05
PE/VTE	45	1.29	6	0.4	9	0.36	20	2	18	1.45
Urinoma/prolonged leak	–	–	1	0.07	2	0.08	–	–	2	0.16
Wound infection/seroma or dehiscence/hernia	7	20	15	1	2	0.08	9	0.9	29	2.33
Miscellaneous	42	1.21	54	3.6	24	0.97	–	–	132	11

Note: One patient may have had more than one complication

USC University of Southern California, *PE* pulmonary embolism, *VTE* venous thromboembolic event. Miscellaneous includes Peyronie's disease, unknown hernia, cholecystitis, hematuria, ulcer, gout, acute urinary retention, clot retention, congestive heart failure, renal failure, diverticulitis, ulcer, ARDS, pneumothorax, arrhythmia

[a]Combination of two previously published cohorts

[b]Authors note bladder neck contracture rate decreased from 8 % to 1.5 % in historic (1983–1991) versus contemporary (1992–2003) cohort. Bladder neck closed to 22–24 Fr instead of 18 Fr

major institutions have reported remarkably similar PSA progression-free probabilities at 5 and 10 years, and some studies now include probabilities up to 25 years (Table 7.2) [38–45].

In a single-surgeon series by Scardino, 1,746 consecutive patients with clinical stage T1–T3 N0-X cancer underwent RP and were followed closely postoperatively with serum PSA levels (mean follow-up 72 months) [38]. Progression was defined as a rising serum PSA>0.2 ng/mL, or clinical evidence of local or distant recurrence, or initiation of adjuvant radiotherapy or androgen deprivation therapy. At 5, 10, and 15 years, the actuarial probabilities of progression-free survival were 82 %, 77 %, and 75 %, respectively.

However, PSA recurrence alone has a highly variable natural history and sometimes poses limited threat to the longevity of many patients.

Several of these studies now have sufficient follow-up data to report long-term prostate cancer-specific mortality (PCSM) after RP in the PSA screening era [40, 41, 46]. Once the prostate has been removed, the most powerful prognostic factor is pathologic stage. Eggener et al. performed a multi-institution study using clinical and pathologic data and follow-up information from 11,521 patients treated at five academic centers from 1987 to 2005 to predict 15-year PCSM (Table 7.3) [46]. A nomogram was then created and validated on a cohort of 12,389

Table 7.2 Freedom from biochemical progression after radical prostatectomy

Series	N	Clinical stage	Year of RP	Biochemical recurrence-free survival				
				5-years	10-years	15-years	20-years	25-years
Bianco et al. [38]	1,746	T1–T3[a]	1983–2003	82	77	75	–	–
Hull et al. [39]	1,000	T1–T2[b]	1993–1998	78	75	–	–	–
Mullins et al. [40]	4,569	T1–T3[c]	1982–2011	–	82	78	74	68
Porter et al. [41]	787	T1–T3[d]	1954–1994	85	71	61	59	55
Roehl et al. [42]	3,478	T1–T2[c]	1983–2003	80	68	–	–	–
Trapasso et al. [43]	601	T1–T2[b]	1972–1992	69	47	–	–	–
Walz et al. [44]	293	T3[c]	1987–2003	52	44	–	–	–
Zinke et al. [45]	3,170	T1–T2[c]	1966–1991	70	52	40	–	–

RP radical prostatectomy, *PSA* prostate-specific antigen
[a] Biochemical progression defined as serum PSA > 0.4 ng/mL from 1983 to 1996; PSA 0.2 ng/mL after 1996
[b] Biochemical progression defined as serum PSA > 0.4 ng/mL
[c] Biochemical progression defined as serum PSA > 0.2 ng/mL
[d] Biochemical progression defined as serum PSA > 0.1 ng/mL

Table 7.3 Probability of death from prostate cancer and competing causes after radical prostatectomy at 10, 15, and 20 years in 23,910 men in combined modeling and validation cohorts by pathologic Gleason score, pathologic stage, and age at diagnosis [46]

	10 years, mean % (95 % CI)				15 years, mean % (95 % CI)				20 years, mean % (95 % CI)			
	PCSM		Competing cause mortality		PCSM		Competing cause mortality		PCSM		Competing cause mortality	
Age less than 60:	–	–	–	–	–	–	–	–	–	–	–	–
Gleason score:	–	–	–	–	–	–	–	–	–	–	–	–
6 or less	0.1	(0.03–0.3)	2.4	(2–3)	0.6	(0.2–1.5)	6	(4.5–8)	1.2	(0.4–3)	11	(7–17)
3 + 4	2.2	(1.5–3.3)	3.2	(2.4–4.4)	4.7	(3–6.8)	6.5	(4.6–8.8)	16	(7.2–29)	14	(8–23)
4 + 3	5.6	(3.4–8.7)	4.9	(3–7.6)	9	(5.5–14)	10	(5.4–16)	9	(5.5–14)	10	(5.4–16)
8 – 10	15	(11–20)	3.3	(1.7–5.9)	31	(23–39)	6.5	(3.5–11)	31	(23–39)	16	(6.5–28)
Organ confined	0.5	(0.3–8.4)	2.6	(2.1–3.2)	0.8	(0.3–1.6)	6.8	(5–9)	0.8	(0.3–1.6)	12	(6.3–19)
EPE	1.7	(0.1–2.5)	3.6	(2.7–4.6)	2.9	(2–4.2)	6.6	(5–8.5)	7	(2–16)	12	(8.2–16)
SVI	8.4	(5.2–12)	2.3	(0.9–4.8)	27	(18–37)	5.3	(2.3–10)	33	(19–47)	5.3	(2.3–10)
LN+	18	(13–24)	2.8	(1.2–5.9)	30	(22–38)	6.5	(3.1–12)	41	(27–55)	16	(5.6–31)
Age 60–69:	–	–	–	–	–	–	–	–	–	–	–	–
Gleason score:	–	–	–	–	–	–	–	–	–	–	–	–
6 or less	0.1	(0.03–0.2)	6	(4.6–6.4)	0.2	(0.01–0.6)	12	(10–14)	0.2	(0.01–0.6)	33	(23–42)
3 + 4	1.7	(1.1–2.5)	6.3	(5.2–7.6)	4.2	(2.8–5.9)	14	(12–17)	9	(4.8–15)	32	(19–45)
4 + 3	4.4	(2.6–7.1)	4.7	(3–6.9)	11	(6.9–16)	11	(6.9–16)	23	(13–34)	34	(9–62)
8 – 10	13	(9.7–17)	7.2	(4.8–10)	26	(20–32)	16	(11–21)	39	(25–53)	26	(17–36)
Organ confined	0.5	(0.3–8.7)	5	(4.2–5.8)	1	(0.5–1.8)	12	(9.7–14)	1.4	(0.7–2.7)	29	(19–40)
EPE	1.9	(1.3–2.7)	6.6	(5.5–7.9)	3.9	(2.8–5.3)	14	(12–16)	6.6	(4.1–9.9)	34	(24–43)
SVI	8.8	(5.8–12)	8.5	(5.6–12)	22	(15–29)	16	(11–23)	26	(18–36)	47	(17–72)
LN+	12	(7.7–17)	7.2	(4–12)	22	(15–30)	13	(8–20)	42	(26–57)	16	(9–26)

(continued)

Table 7.3 (continued)

	10 years, mean % (95 % CI)		15 years, mean % (95 % CI)		20 years, mean % (95 % CI)	
	PCSM	Competing cause mortality	PCSM	Competing cause mortality	PCSM	Competing cause mortality
Age 70–79:	– –	– –	– –	– –	– –	– –
Gleason score:	– –	– –	– –	– –	– –	– –
6 or less	0	11 (6.7–17)	1.2 (0.1–5.8)	22 (13–32)	1.2 (0.1–5.8)	30 (17–44)
3+4	1.3 (0.4–3.6)	16 (11–22)	6.5 (1.9–15)	33 (22–44)	17 (2–44)	61 (29–82)
4+3	6.6 (2–15)	18 (9.7–29)	6.6 (2–15)	23 (11–37)	18 (3–45)	23 (11–37)
8–10	18 (9–31)	11 (4–22)	37 (17–57)	11 (4–22)	37 (17–57)	21 (5–46)
Organ confined	1.4 (0.4–4)	14 (9.2–19)	1.5 (0.4–4)	18 (12–25)	1.5 (0.4–4)	43 (17–68)
EPE	0.5 (0.1–2.6)	12 (7.3–18)	10 (4–19)	27 (18–38)	20 (7–39)	41 (26–56)
SVI	13 (6–23)	22 (13–34)	15 (7–26)	36 (18–55)	15 (7–26)	36 (18–55)
LN+	23 (8–43)	10 (1.5–27)	23 (8–43)	10 (1.5–27)	23 (8–43)	10 (1.5–27)

PCSM prostate cancer-specific mortality, *EPE* extraprostatic extension, *SVI* seminal vesicle invasion, *LN*+ lymph node metastases

From Eggener et al. Predicting 15-year prostate cancer specific mortality after radical prostatectomy. *Journal of Urology* 2011;185:869–75. Reprinted with kind permission from Elsevier Limited

patients treated at a separate institution during the same period with a concordance index of 0.92. A total of 788 patients from the modeling cohort received postoperative radiotherapy, and 1,045 men received androgen deprivation therapy for BCR or clinical progression. The overall 15-year PCSM rate was 7 %. The PCSM risk in men with pathologic Gleason scores 8–10 cancer was generally 31 % or greater at 15–20 years, which was substantially greater than the risk of death from competing causes, even at age 70 years or more. Seminal vesicle invasion and lymph node metastases were also associated with an increased risk of PCSM.

But in patients with tumors graded Gleason 6 or less, the PCSM risk at 15–20 years was negligible (1.2 % or less), and substantially less than death from competing causes regardless of age at diagnosis [46]. These observations were supported by data from the PIVOT trial, which randomized men with PSA-screening detected cancers to RP versus observation [47]. Men with low-risk prostate cancer who underwent RP were not found to have a significant reduction in PCSM, compared with men who had been randomized to observation.

Clearly, few patients, including those with adverse pathologic features, will die from prostate cancer within 15 years of RP. This finding documents the effectiveness of RP and also the lesser lethality of cancers detected by early screening. Although surgery remains an excellent treatment option, appropriate patient selection must be a primary factor in the decision to treat at all.

Conclusion

RP reliably eradicates the disease in most men with clinically localized prostate cancer, and the procedure remains the gold standard treatment in this population of patients. The operation is technically complex, but experienced surgeons can perform it consistently with minimal perioperative morbidity. Urinary continence and erectile function are highly sensitive to the details of surgical technique and the experience of the surgeon. Careful attention must be given to assessing the patient's disease and deciding the best surgical approach, to maximize both cancer control and long-term functional outcomes.

References

1. Millin T. Retropubic prostatectomy. J Urol. 1948;59(3):267–80. PubMed PMID: 18903535.
2. Wein AJ, Kavoussi LR, Novick AC, Partin AW, Peters CA. Campbell-Walsh Urology. 10th ed. Saint Louis, MO: Saunders; 2011. p. 5688.
3. Begg CB, Riedel ER, Bach PB, Kattan MW, Schrag D, Warren JL, et al. Variations in morbidity after radical prostatectomy. N Engl J Med. 2002;346(15):1138–44. PubMed PMID: 11948274.
4. Bianco Jr FJ, Vickers AJ, Cronin AM, Klein EA, Eastham JA, Pontes JE, et al. Variations among experienced surgeons in cancer control after open radical prostatectomy. J Urol. 2010;183(3):977–82. PubMed PMID: 20083278. Pubmed Central PMCID: 3244752.
5. Catalona WJ, Carvalhal GF, Mager DE, Smith DS. Potency, continence and complication rates in 1,870 consecutive radical retropubic prostatectomies. J Urol. 1999;162(2):433–8. PubMed PMID: 10411052.
6. Maffezzini M, Seveso M, Taverna G, Giusti G, Benetti A, Graziotti P. Evaluation of complications and results in a contemporary series of 300 consecutive radical retropubic prostatectomies with the anatomic approach at a single institution. Urology. 2003; 61(5):982–6. PubMed PMID: 12736020.
7. Coakley FV, Eberhardt S, Kattan MW, Wei DC, Scardino PT, Hricak H. Urinary continence after radical retropubic prostatectomy: relationship with membranous urethral length on preoperative endorectal magnetic resonance imaging. J Urol. 2002;168(3):1032–5. PubMed PMID: 12187216.
8. Greene KL, Albertsen PC, Babaian RJ, Carter HB, Gann PH, Han M, et al. Prostate specific antigen best practice statement: 2009 update. J Urol. 2013;189(1 Suppl):S2–11. PubMed PMID: 23234625.
9. Levran Z, Gonzalez JA, Diokno AC, Jafri SZ, Steinert BW. Are pelvic computed tomography, bone scan and pelvic lymphadenectomy necessary in the staging of prostatic cancer? Br J Urol. 1995;75(6):778–81. PubMed PMID: 7542138.
10. Messing EM, Manola J, Yao J, Kiernan M, Crawford D, Wilding G, et al. Immediate versus deferred androgen deprivation treatment in patients with node-positive prostate cancer after radical prostatectomy and pelvic lymphadenectomy. Lancet Oncol. 2006;7(6):472–9. PubMed PMID: 16750497. Epub 2006/06/06. eng.
11. Masterson TA, Bianco Jr FJ, Vickers AJ, DiBlasio CJ, Fearn PA, Rabbani F, et al. The association between total and positive lymph node counts, and disease progression in clinically localized prostate cancer. J Urol. 2006;175(4):1320–4. PubMed PMID: 16515989. Pubmed Central PMCID: PMC1950746. discussion 4–5. Epub 2006/03/07. eng.
12. Han M, Partin AW, Pound CR, Epstein JI, Walsh PC. Long-term biochemical disease-free and cancer-specific survival following anatomic radical retropubic prostatectomy. The 15-year Johns Hopkins experience. Urol Clin North Am. 2001;28(3):555–65.
13. Schumacher MC, Burkhard FC, Thalmann GN, Fleischmann A, Studer UE. Good outcome for patients with few lymph node metastases after radical retropubic prostatectomy. Eur Urol. 2008;54(2):344–52. PubMed PMID: 18511183. Epub 2008/05/31. eng.
14. Briganti A, Chun FK, Salonia A, Zanni G, Scattoni V, Valiquette L, et al. Validation of a nomogram predicting the probability of lymph node invasion among patients undergoing radical prostatectomy and an extended pelvic lymphadenectomy. Eur Urol. 2006;49(6):1019–26. PubMed PMID: 16530933. discussion 26–7. Epub 2006/03/15. eng.
15. Partin AW, Kattan MW, Subong EN, Walsh PC, Wojno KJ, Oesterling JE, et al. Combination of prostate-specific antigen, clinical stage, and Gleason score to predict pathological stage of localized prostate cancer. A multi-institutional update. JAMA. 1997;277(18):1445–51. PubMed PMID: 9145716. Epub 1997/05/14. eng.
16. Stephenson AJ, Scardino PT, Eastham JA, Bianco Jr FJ, Dotan ZA, Fearn PA, et al. Preoperative nomogram predicting the 10-year probability of prostate cancer recurrence after radical prostatectomy. J Natl Cancer Inst. 2006;98(10):715–7. PubMed PMID: 16705126. Pubmed Central PMCID: 2242430. Epub 2006/05/18. eng.
17. Heidenreich A, Varga Z, Von Knobloch R. Extended pelvic lymphadenectomy in patients undergoing radical prostatectomy: high incidence of lymph node metastasis. J Urol. 2002;167(4):1681–6. PubMed PMID: 11912387. Epub 2002/03/26. eng.
18. Masterson TA, Serio AM, Mulhall JP, Vickers AJ, Eastham JA. Modified technique for neurovascular bundle preservation during radical prostatectomy: association between technique and recovery of erectile function. BJU Int. 2008;101(10):1217–22. PubMed PMID: 18279446. Pubmed Central PMCID: 2568897.
19. Walz J, Graefen M, Huland H. Basic principles of anatomy for optimal surgical treatment of prostate cancer. World J Urol. 2007;25(1):31–8. PubMed PMID: 17333199. Epub 2007/03/03. eng.
20. Walz J, Burnett AL, Costello AJ, Eastham JA, Graefen M, Guillonneau B, et al. A critical analysis of the current knowledge of surgical anatomy related to optimization of cancer control and preservation of continence and erection in candidates for radical prostatectomy. Eur Urol. 2010;57(2):179–92. PubMed PMID: 19931974. Epub 2009/11/26. eng.
21. Canto EI, Nath RK, Slawin KM. Cavermap-assisted sural nerve interposition graft during radical prostatectomy. Urol Clin North Am. 2001;28(4):839–48. PubMed PMID: 11791500.
22. Secin FP, Koppie TM, Scardino PT, Eastham JA, Patel M, Bianco FJ, et al. Bilateral cavernous nerve interposition grafting during radical retropubic prostatectomy: Memorial Sloan-Kettering Cancer Center

experience. J Urol. 2007;177(2):664–8. PubMed PMID: 17222654. Epub 2007/01/16. eng.

23. Ohori M, Scardino PT, Lapin SL, Seale-Hawkins C, Link J, Wheeler TM. The mechanisms and prognostic significance of seminal vesicle involvement by prostate cancer. Am J Surg Path. 1993;17(12):1252–61. PubMed PMID: 8238732.

24. Licht MR, Klein EA, Tuason L, Levin H. Impact of bladder neck preservation during radical prostatectomy on continence and cancer control. Urology. 1994;44(6):883–7. PubMed PMID: 7527169. Epub 1994/12/01. eng.

25. Hedican SP, Walsh PC. Postoperative bleeding following radical retropubic prostatectomy. J Urol. 1994;152(4):1181–3. PubMed PMID: 8072090. Epub 1994/10/01. eng.

26. Vickers AJ, Bianco FJ, Serio AM, Eastham JA, Schrag D, Klein EA, et al. The surgical learning curve for prostate cancer control after radical prostatectomy. J Natl Cancer Inst. 2007;99(15):1171–7. PubMed PMID: 17652279. Epub 2007/07/27. eng.

27. Eastham JA, Kattan MW, Rogers E, Goad JR, Ohori M, Boone TB, et al. Risk factors for urinary incontinence after radical prostatectomy. J Urol. 1996;156(5):1707–13. PubMed PMID: 8863576.

28. Vickers AJ, Bianco FJ, Gonen M, Cronin AM, Eastham JA, Schrag D, et al. Effects of pathologic stage on the learning curve for radical prostatectomy: evidence that recurrence in organ-confined cancer is largely related to inadequate surgical technique. Eur Urol. 2008;53(5):960–6. PubMed PMID: 18207316. Pubmed Central PMCID: 2637145.

29. Vickers A, Savage C, Bianco F, Mulhall J, Sandhu J, Guillonneau B, et al. Cancer control and functional outcomes after radical prostatectomy as markers of surgical quality: analysis of heterogeneity between surgeons at a single cancer center. Eur Urol. 2011;59(3):317–22. PubMed PMID: 21095055. Pubmed Central PMCID: 3060298. Epub 2010/11/26. eng.

30. Augustin H, Hammerer P, Graefen M, Palisaar J, Noldus J, Fernandez S, et al. Intraoperative and perioperative morbidity of contemporary radical retropubic prostatectomy in a consecutive series of 1243 patients: results of a single center between 1999 and 2002. Eur Urol. 2003;43(2):113–8. PubMed PMID: 12565767.

31. Dorin RP, Daneshmand S, Lassoff MA, Cai J, Skinner DG, Lieskovsky G. Long-term outcomes of open radical retropubic prostatectomy for clinically localized prostate cancer in the prostate-specific antigen era. Urology. 2012;79(3):626–31. PubMed PMID: 22245303. Epub 2012/01/17. eng.

32. Kundu SD, Roehl KA, Eggener SE, Antenor JA, Han M, Catalona WJ. Potency, continence and complications in 3,477 consecutive radical retropubic prostatectomies. J Urol. 2004;172(6 Pt 1):2227–31. PubMed PMID: 15538237.

33. Lepor H, Kaci L. Contemporary evaluation of operative parameters and complications related to open radical retropubic prostatectomy. Urology. 2003;62(4):702–6. PubMed PMID: 14550447.

34. Lepor H, Nieder AM, Ferrandino MN. Intraoperative and postoperative complications of radical retropubic prostatectomy in a consecutive series of 1,000 cases. J Urol. 2001;166(5):1729–33. PubMed PMID: 11586211.

35. Lerner SE, Blute ML, Lieber MM, Zincke H. Morbidity of contemporary radical retropubic prostatectomy for localized prostate cancer. Oncology. 1995;9(5):379–82. discussion 82, 85–6, 89. PubMed PMID: 7547200.

36. Cisek LJ, Walsh PC. Thromboembolic complications following radical retropubic prostatectomy. Influence of external sequential pneumatic compression devices. Urology. 1993;42(4):406–8. PubMed PMID: 8212439.

37. Pound CR, Partin AW, Eisenberger MA, Chan DW, Pearson JD, Walsh PC. Natural history of progression after PSA elevation following radical prostatectomy. JAMA. 1999;281(17):1591–7. PubMed PMID: 10235151. Epub 1999/05/11. eng.

38. Bianco Jr FJ, Scardino PT, Eastham JA. Radical prostatectomy: long-term cancer control and recovery of sexual and urinary function ("trifecta"). Urology. 2005;66(5 Suppl):83–94. PubMed PMID: 16194712.

39. Hull GW, Rabbani F, Abbas F, Wheeler TM, Kattan MW, Scardino PT. Cancer control with radical prostatectomy alone in 1,000 consecutive patients. J Urol. 2002;167(2 Pt 1):528–34. PubMed PMID: 11792912.

40. Mullins JK, Feng Z, Trock BJ, Epstein JI, Walsh PC, Loeb S. The impact of anatomical radical retropubic prostatectomy on cancer control: the 30-year anniversary. J Urol. 2012;188(6):2219–24. PubMed PMID: 23083655. Epub 2012/10/23. eng.

41. Porter CR, Kodama K, Gibbons RP, Correa Jr R, Chun FK, Perrotte P, et al. 25-year prostate cancer control and survival outcomes: a 40-year radical prostatectomy single institution series. J Urol. 2006;176(2):569–74. PubMed PMID: 16813891. Epub 2006/07/04. eng.

42. Roehl KA, Han M, Ramos CG, Antenor JA, Catalona WJ. Cancer progression and survival rates following anatomical radical retropubic prostatectomy in 3,478 consecutive patients: long-term results. J Urol. 2004;172(3):910–4. PubMed PMID: 15310996.

43. Trapasso JG, deKernion JB, Smith RB, Dorey F. The incidence and significance of detectable levels of serum prostate specific antigen after radical prostatectomy. J Urol. 1994;152(5 Pt 2):1821–5. PubMed PMID: 7523728.

44. Walz J, Joniau S, Chun FK, Isbarn H, Jeldres C, Yossepowitch O, et al. Pathological results and rates of treatment failure in high-risk prostate cancer patients after radical prostatectomy. BJU Int. 2011;107(5):765–70. PubMed PMID: 20875089.

45. Zincke H, Oesterling JE, Blute ML, Bergstralh EJ, Myers RP, Barrett DM. Long-term (15 years) results after radical prostatectomy for clinically localized (stage T2c or lower) prostate cancer. J Urol. 1994;152(5 Pt 2):1850–7. PubMed PMID: 7523733.

46. Eggener SE, Scardino PT, Walsh PC, Han M, Partin AW, Trock BJ, et al. Predicting 15-year prostate cancer specific mortality after radical prostatectomy.

J Urol. 2011;185(3):869–75. PubMed PMID: 21239008. Epub 2011/01/18. eng.

47. Wilt TJ, Brawer MK, Jones KM, Barry MJ, Aronson WJ, Fox S, et al. Radical prostatectomy versus observation for localized prostate cancer. N Engl J Med. 2012;367(3):203–13. PubMed PMID: 22808955. Pubmed Central PMCID: 3429335. Epub 2012/07/20. eng.

Salvage Robotic-Assisted Laparoscopic Radical Prostatectomy

Samuel D. Kaffenberger, Michael S. Cookson, and Joseph A. Smith Jr.

Abbreviations

SRP	Salvage radical prostatectomy
sRALP	Salvage robotic-assisted laparoscopic prostatectomy
PSA	Prostate-specific antigen
BCR	Biochemical recurrence
RALP	Robotic-assisted laparoscopic prostatectomy

Introduction

Recurrence of prostate cancer after failed nonsurgical local therapy remains a significant clinical problem, with rates of relapse ranging from 20 to 60 % depending on the modality utilized, patient clinical and disease characteristics, and length of follow-up [1–3]. A high proportion of these patients will have clinically localized recurrence of disease, lending to the possibility of potentially curative salvage therapies like salvage radical prostatectomy (SRP) [4]. In patients who are

S.D. Kaffenberger, M.D.
M.S. Cookson, M.D., M.M.H.C.
J.A. Smith Jr., M.D. (✉)
Department of Urologic Surgery, Vanderbilt University Medical Center, A-1302 Medical Center North, Nashville, TN, USA
e-mail: Joseph.Smith@Vanderbilt.edu

poor surgical candidates or who have short life expectancies, consideration must be given to salvage cryotherapy or androgen deprivation therapy. Although not proven, it has been suggested that SRP results in superior cancer-free survival when compared to salvage cryotherapy [5]. While results have improved in later-generation cryoablation systems, long-term oncologic results are still pending [6].

Despite the excellent oncologic outcomes of open SRP, it is not commonly performed [3]. In part, this is due to limited life expectancy in an often-comorbid elderly patient population; however, the pronounced difficulty and morbidity of open SRP are certainly contributing factors. Historically, open SRP has been marked by significant risk of major complications, including rectal injury rates of over 15 % and high rates of anastomotic stricture [7, 8]. There have been vast improvements in outcomes of open SRP in more contemporary series with rectal injury rates declining to 2–5 % [9–11].

The rapid adoption of minimally invasive radical prostatectomy in the USA has led to the exploratory utilization of robotics in the salvage setting at a number of centers [12–19]. Although experience is evolving, salvage robotic-assisted laparoscopic prostatectomy (sRALP) appears to be a compelling alternative treatment to open SRP for certain patients with recurrent prostate cancer after primary therapy. Like its open counterpart, careful patient selection and surgical experience will significantly influence perioperative and oncologic outcomes.

J.A. Eastham and E.M. Schaeffer (eds.), *Radical Prostatectomy: Surgical Perspectives*,
DOI 10.1007/978-1-4614-8693-0_8, © Springer Science+Business Media New York 2014

Background

The first published case of sRALP was in 2008. Since then, five series have been published of 83 patients in total [13–17, 19]. In our initial experience of 45 cases, sRALP appears feasible, effective, and safe in properly selected patients. In fact, it has emerged as our preferred approach for the performance of salvage radical prostatectomy. While pure laparoscopic salvage radical prostatectomy series have been published, the robotic platform is ideally suited for the performance of minimally invasive radical prostatectomy in the salvage setting [20]. The dexterity of the robotic instruments, precise tissue handling and suturing, and three-dimensional magnification of the operative field all facilitate this challenging operation.

Patient Selection

Proper patient selection is particularly crucial for any salvage operation to maximize the chance of improving survival while minimizing unnecessary and morbid procedures. Patients should have a life expectancy of at least 10–15 years and should have biopsy-proven localized disease, clinical stage ≤T3, with no evidence of distant metastases on preoperative imaging. Other disease characteristics to consider which may reflect systemic rather than local disease are elevated pre-sRALP prostate specific antigen (PSA), rapid PSA doubling time, short time from primary therapy to recurrence, and high pre-sRALP biopsy Gleason score. While none of these are an absolute contraindication for the performance of sRALP, pre-sRALP PSA and biopsy Gleason score have both been shown to be predictive of biochemical recurrence (BCR) and development of metastatic disease in the salvage setting [21]. Multiparametric magnetic resonance imaging may be useful for enhanced local staging, although we do not routinely perform this test.

Preoperative Patient Counseling and Preparation

Patients should be well informed of the risks inherent to the operation, including the high risk of erectile dysfunction, the considerably increased risk of incontinence compared to surgery in a non-irradiated patient, as well as the standard risks of bleeding and infection. The small but increased chance of rectal injury should also be discussed. Preoperative mechanical bowel preparation is performed with one bottle of magnesium citrate the day prior to surgery and a clear liquid diet until midnight the night before surgery. Full antimicrobial (Nichols) bowel preparation is an option.

Operative Technique

The surgical technique for sRALP does not differ greatly from that of standard robotic-assisted laparoscopic prostatectomy (RALP) and the steps that are not significantly altered in the post-radiation setting will be only briefly described. We utilize the six-port transperitoneal approach for both standard RALP and sRALP. The patient is placed in the dorsal lithotomy position and the arms are tucked and padded. The patient is then tilted to a steep Trendelenburg position before prepping and draping to ensure that there is no sliding on the bed. After confirming stability on the bed, the patient is then leveled out for insufflation and port placement. A Foley catheter is placed on the field and the bladder is drained. We do not routinely administer subcutaneous heparin or enoxaparin prior to RALP or sRALP. After receiving a single intravenous dose of a first-generation cephalosporin, a 12 mm supra-umbilical incision is created and a Veress needle is utilized to insufflate the abdomen. A 12 mm supra-umbilical trocar is placed for the camera and the three robotic trocars and two assistance ports are placed as per a standard RALP. The patient is placed in steep Trendelenburg position and adhesions are taken down as necessary.

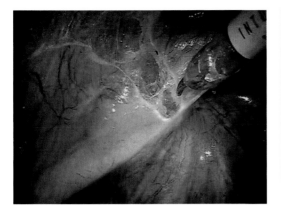

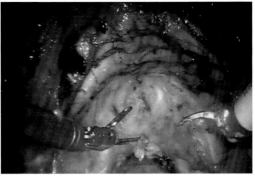

Fig. 8.2 Markedly fibrotic and thickened endopelvic fascia in a patient undergoing sRALP after external beam radiation therapy

Fig. 8.1 Incising the peritoneum lateral to the right medial umbilical ligament down to the level of the vas deferens and internal ring on the right

Exposure of the Prostate, Dissection of the Bladder Neck and Seminal Vesicles

The initial exposure of the prostate is identical between salvage and non-salvage RALP. The peritoneum is incised lateral to each medial umbilical ligament and the incision is extended to the vasa deferentia at the level of the internal inguinal ring on each side of the pelvis (Fig. 8.1). The medial umbilical ligaments and urachus are divided high on the anterior abdominal wall and the space of Retzius is developed. The fourth arm is utilized to place cranial and posterior tension on the bladder. The endopelvic fascia, which is often markedly fibrotic and thickened in the salvage setting, is carefully incised (Figs. 8.2 and 8.3). The fatty tissue overlying the prostate is dissected off and the superficial dorsal vein branches are divided with electrocautery. Ligation of the deep dorsal venous complex is omitted at this point in the procedure to allow for improved mobility during the apical dissection.

The bladder neck is then identified and incised with a combination of sharp dissection and electrocautery as per a standard RALP (Fig. 8.4). Once the posterior bladder neck has been incised, the vasa deferentia are identified and divided (Fig. 8.5). The fourth arm is utilized to provide anterior tension on the distal vas deferens, elevating the prostate. The third arm can be utilized to grasp the proximal vas deferens to facilitate dissection of the seminal vesicles (Fig. 8.6). 30–35 % of patients undergoing salvage radical prostatectomy will have seminal vesicle involvement so careful and wide excision of the seminal vesicles is prudent [19, 21].

Development of the Posterior Plane and Control of the Pedicle

The plane posterior to Denonvilliers' fascia is generally well preserved in patients after primary radiation therapy, especially when compared to the interfascial plane above Denonvilliers' fascia (Fig. 8.7). Dissection in this plane also permits wide excision of the posterior prostate in the case of disease extension. Even locally extensive tumors rarely penetrate Denonvilliers' fascia. The fourth arm is utilized to retract the prostate and seminal vesicles anteriorly and cranially. Tension is placed on Denonvilliers' fascia with the third arm and the fascia should be incised sharply, exposing the perirectal fat (Fig. 8.8). This plane should be developed caudally towards the posterior prostatic apex without the use of cautery and is greatly facilitated by the improved visualization afforded by robotic-assistance, which allows an easier and safer posterior dissection (Fig. 8.9). This step should proceed

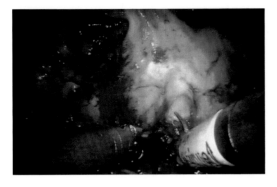

Fig. 8.3 Intraoperative view demonstrating incision of the thickened right endopelvic fascia

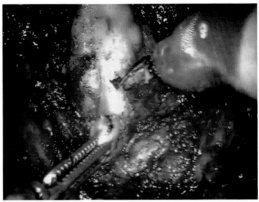

Fig. 8.6 After dissection and division of the right vas deferens, the fourth arm is used to provide anterior retraction on the distal stump (out of the picture) and the third arm utilizes the proximal stump of the vas deferens as a handle to aid in the dissection of the right seminal vesicle

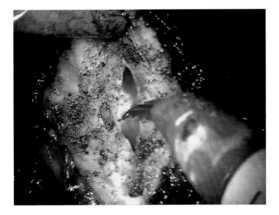

Fig. 8.4 The anterior bladder neck has been incised utilizing a combination of cautery and sharp dissection

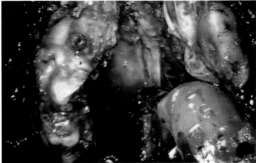

Fig. 8.7 Denonvilliers' fascia is placed on tension by the third arm and incised sharply. The fourth arm is providing anterior and cranial retraction on the prostate and seminal vesicles (out of the picture)

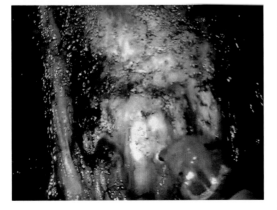

Fig. 8.5 The posterior bladder neck is incised and both vasa deferentia are identified

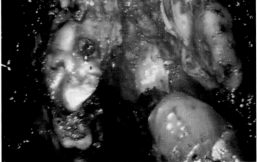

Fig. 8.8 The perirectal fat is exposed after incision of Denonvilliers' fascia, indicating the correct posterior plane in the salvage setting

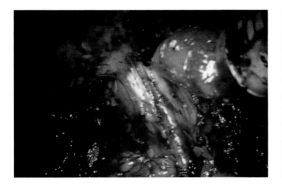

Fig. 8.9 The posterior plane is almost completely developed. The rectum is tented up as the last remaining attachments between the posterior prostatic apex and the rectum are divided sharply

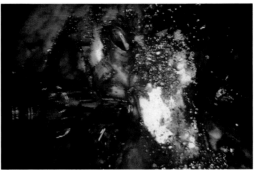

Fig. 8.11 Intraoperative view demonstrating marked apical fibrosis in patient who had previously received brachytherapy

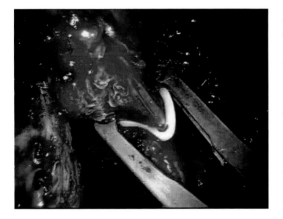

Fig. 8.10 The right prostatic pedicle is isolated and controlled with Hem-o-lok clips (Teleflex Medical, Research Triangle Park, NC)

cautiously as dense adhesions may be present. While some have advocated for nerve-sparing sRALP, we generally perform a wide excision of the lateral prostatic fascia and neurovascular bundle in this setting to optimize the chance of cure [15, 17, 19]. 38–45 % of patients undergoing salvage radical prostatectomy will have extra-prostatic extension on final pathologic analysis. Furthermore, erectile function in a post-radiation cohort is often poor even before surgery [19, 21]. The pedicles are then isolated via anterior retraction on the prostate and seminal vesicles and divided with Hem-o-lok clips (Teleflex Medical, Research Triangle Park, NC) and scissors (Fig. 8.10).

Apical Dissection and Division of the Urethra

Prior to division of the dorsal venous complex, we will completely free the lateral margins of the prostate to allow full mobilization of the prostate. This improves visualization of the posterior prostatic apex, which is often the most adherent after radiation therapy—particularly with brachytherapy (Fig. 8.11). The fourth arm is used to pull the prostate posteriorly and cranially to aid in the definition of tissue planes which can be quite obliterated and fibrotic. The three-dimensional magnification of the operative field afforded by robotic-assistance is again extremely helpful around the apex. In the salvage setting we do not ligate the dorsal venous complex prior to its division in order to improve mobility and visualization during dissection of the prostatic apex. Bleeding is usually limited due to tissue fibrosis and loss of vascularity as well as the effect of the pneumoperitoneum. Following division of the dorsal venous complex, the urethra is sharply divided, the catheter is removed, and any remaining apical prostatic tissue should be meticulously dissected free (Fig. 8.12). This can be quite difficult in the salvage setting and care must be taken to decrease the chance of a positive apical margin. At times, the apical and periprostatic fibrosis may obscure the true boundaries of the prostate and additional margins can be sent off as needed.

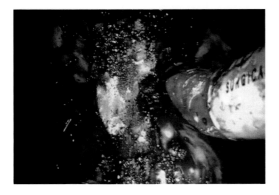

Fig. 8.12 Intraoperative view after division of the dorsal venous complex and urethra demonstrating dissection of the posterior apical prostatic tissue. Note the marked peri-apical fibrosis

After completion of the apical dissection, division of the urethra and posterior attachments, a figure-of-eight with 2-0 polyglactin (vicryl) suture on an SH needle can be placed on the distal dorsal venous complex for hemostatic purposes.

Node Dissection

In the significant majority of patients undergoing sRALP, we perform an extended bilateral pelvic lymphadenectomy [19]. The possibility for incremental survival gain and improved staging information must be balanced against the potential of increased perioperative morbidity. Especially when external beam irradiation has been used, there can be considerable fibrosis along the iliac vessels. Although pelvic node dissection is feasible in virtually any patient, the incremental gain in terms of either survival or staging is minimal. Therefore, if node dissection seems excessively hazardous because of scarring from irradiation or prior mesh hernia repair, we may omit it.

Vesicourethral Anastomosis

Completion of a secure mucosal-to-mucosal anastomosis is critical, especially in the salvage setting. A distinct advantage of the robot is the facility with which a running, water-tight anastomosis can be obtained. This limits postoperative

morbidity from a prolonged urine leak, but also minimizes the risk of bladder neck contracture.

The anastomosis is performed with a running single-suture technique using the robotic fourth arm to help monitor tissue approximation. Alternatively, a barbed suture can be used. Regardless, the key is to have complete mucosal-to-mucosal tissue approximation.

Undocking of the Robot

Following completion of the vesicourethral anastomosis, the bladder is filled to assess the integrity of the anastomosis and a surgical drain can be placed through the left lateral robotic trocar incision site. We generally only leave a drain if a lymph node dissection has been performed. The robot is undocked, the table is leveled, and the trocars and specimen are removed. The fascia of the 12 mm assistant port and supra-umbilical camera port sites are closed with #1 absorbable polyglactin (vicryl) suture after utilizing the camera to inspect the anterior abdominal wall and port sites for bleeding. The skin is then closed and the patient is awakened and taken to the recovery room.

Postoperative Care

Patients undergoing sRALP are managed postoperatively according to our standardized robotic prostatectomy pathway, which includes early ambulation, a full liquid diet on the morning of postoperative day 1, intravenous ketorolac to reduce the utilization of narcotics for pain control, and an aggressive bowel regimen [22]. Surgical drains are generally removed on the first postoperative day, unless the output is greater than 200 cc over 24 h, in which case patients will go home with the drain and have it removed once the output approximates this threshold. Salvage status alone should not significantly prolong hospital stay. In our experience, 94 % of patients undergoing sRALP are discharged on the first postoperative day [19]. The Foley catheter is left indwelling for at least

2 weeks because of the poor healing of irradiated tissue. A cystogram prior to catheter removal is performed only if the anastomosis was technically difficult or if there is clinical suspicion of incomplete healing.

Complications

Fortunately, despite the complexity of this procedure, major complications are rare. A key advantage of the robotic platform is low blood loss. In published sRALP series, median estimated blood loss has ranged from 75–150 cc with no blood transfusions or conversions from laparoscopic to open in 83 patients [13–17, 19]. Anastomotic strictures are also uncommon, with rates ranging from 0 to 17 % in sRALP series and most reporting rates between 7 % and 9 % [14–17, 19]. This compares favorably to open series, with stricture rates after SRP reported as high as 22–30 % [9, 10]. A small percentage (0–33 %) of patients develop anastomotic leaks requiring prolonged catheterization. One pulmonary embolism and one deep vein thrombosis, both of which were treated medically, have been reported [17, 19]. One enterotomy during lysis of adhesions which was repaired primarily without complication has also been reported [16]. Of the 83 patients undergoing sRALP in published series, only one rectal injury (1 %) was reported [19].

If there is concern as to the integrity of the rectal wall, it can be evaluated by exam, rectal insufflation after filling the pelvis with saline, and rectal transillumination with a sigmoidoscope as has been advocated by Chauhan et al. [17] (Fig. 8.13). We do not routinely perform these tests unless there is concern for a rectal injury. If a rectal injury is identified, we recommend primary, multilayer closure, tissue interposition, as well as general surgery consultation and strong consideration for fecal diversion given the increased risk for rectourethral fistula in the postradiation setting.

Oncologic Outcomes

Although published sRALP series are early in their experience with median follow-up ranging from 4 to 18 months, early oncologic outcomes are encouraging. Of the 83 sRALP patients in the literature, 18 (22 %) had positive margins which is in line with contemporary open SRP series, which have ranged from 11 to 33 % [11, 13–17, 19, 21, 23]. Margin status is reported to be a predictor of BCR after primary radical prostatectomy as well as in the salvage setting [23, 24]. However, given the heterogeneous patient populations, differing pathologic analyses, and differing rates of neoadjuvant androgen deprivation therapy, comparisons between series are difficult.

a   **b**

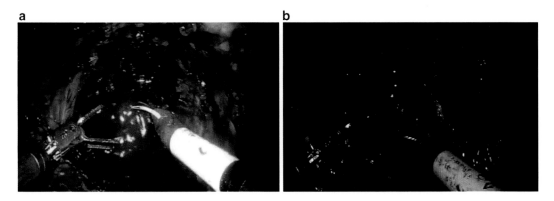

Fig. 8.13 (**a**) A lighted, flexible sigmoidoscope is placed into the rectum to evaluate for defects in the rectal wall. (**b**) The robotic camera light is turned off. No transillumination is apparent, indicating an intact rectal wall

Of the 74 patients in the literature undergoing sRALP who received a bilateral pelvic node dissection, 4 (5 %) were detected to have positive nodes [14–17, 19]. In our experience with 16 months of median follow-up, 6 patients (18 %) had BCR, the majority of whom had biochemical persistence after sRALP. This is comparable to the approximately 25 % BCR at 16 months reported by Chade et al. in a large multi-institutional study of 404 patients undergoing open SRP [21]. Further follow-up will be required to determine the continued oncologic efficacy of this procedure.

Functional Outcomes

Early experience and short follow-up limit some of the conclusions on functional recovery that can be ascertained from the available data on sRALP. In general, functional outcomes are worse in the salvage population than in the primary radical prostatectomy population for both open SRP and sRALP. Continence rates (0–1 pad per day) in sRALP series have ranged from 33 to 80 % [14–17, 19]. In our experience, 39 % of patients returned to continence (0–1 pads per day), and although this is less than some rates reported in contemporary open SRP series, 35 % of our patients have follow-up of less than 1 year [9–11]. Of the two groups reporting pad-free rates on 24 total patients, 60 % and 71 % were pad-free at the end of their respective follow-up [15, 17]. It is expected that continence rates in most series will improve with continued follow-up.

Erectile function in the salvage setting is universally poor. The majority of patients have impaired erectile preoperatively—only 21 % of patients were able to obtain an erection sufficient for penetration without the assistance of medication pre-sRALP in our series [19]. Moreover, few patients have nerve-sparing procedures performed. Of the 17 patients able to obtain erections preoperatively with or without pharmacologic assistance, only 5 (29 %) were able to obtain erections sufficient for intercourse with additional therapy beyond phosphodiesterase type 5 inhibitors. High rates of impotence have been a consistent finding in other sRALP series [14–17].

The short follow-up of our series and others may underestimate return to potency, but even in modern open SRP series with long-term follow-up, potency rates are invariably poor [9, 11, 21].

Summary

sRALP, as in open SRP, can be a difficult procedure. Given the fibrosis and obliterated tissue planes as well as increased potential for serious complications, it is not advised for the novice robotic surgeon. While the benefits of robotics in the primary setting are contested, we feel that use of the robotic platform in the salvage setting greatly facilitates the performance of radical prostatectomy. sRALP is safe, with some outcomes favorable to open, salvage radical prostatectomy series. Primary advantages are the improved visualization of the posterior prostatic plane, low complication rates including the decreased development of anastomotic stricture, low blood loss, and short length of stay.

Despite the advantages of the robot in the salvage setting, sRALP is a procedure with the potential for significant morbidity and long-term quality of life compromise. Furthermore, although oncologic outcomes are favorable for some patients, a substantial number develop BCR. Performance of a technically proficient operation is essential but must be completed with proper selection of patients most likely to benefit from surgery.

References

1. Zelefsky MJ, Kuban DA, Levy LB, Potters L, Beyer DC, Blasko JC, et al. Multi-institutional analysis of long-term outcome for stages T1-T2 prostate cancer treated with permanent seed implantation. Int J Radiat Oncol Biol Phys. 2007;67(2):327–33.
2. Zietman AL, Coen JJ, Dallow KC, Shipley WU. The treatment of prostate cancer by conventional radiation therapy: an analysis of long-term outcome. Int J Radiat Oncol Biol Phys. 1995;32(2):287–92.
3. Agarwal PK, Sadetsky N, Konety BR, Resnick MI, Carroll PR. Treatment failure after primary and salvage therapy for prostate cancer: likelihood, patterns of care, and outcomes. Cancer. 2008;112(2):307–14.
4. Zagars GK, Pollack A, von Eschenbach AC. Prostate cancer and radiation therapy—the message conveyed

by serum prostate-specific antigen. Int J Radiat Oncol Biol Phys. 1995;33(1):23–35.

5. Pisters LL, Leibovici D, Blute M, Zincke H, Sebo TJ, Slezak JM, et al. Locally recurrent prostate cancer after initial radiation therapy: a comparison of salvage radical prostatectomy versus cryotherapy. J Urol. 2009;182(2):517–25. discussion 25–7.

6. Mouraviev V, Spiess PE, Jones JS. Salvage cryoablation for locally recurrent prostate cancer following primary radiotherapy. Eur Urol. 2012;61(6):1204–11.

7. Chen BT, Wood Jr DP. Salvage prostatectomy in patients who have failed radiation therapy or cryotherapy as primary treatment for prostate cancer. Urology. 2003;62 Suppl 1:69–78.

8. Rogers E, Ohori M, Kassabian VS, Wheeler TM, Scardino PT. Salvage radical prostatectomy: outcome measured by serum prostate specific antigen levels. J Urol. 1995;153(1):104–10.

9. Stephenson AJ, Scardino PT, Bianco Jr FJ, DiBlasio CJ, Fearn PA, Eastham JA. Morbidity and functional outcomes of salvage radical prostatectomy for locally recurrent prostate cancer after radiation therapy. J Urol. 2004;172(6 Pt 1):2239–43.

10. Ward JF, Sebo TJ, Blute ML, Zincke H. Salvage surgery for radiorecurrent prostate cancer: contemporary outcomes. J Urol. 2005;173(4):1156–60.

11. Heidenreich A, Richter S, Thuer D, Pfister D. Prognostic parameters, complications, and oncologic and functional outcome of salvage radical prostatectomy for locally recurrent prostate cancer after 21st-century radiotherapy. Eur Urol. 2010;57(3):437–43.

12. Hu JC, Gu X, Lipsitz SR, Barry MJ, D'Amico AV, Weinberg AC, et al. Comparative effectiveness of minimally invasive vs open radical prostatectomy. JAMA. 2009;302(14):1557–64.

13. Jamal K, Challacombe B, Elhage O, Popert R, Kirby R, Dasgupta P. Successful salvage robotic-assisted radical prostatectomy after external beam radiotherapy failure. Urology. 2008;72(6):1356–8.

14. Kaouk JH, Hafron J, Goel R, Haber GP, Jones JS. Robotic salvage retropubic prostatectomy after radiation/brachytherapy: initial results. BJU Int. 2008;102(1):93–6.

15. Boris RS, Bhandari A, Krane LS, Eun D, Kaul S, Peabody JO. Salvage robotic-assisted radical prosta-

tectomy: initial results and early report of outcomes. BJU Int. 2009;103(7):952–6.

16. Eandi JA, Link BA, Nelson RA, Josephson DY, Lau C, Kawachi MH, et al. Robotic assisted laparoscopic salvage prostatectomy for radiation resistant prostate cancer. J Urol. 2010;183(1):133–7.

17. Chauhan S, Patel MB, Coelho R, Liss M, Rocco B, Sivaraman AK, et al. Preliminary analysis of the feasibility and safety of salvage robot-assisted radical prostatectomy after radiation failure: multi-institutional perioperative and short-term functional outcomes. J Endourol. 2011;25(6):1013–9.

18. Rocco B, Cozzi G, Spinelli MG, Grasso A, Varisco D, Coelho RF, et al. Current status of salvage robot-assisted laparoscopic prostatectomy for radiorecurrent prostate cancer. Curr Urol Rep. 2012;13(3): 195–201 [Review].

19. Kaffenberger SD, Keegan KA, Bansal NK, Morgan TM, Tang DH, Barocas DA, et al. Salvage robotic assisted laparoscopic radical prostatectomy: a single institution, 5-year experience. J Urol. 2013;189(2):507–13.

20. Nunez-Mora C, Garcia-Mediero JM, Cabrera-Castillo PM. Radical laparoscopic salvage prostatectomy: medium-term functional and oncological results. J Endourol. 2009;23(8):1301–5.

21. Chade DC, Shariat SF, Cronin AM, Savage CJ, Karnes RJ, Blute ML, et al. Salvage radical prostatectomy for radiation-recurrent prostate cancer: a multi-institutional collaboration. Eur Urol. 2011;60(2):205–10.

22. Kaufman MR, Baumgartner RG, Anderson LW, Smith Jr JA, Chang SS, Herrell SD, et al. The evidence-based pathway for peri-operative management of open and robotically assisted laparoscopic radical prostatectomy. BJU Int. 2007;99(5):1103–8 [Review validation studies].

23. Sanderson KM, Penson DF, Cai J, Groshen S, Stein JP, Lieskovsky G, et al. Salvage radical prostatectomy: quality of life outcomes and long-term oncological control of radiorecurrent prostate cancer. J Urol. 2006;176(5):2025–31. discussion 31–2.

24. Grossfeld GD, Chang JJ, Broering JM, Miller DP, Yu J, Flanders SC, et al. Impact of positive surgical margins on prostate cancer recurrence and the use of secondary cancer treatment: data from the CaPSURE database. J Urol. 2000;163(4):1171–7. quiz 295.

Open Salvage Radical Prostatectomy for Recurrence of Prostate Cancer after Radiation Therapy

9

James A. Eastham

Abbreviations

DVC	Dorsal vein complex
NVB	Neurovascular bundle
PCNA	Proliferative cell nuclear antigen
PLND	Pelvic lymph node dissection
PSA	Prostate-specific antigen
RP	Radical prostatectomy
RT	Radiation therapy

Introduction

The management of patients with a rising serum prostate-specific antigen (PSA) level after definitive local therapy is one of the most perplexing problems faced by urologists and oncologists [1, 2]. Because radiation therapy (RT) spares some PSA-producing nonneoplastic prostate epithelial cells, the first question to consider is whether the rise in PSA is temporary and benign, or whether it originates from local recurrence of cancer or from distant metastases or both. Local recurrence after RT is associated with a poor

J.A. Eastham, M.D. (✉)
Sidney Kimmel Center for Prostate and Urologic
Cancers, Memorial Sloan-Kettering Cancer Center,
353 East 68th Street, Suite 617B, New York,
NY 10021, USA
e-mail: easthamj@mskcc.org

prognosis, although additional treatment to the primary site may be curative. While the risk of death varies for patients with disease relapse after RT, many will develop local progression or metastasis, or die of their disease [3, 4]. By the time a relapse becomes clinically (rather than just biochemically) evident, the cancer has usually progressed beyond the point where local salvage therapy might be beneficial. The challenge to the clinician, therefore, is to detect local recurrence while the cancer is still curable.

There are a number of treatment options for men with local recurrence of prostate cancer after RT, including expectant management, hormonal therapy (continuous or intermittent) or further local (i.e., salvage) therapy with high-intensity focused ultrasound, brachytherapy, cryoablation, or radical prostatectomy (RP). Salvage RP is technically challenging but provides excellent local control [5–9] and can eradicate the disease in a high proportion of patients whose cancer is confined to the prostate or immediate periprostatic tissue. While the majority of patients undergoing salvage RP have pathologically advanced cancer (including seminal vesicle invasion and/or lymph node metastases), comparisons between similar pathologic stages show that outcomes after salvage RP are similar to those after standard RP. As with standard RP, patient selection is of utmost importance in planning appropriate treatment.

J.A. Eastham and E.M. Schaeffer (eds.), *Radical Prostatectomy: Surgical Perspectives*,
DOI 10.1007/978-1-4614-8693-0_9, © Springer Science+Business Media New York 2014

Post-radiation Prostate Biopsy

Local recurrence after RT is defined as a rising PSA level in conjunction with a positive needle biopsy of the prostate at least 18–24 months after completion of RT [10]. A biopsy taken earlier may not be reliable, as a percentage of tumors will continue to regress during that time, and even beyond. There is no set interval beyond which residual tumor seen on biopsy is both viable and biologically significant. Interestingly, studies have shown that clinically significant post-RT local recurrence usually occurs at the site of primary tumor, suggesting that radiation resistance, rather than development of a new cancer, is the most likely cause of local failure after RT [11].

Because radiation-induced atypia may be difficult to distinguish from residual cancer exhibiting severe radiation changes [12, 13], care must be taken when evaluating post-RT prostate biopsies. To investigate radiation-related histologic changes within the prostate, Gaudin et al. reviewed prostate needle biopsies from 137 patients obtained at a median of 36 months after three-dimensional conformal RT [13]. The most common histopathologic changes to benign prostate tissue were glandular atrophy, cytologic atypia, and basal cell prominence. The benign glands were intensely immunoreactive with antibodies to high-molecular-weight cytokeratin (34 [beta] E12), and showed either negative or weakly positive reactions to PSA. The changes in benign prostate tissues were similar whether patients were treated with RT only or with neoadjuvant androgen deprivation therapy in addition to RT. In contrast, for prostate cancer treated with RT, some patients showed no apparent RT effect while others experienced RT-related changes characterized by poorly formed, PSA-positive/cytokeratin-negative glands as well as residual neoplastic cells containing abundant clear to finely granular cytoplasm (Fig. 9.1). The investigators concluded that (1) the effect of RT on

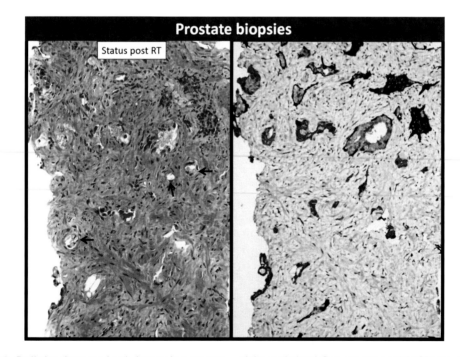

Fig. 9.1 Radiation therapy-related changes in a prostate needle biopsy are characterized by a diminution in the number of neoplastic glands, which are often poorly formed and haphazardly arranged within the prostatic stroma (*left*). Immunohistochemistry with triple stain that combines two basal cell markers (p63 and high molecular weight cytokeratin [clone 34betaE12] in *brown*) and alpha-methylacyl-CoA racemase (AMACR) (in *pink/red*). The glands with no *brown* and only *red-pink* are cancerous glands, while those with the both *red-pink* plus a *brown* rim are benign (*right*). Figure courtesy of Samson W. Fine, MD, of the MSKCC Department of Pathology, Surgical Pathology Diagnostic Services, Genitourinary Pathology. Used with permission

prostate cancer is variable, with some cases showing profound therapy-related changes and others showing no apparent therapy effect, and (2) post-RT benign prostate glands show profound histopathologic changes that may be confused with prostate cancer. This distinction is critical because a biopsy showing only prostate cancer with profound RT-related changes likely identifies a subset of tumors with little or no biological activity. Crook et al. studied irradiated prostate cancer and correlated the degree of RT effect to proliferative cell nuclear antigen (PCNA) immunohistochemistry [14]. They found that prostate cancer with marked therapy effect showed significantly less PCNA immunoreactivity than prostate cancer with little or no therapy effect (17 % versus 61 %). No local progression was observed in patients whose biopsies showed marked RT effect, suggesting that such patients are at low risk for local failure and are unlikely to require additional local (i.e., salvage) therapy.

Salvage Radical Prostatectomy

Early recurrence of prostate cancer is likely to be organ confined and therefore amenable to salvage therapy. Although salvage RP has been used successfully to eradicate locally recurrent prostate cancer after definitive RT, complications are common [6, 9, 15–17]. Accordingly, the procedure should only be performed by experienced urologic surgeons. Patient selection should be limited to those in excellent health, with a life expectancy of at least 10 years, whose cancer (whether initial org recurrent) is clinically organ-confined and potentially curable. Patients should have no evidence of metastatic disease, no evidence of lymph node involvement before RT, and no evidence of severe radiation cystitis or proctitis. Salvage RP is technically feasible using current surgical techniques, with satisfactory immediate intraoperative and postoperative outcomes [15]. The majority of patients can be treated via a retropubic approach; rarely is a combined abdominoperineal approach required. The rate of major complications has decreased from 33 to 13 % for patients treated before and after 1993 ($p=0.02$) and rectal injury

has been encountered in only 1 of 60 patients (2 %) since 1993.

Salvage RP can be safely performed after failed external beam RT, brachytherapy, or combinations of these techniques. Short-term and long-term complications are more common after salvage RP than standard RP, partly because the normal anatomic planes are lost as a consequence of radiation. According to published series, up to 15 % of patients experienced rectal injuries although recent reports suggest the incidence in closer to 2 % [15]. Other early complications of surgery include ureteral transection, prolonged anastomotic leakage, and/or pulmonary embolism. Later complications include development of an anastomotic stricture or persistent urinary incontinence. The overall anastomotic stricture rate is as high as 30 % [15], and most patients who develop an anastomotic stricture will require multiple interventions. The development of an anastomotic stricture appears less likely in patients undergoing minimally invasive salvage RP than those undergoing an open procedure [15–19]. A review of published series suggests that the recovery of continence after salvage RP (both open and minimally invasive) has improved over time [6, 9, 15, 20], likely reflecting not only an improvement in surgical technique but also better targeted radiation therapies resulting in better preservation of the urinary sphincter.

Erectile dysfunction has been considered almost inevitable after salvage RP, but in selected cases this may be prevented by preservation of one or both neurovascular bundles. Stephenson et al. reported on a series of 100 consecutive patients with biopsy-confirmed, locally recurrent prostate cancer treated with salvage RP between 1984 and 2003. While overall postsurgical potency in that series was low (16 % [95 % CI, 4–28 %]), many patients had erectile dysfunction prior to salvage RP [15]. For men who were potent preoperatively, the 5-year recovery of potency was 45 % (95 % CI, 16–75 %). Of seven patients who underwent bilateral nerve-sparing procedures, five (71 %) recovered functional erections. Importantly, none of the seven had a positive surgical margin in the area where the neurovascular bundle was preserved.

Data on patterns of recurrence (local or metastatic) after salvage RP have been fairly limited. Several recent series, however, have demonstrated excellent oncologic outcomes after salvage RP (>90 % cancer-specific survival at 5 years) [5, 6, 8, 9, 20]. In a retrospective study by Paparel et al. of 146 patients treated with salvage RP at a single institution [8], the 5-year recurrence-free probability was 54 % (95 % CI, 44–63 %). Clinical local recurrence occurred in only one patient, who also had bone metastases. Sixteen patients died of prostate cancer and 19 died of other causes. The 5-year cumulative incidence of death due to prostate cancer was 4 % (95 % CI, 2–11 %). Serum PSA level and biopsy Gleason score before salvage RP were found to be significantly associated with death from prostate cancer ($p < 0.0005$ and $p = 0.002$, respectively).

Technique of Open Salvage Radical Prostatectomy

Salvage RP is curative only if the entire cancer is removed. Accurate preoperative assessment of the cancer allows the surgeon to plan an operation tailored to the size, location, and extent of the patient's cancer, as well as the prostatic and periprostatic anatomy. Consideration of additional factors such as PSA levels, clinical stage, and the results of systematic needle biopsy increase the likelihood of successful treatment. Information about the location of positive biopsies, the length of cancer in each core, and the Gleason grade can help to characterize the location and extent of cancer within the prostate and surrounding tissues. Knowledge of the presence and location of any extraprostatic extension allows the surgeon to modify the operation by performing a wider excision in the involved area to decrease the risk of a positive surgical margin.

Patient Positioning and Initial Incision

The patient should be in a supine position (see Fig. 7.2), with the table flexed as needed to gain access to the pelvis. Sharply incise the transver-

salis fascia through an 8-cm suprapubic midline incision extending toward the umbilicus, and enter the retropubic space. Take care not to sweep perivesical lymph nodes cephalad as the lateral pelvic sidewalls are exposed. A self-retaining Turner Warwick retractor is effective in providing adequate pelvic exposure, although alternative retractors can be used as well. Insert an 18 Fr Foley catheter and fill the balloon with 10–15 cm^3 of sterile water.

Pelvic Lymph Node Dissection

Patients undergoing salvage RP are at increased risk of nodal involvement compared to those undergoing standard RP [5, 6, 8, 9], and a pelvic lymph node dissection (PLND) at the time of RP is recommended for all such patients. There have been no prospective studies demonstrating the appropriate anatomical limits of a PLND for prostate cancer. However, lymphatic drainage of the prostate is known to be highly variable and involves regions not sampled during an obturator-only PLND [21]. Some surgeons resect only the external iliac lymph nodes unless imaging suggests abnormal lymph nodes in other regions, while other surgeons routinely perform a more extensive dissection that includes the obturator, external iliac, and hypogastric areas. When such an extended PLND is performed, not only are more nodes retrieved, but the lymph nodes from most of the potential landing zones are removed— significantly increasing the number of patients found to have lymph node invasion [21–23]. The extended dissection yields a higher lymph node count and detects more positive lymph nodes than a lymphadenectomy that is limited to the nodal tissue between the external iliac vein and top of the obturator nerve (external iliac area).

Mobilization of the Prostate and Control of the Dorsal Vein Complex

Mobilize the prostate by incising the endopelvic fascia laterally in the groove between the prostate and the levator ani muscles. Extend the fascial incision sharply toward the pelvis where the fascia

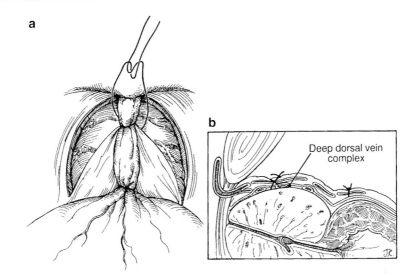

Fig. 9.2 The superficial dorsal vein complex (DVC) is suture ligated at the bladder neck, approximately 1 cm cephalad to the junction of the prostate and bladder (**a, b**). A deeper suture is placed around the superficial and deep DVC midway toward the apex, extending from one cut edge of endopelvic fascia to the other. Using a Babcock clamp to "bunch" this tissue together can facilitate placement of this suture. These sutures limit back bleeding on transection of the DVC. From Scardino PT, Linehan WM. Comprehensive Textbook of Genitourinnary Oncology. © 2011 Wolters Kluwer Health, used with permission

condenses into the puboprostatic ligaments. Blunt dissection is inadequate during this procedure, as tissues are typically fused together. Using sharp dissection, further mobilize the prostate from the levator ani muscles. The puboprostatic ligaments need not be divided if the apex of the prostate is adequately exposed.

To prevent significant back bleeding, ligate the superficial dorsal vein complex at the bladder neck and suture-ligate the deep dorsal vein complex at the mid-prostate using a 0-polyglactin absorbable suture on a CT-1 needle (Fig. 9.2). The first suture marks the site of division of the bladder neck later in the operation. The suture at the level of the mid-prostate traverses the anterior surface of the gland from one cut edge of endopelvic fascia to the other. Placement of this stitch is facilitated by use of either a Babcock or Allis clamp to bunch the deep dorsal venous complex followed by a figure-of-eight suture beneath the closed clamp. This suture should not be placed too far laterally as this may injure the periprostatic veins and increase bleeding.

Next, pass a right-angle clamp through the fascia beneath the entire dorsal vein complex anterior to the urethra just distal to the prostatic apex (Fig. 9.3a). This clamp will be used to grasp a 22-gauge stainless steel wire looped on the end. Grasp the small loop in the wire with the right-angled clamp and bring it beneath the dorsal vein complex, then grasp the two ends of the wire with a Kelly or Cocker clamp. Use a third suture of 0-polyglactin absorbable suture on a CT-1 needle to control the deep dorsal venous complex at the pelvic floor. The wire (which has been placed anterior to the urethra) can be used as a guide to set the proper depth of this suture. Pass a second throw of this suture approximately halfway above the first throw, and then pass a third and final throw through the periosteum on the underside of the pubic bone. The final throw helps to crush the superficial dorsal veins between the pubis and the main dorsal vein complex. It also fixes the urethra in the pelvis, which may reduce urethral hypermobility.

The wire serves as a template when the complex is transected sharply with a No. 15 surgical blade on a long knife handle between the mid-prostate and pelvic floor dorsal venous complex sutures (Fig. 9.3b). Adjusting the upward tension on the wire and downward traction on the

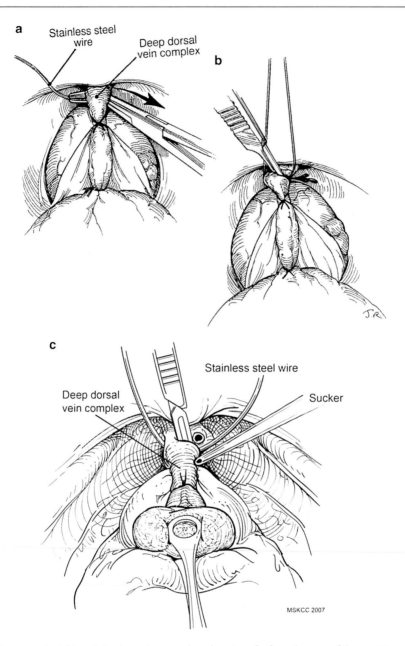

Fig. 9.3 A long-nosed right-angled clamp is passed through the fascia between the urethra and dorsal vein complex (DVC) and grasps a stainless steel wire that is looped on the end (**a**). The wire serves as a guide to allow a square transection of the DVC and its surrounding fascia (**b**). A sucker tip can be used to retract the apex of the prostate (**c**). By this maneuver the DVC can be divided close to or far from the apex of the prostate, as the surgeon chooses, with care to avoid a positive anterior surgical margin. A&B from Scardino PT, Linehan WM. Comprehensive Textbook of Genitourinnary Oncology. © 2011 Wolters Kluwer Health, used with permission. C used with permission from Memorial Sloan-Kettering Cancer Center

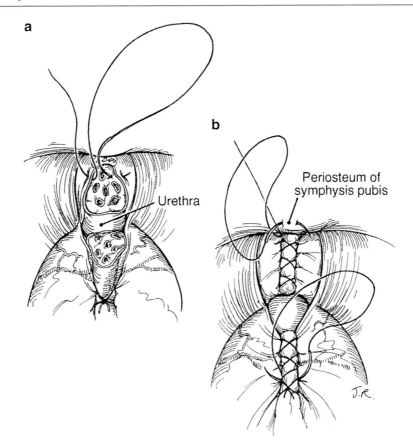

Fig. 9.4 Bleeding from the transected dorsal vein complex is controlled by oversewing the cut edges of the lateral pelvic fascia with a continuous suture (**a**), the last pass of which is brought through the periosteum of the pubis (**b**) to compress the superficial venous complex above the lateral pelvic fascia and to fix the fascia to the periosteum, simulating the function of the puboprostatic ligaments. Back bleeding from the ventral prostate is controlled with clips or with a continuous hemostatic suture, taking care not to draw the neurovascular bundles medially. From Scardino PT, Linehan WM. Comprehensive Textbook of Genitourinnary Oncology. © 2011 Wolters Kluwer Health, used with permission

prostate with a sponge stick will enable division of the dorsal vein complex sufficiently far from the apex to minimize the risk of a positive anterior surgical margin. The dorsal vein complex must be divided sufficiently distal to the anterior prostate to avoid an anterior positive margin. A sucker tip placed on the prostatic apex can be used to further expose this area (Fig. 9.3c). Using a surgical wire to divide the dorsal vein complex will facilitate the anterior dissection of the prostate. To control bleeding from the dorsal vein complex, sew together the incised edges of the lateral pelvic fascia on either side of the complex using a continuous 00-polyglactin absorbable suture on a CT-2 needle (Fig. 9.4a). Finally, sew

the suture through the periosteum of the pubis, compressing the superficial veins between the fascia and the pubic bone (Fig. 9.4b).

Lateral Dissection (Neurovascular Bundle)

Approaching the neurovascular bundles (NVB) laterally allows wide exposure of the apex so that the apical tissue can be completely resected. The fascia over the NVB can be incised more medially or laterally to the nerve, depending on the extent or location of the cancer and whether the nerves are to be preserved. In general, most

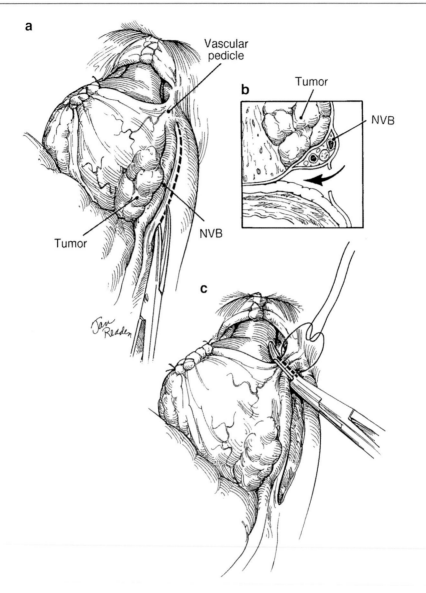

Fig. 9.5 Resection of the neurovascular bundle (NVB). Should the cancer lie close to the NVB, all or part of the bundle should be resected to assure complete removal of the cancer. A plane of dissection is chosen laterally. If the entire bundle is to be resected, dissection begins over the lateral rectal wall in the fat beneath the NVB (**a**, **b**). The incision is extended distally and the NVB is secured with clips or ties and divided distal to the apex of the prostate (**c**)

patients undergoing salvage RP are not candidates for NVB preservation. For most patients, therefore, the initial incision will be made lateral to the NVB (Fig. 9.5). This incision should be extended sharply, because blunt dissection with a Kitner ("peanut") dissector or with a finger is rarely successful and risks avulsion of prostatic tissue or injury to the rectum. Typically there is little scarring laterally and a plane beneath the

NVB can be developed from the apex to the lateral vascular pedicle of the prostate.

When NVB preservation is feasible, the initial opening of the lateral prostatic fascia should be made medial to the NVB and the structures mobilized sharply off the gland (Fig. 9.6a, b). As the NVB is mobilized, small venous branches off the NVB can be identified, isolated, and divided between small hemoclips placed parallel to the

Fig. 9.6 Preservation of left neurovascular bundle (NVB). After the dorsal vein complex has been divided, the prostate is rotated to the right and the levator muscles are bluntly dissected away. The lateral pelvic fascia is then incised in the groove between the prostate and the NVB. The NVB is most easily dissected away from the apical third of the prostate (**a, b**). The small branches of the vascular pedicle to the apex must be divided. The posterior layer of Denonvilliers' fascia is then incised, releasing the NVB from the prostate and urethra (**c–e**) so that the nerves will not be tethered when the urethral anastomotic sutures are tied

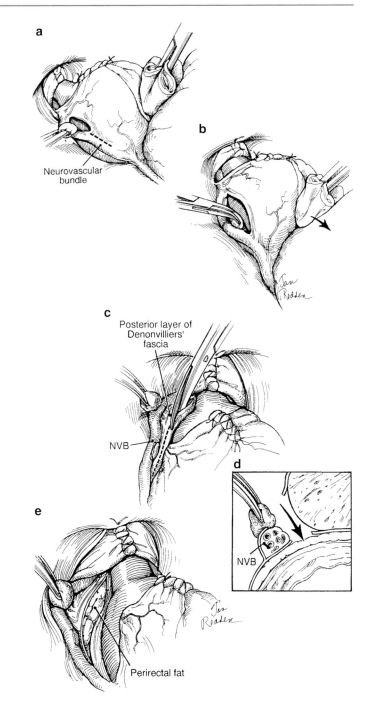

NVB. This will reduce bleeding and further the mobilization of the NVB off the gland. These vascular branches are particularly common near the apex of the prostate. Once the NVB has been mobilized off the prostate, sharply divide the firm, fibrous layer of Denonvilliers' fascia (Fig. 9.6c, e). It must be deliberately incised, releasing the NVB laterally and allowing a deep plane of dissection along the fat of the anterior rectal wall. The risk of a positive surgical margin will be greatly increased unless this layer of fascia is included in the excised specimen.

The thick lateral vascular pedicle supplying the prostate is encountered toward the base of the prostate (Fig. 9.7). Isolate the lateral vascular pedicle

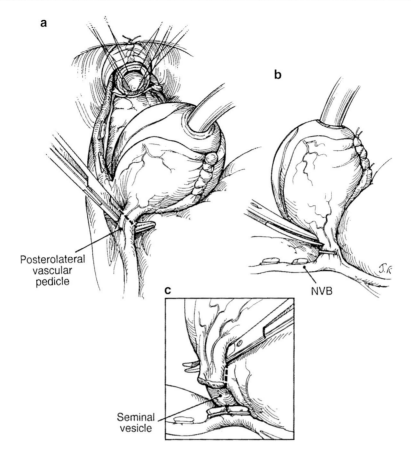

Fig. 9.7 The lateral vascular pedicle of the prostate is isolated with a right-angled clamp (**a**), controlled with clips
(**b**) and divided to expose the lateral aspect of the seminal

vesicle. Further exposure is gained by division of the vascular bands between the bladder neck and the seminal
vesicles and prostate (**c**)

with a right-angle clamp and control with clips or
ties. Full division of the lateral pedicle will expose
the lateral edge of the seminal vesicle (Fig. 9.7c).

Division of the Urethra, Placement
of Anastomotic Sutures, Dissection
of the Prostate Off the Rectum,
and Division/Reconstruction
of the Bladder

Once the apex is completely mobilized, sharply
divide the anterior two-thirds of the urethra at the
apex of the gland (Fig. 9.8a). Using 00-Monocryl
sutures on a UR-6 needle, place the first four anastomotic sutures at the 1, 3, 9, and 11 o'clock positions in the urethral stump (Fig. 9.8b–d). The

urethra may be thin; in such cases after the urethral
stitch is placed a second bite of the fascia of the
dorsal venous complex may be included to provide
support when these anastomotic sutures are ultimately tied (Fig. 9.8c). Remove the catheter and
place the final two anastomotic sutures at the 5 and
7 o'clock positions (Fig. 9.9a). Once the posterior
anastomotic sutures are placed, divide the posterior urethra (Fig. 9.9b). Connect the previous (lateral) incisions in Denonvilliers' fascia beneath the
divided urethra, staying several millimeters away
from the prostatic apex. Sharply dissect the prostate off the rectum beneath Denonvilliers' fascia.
To reduce the incidence of positive posterolateral
margins, deep dissection beneath Denonvilliers'
fascia posteriorly should be performed. Blunt dissection is to be avoided because often the prostate

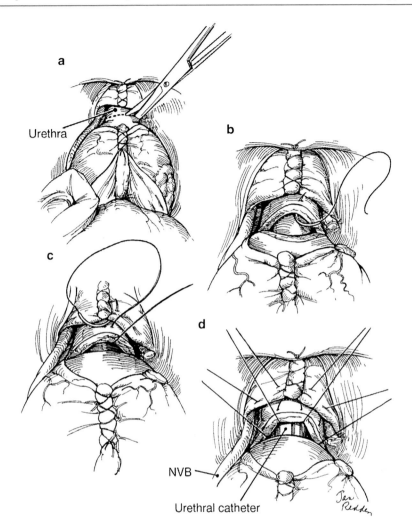

Fig. 9.8 Close-up views of urethra at the prostatic apex, illustrating the site of anterior division (**a**, **b**) and the placement of the anterior anastomotic sutures beneath the mucosa of the urethra and then separately through the thick layer of lateral pelvic fascia (**c**, **d**) that was oversewn to control the dorsal vein complex (*NVB* neurovascular bundle)

is fused to the rectum and requires sharp dissection to separate these structures. Continue this dissection until the seminal vesicles are identified. Denonvilliers' fascia should be left intact over the seminal vesicles. The fascial layer can be incised near the tips of the seminal vesicles.

Seminal Vesicles

Control of bleeding and exposure of the seminal vesicle is improved if the vascular band of tissue between the bladder and the base of the prostate and seminal vesicles is deliberately isolated, clipped, and divided (Fig. 9.10). This ensures a wide lateral margin around the base of the prostate. The seminal vesicles can then be sharply dissected from the bladder base. As the mobilization of the seminal vesicles continues, the vascular pedicle at the tip of the seminal vesicles can be exposed, clipped, and divided, ending with the identification and division of the ampulla of each vas deferens. In some cases this dissection is easier if the vas deferens is divided first. The artery to

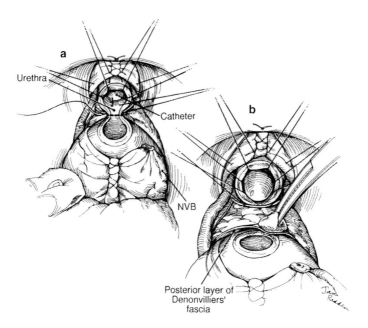

Fig. 9.9 The remaining urethra and posterior layer of Denonvilliers' fascia beneath it are divided. Two posterior anastomotic sutures are placed at 5 and 7 o'clock through the fascia and urethra (**a**). The correct plane of dissection adjacent to the rectum is difficult to identify; the dissection should be performed sharply (**b**) (*NVB* neurovascular bundle)

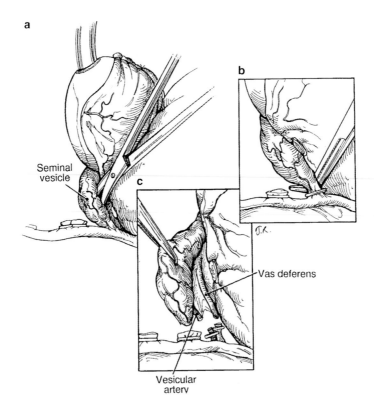

Fig. 9.10 (**a**) The seminal vesicles are typically approached laterally and the plane between the vesicles and the bladder developed with scissors. (**b**) The major blood supply to the seminal vesicles lies anterior and lateral. When these vessels are clipped and divided close to the wall of the vesicle, it is easier to identify the large artery that enters at the apex of the seminal vesicle. (**c**) The ampullae of the vas are clipped to include the vasal arteries and divided

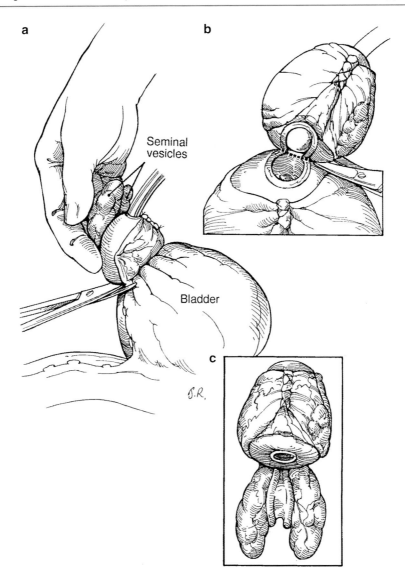

Fig. 9.11 The seminal vesicles and vasa dissected off the posterior wall of the bladder (**a**). The bladder neck is divided anteriorly (**b**), and the Foley catheter balloon is withdrawn through this incision. No attempt is made to spare the bladder neck. Small vessels are controlled with the electrocautery. The ureteral orifices are identified prior to division of the posterior bladder neck. The resected specimen (**c**) is closely palpated and examined to determine the completeness of resection. Any margin suspicious for cancer can be tagged with a suture and the entire specimen sent to pathology for frozen section evaluation

the vas deferens must be carefully secured. Meticulous control of the small vessels surrounding the seminal vesicles laterally and anteriorly will substantially reduce blood loss during the operation. The seminal vesicles and vasa deferentia can then be mobilized, within their fascia, all the way to the bladder neck. Finally, the bladder neck should be divided well away from the pros-

tate (Fig. 9.11). Tapering the bladder neck into the prostatic urethra does not improve the rate of long-term continence but does increase the risk of positive surgical margins.

Once the prostate has been removed, the divided bladder neck must be reconstructed (Fig. 9.12). Evert the mucosa anteriorly with fine absorbable sutures, and close the bladder neck

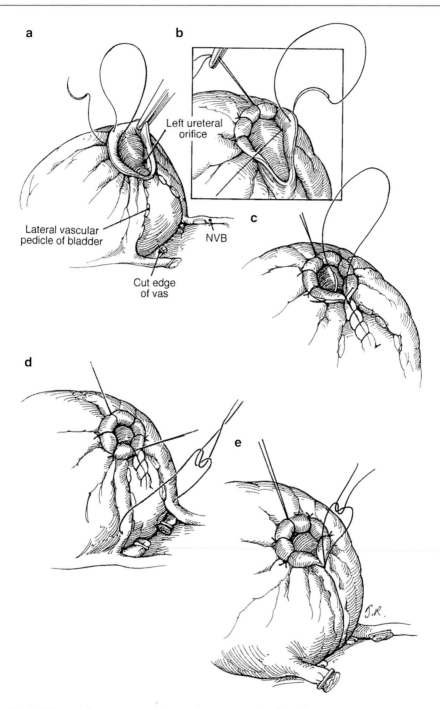

Fig. 9.12 The bladder neck is reconstructed by everting the mucosa anteriorly (**a**, **b**) and closing the bladder posteriorly with a running suture, creating a "tennis-racket" closure (**c**). The suture closest to the trigone should include muscle but little mucosa to avoid tethering the ureteral orifices. In a separate layer, the lateral vascular pedicles of the bladder are brought together in the midline to reinforce the closure and assure hemostasis (**d**, **e**), creating a cone shape to the reconstructed bladder neck

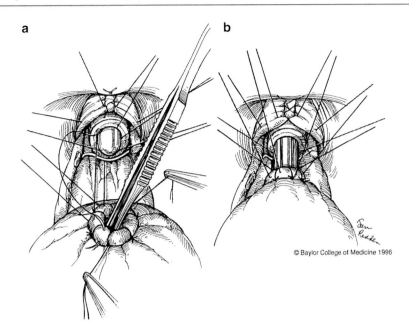

Fig. 9.13 The sutures already placed through the urethra are now placed through the bladder neck (**a**) to provide a mucosa-to-mucosa anastomosis (**b**)

posteriorly with a running 00 polyglactin absorbable suture until it is approximately 26–30 Fr in diameter. The mucosa must be fully everted 360° around the reconstructed bladder neck. Once the bladder neck reconstruction is complete, place the previously placed urethral sutures through the reconstructed bladder neck (Fig. 9.13). All sutures are placed such that the knots are tied on the outside of the lumen. Pass a new Foley catheter (18 Fr, 5-mL balloon) through the urethra and into the bladder, inflate the balloon with 15 mL of sterile water, and tie the sutures.

Management of Rectal Injury

Injury most often occurs during the apical dissection when the surgeon is unsure of the depth of incision. If a rectal injury occurs, it should not be repaired until after the prostatectomy has been completed. The injury is then closed in two inverted layers, and the closure must be air-tight. Once the injury is closed, insert a rectal tube or rigid sigmoidoscope, fill the pelvis with water, then inflate the rectum with air. If bubbles are

seen, place additional sutures. To reduce the potential of fistula formation, omentum should be placed between the rectum and vesicourethral anastomosis. Mobilize the omentum by opening the peritoneum in the rectovesical cul-de-sac and delivering a segment of omentum through the opening. A colostomy should be strongly considered after intraoperative consultation with a colorectal surgeon.

Conclusion

Salvage RP, while technically challenging, provides excellent local control of radiation-recurrent prostate cancer and is the only treatment option associated with long-term cancer-specific survival. It can eradicate the disease in a high proportion of patients treated when the cancer is confined to the prostate or immediate periprostatic tissue. Although rates of major complications have decreased significantly in the past two decades, the development of postoperative urinary incontinence and anastomotic strictures continues to challenge urologic surgeons. Accordingly, as with standard RP, patient selection is of utmost importance. Improving our ability to better identify patients with radiation-recurrent prostate cancer earlier in the course of their disease is paramount.

References

1. Djavan B, Moul JW, Zlotta A, Remzi M, Ravery V. PSA progression following radical prostatectomy and radiation therapy: new standards in the new Millennium. Eur Urol. 2003;43(1):12–27.

2. Darwish OM, Raj GV. Management of biochemical recurrence after primary localized therapy for prostate cancer. Front Oncol. 2012;2:48.

3. Kaplan ID, Prestidge BR, Bagshaw MA, Cox RS. The importance of local control in the treatment of prostatic cancer. J Urol. 1992;147(3 Pt 2):917–21.

4. Zelefsky MJ, Shi W, Yamada Y, Kollmeier MA, Cox B, Park J, et al. Postradiotherapy 2-year prostate-specific antigen nadir as a predictor of long-term prostate cancer mortality. Int J Radiat Oncol Biol Phys. 2009;75(5):1350–6.

5. Chade DC, Shariat SF, Cronin AM, Savage CJ, Karnes RJ, Blute ML, et al. Salvage radical prostatectomy for radiation-recurrent prostate cancer: a multi-institutional collaboration. Eur Urol. 2011;60(2):205–10.

6. Chade DC, Eastham J, Graefen M, Hu JC, Karnes RJ, Klotz L, et al. Cancer control and functional outcomes of salvage radical prostatectomy for radiation-recurrent prostate cancer: a systematic review of the literature. Eur Urol. 2012;61(5):961–71.

7. Rogers E, Ohori M, Kassabian VS, Wheeler TM, Scardino PT. Salvage radical prostatectomy: outcome measured by serum prostate specific antigen levels. J Urol. 1995;153(1):104–10.

8. Paparel P, Cronin AM, Savage C, Scardino PT, Eastham JA. Oncologic outcome and patterns of recurrence after salvage radical prostatectomy. Eur Urol. 2009;55(2):404–10.

9. Heidenreich A, Richter S, Thuer D, Pfister D. Prognostic parameters, complications, and oncologic and functional outcome of salvage radical prostatectomy for locally recurrent prostate cancer after 21st-century radiotherapy. Eur Urol. 2010;57(3):437–43.

10. Crook JM, Perry GA, Robertson S, Esche BA. Routine prostate biopsies following radiotherapy for prostate cancer: results for 226 patients. Urology. 1995;45(4):624–31. discussion 631–632.

11. Arrayeh E, Westphalen AC, Kurhanewicz J, Roach III M, Jung AJ, Carroll PR, et al. Does local recurrence of prostate cancer after radiation therapy occur at the site of primary tumor? Results of a longitudinal MRI and MRSI study. Int J Radiat Oncol Biol Phys. 2012;82(5):e787–93.

12. Bostwick DG, Egbert BM, Fajardo LF. Radiation injury of the normal and neoplastic prostate. Am J Surg Pathol. 1982;6(6):541–51.

13. Gaudin PB, Zelefsky MJ, Leibel SA, Fuks Z, Reuter VE. Histopathologic effects of three-dimensional conformal external beam radiation therapy on benign and malignant prostate tissues. Am J Surg Pathol. 1999;23(9):1021–31.

14. Crook JM, Bahadur YA, Robertson SJ, Perry GA, Esche BA. Evaluation of radiation effect, tumor differentiation, and prostate specific antigen staining in sequential prostate biopsies after external beam radiotherapy for patients with prostate carcinoma. Cancer. 1997;79(1):81–9.

15. Stephenson AJ, Scardino PT, Bianco Jr FJ, DiBlasio CJ, Fearn PA, Eastham JA. Morbidity and functional outcomes of salvage radical prostatectomy for locally recurrent prostate cancer after radiation therapy. J Urol. 2004;172(6 Pt 1):2239–43.

16. Vallancien G, Gupta R, Cathelineau X, Baumert H, Rozet F. Initial results of salvage laparoscopic radical prostatectomy after radiation failure. J Urol. 2003;170(5):1838–40.

17. Boris RS, Bhandari A, Krane LS, Eun D, Kaul S, Peabody JO. Salvage robotic-assisted radical prostatectomy: initial results and early report of outcomes. BJU Int. 2009;103(7):952–6.

18. Nunez-Mora C, Garcia-Mediero JM, Cabrera-Castillo PM. Radical laparoscopic salvage prostatectomy: medium-term functional and oncological results. J Endourol. 2009;23(8):1301–5.

19. Zugor V, Labanaris AP, Porres D, Heidenreich A, Witt JH. Robot-Assisted Radical Prostatectomy for the Treatment of Radiation-Resistant Prostate Cancer: Surgical, Oncological and Short-Term Functional Outcomes. Vanderbilt paper. J Urol 2013. Aug. 31, http/pubmed/24008772.

20. Nguyen PL, D'Amico AV, Lee AK, Suh WW. Patient selection, cancer control, and complications after salvage local therapy for postradiation prostate-specific antigen failure: a systematic review of the literature. Cancer. 2007;110(7):1417–28.

21. Bader P, Burkhard FC, Markwalder R, Studer UE. Is a limited lymph node dissection an adequate staging procedure for prostate cancer? J Urol. 2002;168(2):514–8. discussion 8.

22. Briganti A, Blute ML, Eastham JH, Graefen M, Heidenreich A, Karnes JR, et al. Pelvic lymph node dissection in prostate cancer. Eur Urol. 2009;55(6):1251–65.

23. Touijer K, Rabbani F, Otero JR, Secin FP, Eastham JA, Scardino PT, et al. Standard versus limited pelvic lymph node dissection for prostate cancer in patients with a predicted probability of nodal metastasis greater than 1%. J Urol. 2007;178(1):120–4.

Challenging Cases in Robotic Radical Prostatectomy

10

Gautam Jayram and Mohamad E. Allaf

Introduction

Although recent warnings regarding global PSA screening are anticipated to decrease the number of men treated for indolent prostate cancer, there are still close to 200,000 men diagnosed with the disease yearly [1]. Radical prostatectomy (RP) continues to be a common and effective treatment strategy for localized prostate cancer. The introduction of robotic technology has facilitated a minimally invasive approach to RP, and currently it is estimated that over 80 % of RPs across the USA are performed with robotic-assistance (RARP) [2]. As proficiency with RARP grows, seemingly more men are thought to be candidates for surgical therapy. Robotic surgeons are increasingly faced with a myriad of challenging clinical, preoperative, and intraoperative scenarios, which previously would have necessitated open surgery or non-surgical approaches. In this chapter we describe several such scenarios, and a practical approach for the management of each.

G. Jayram, M.D. (✉)
Brady Urological Institute, Johns Hopkins
Medical Institution, 600 N Wolfe Street Park 2,
Baltimore, MD 21287, USA
e-mail: Gjayram1@jhmi.edu

M.E. Allaf, M.D.
Urology and Oncology, Minimally Invasive
and Robotic Surgery, Brady Urological Institute,
Johns Hopkins Hospital, Baltimore, MD, USA

Obese Patient

Approximately one-third of Americans are now considered obese, double the incidence from 20 years ago [3]. The link between obesity and prostate cancer remains controversial; however, recent studies have shown obesity is associated with poorer pathologic and oncologic outcomes following treatment [4–8]. Obese men are also known to have worse perioperative outcomes following prostatectomy. A recent series of laparoscopic RP demonstrated higher rates of positive margins, urinary incontinence, and erectile dysfunction in obese men (BMI > 30) following surgery compared with non-obese men (BMI < 30). This finding has not correlated uniformly in the robotic literature; however, most series have supported poorer functional recovery and longer operative times in obese patients undergoing RARP [9–11]. In our experience, most obese men have poorer preoperative sexual and urinary parameters, as well as delayed diagnosis due to PSA dilution and/or surgeon reluctance to proceed with aggressive evaluation due to concomitant comorbidity.

Preoperatively, patients should be evaluated closely for cardiopulmonary disease. Coordination with the anesthesia team is critical, as these patients tend to be more hemodynamically sensitive to abdominal insufflation and Trendelenburg position. Further difficulties with intubation and ventilation are common, making preoperative planning with an experienced anesthesia team essential.

Intraoperatively, port placement and robotic positioning are vital to surgical success. The patient should be adequately secured to the operating table such that steep Trendelenburg does not cause the patient to slide once the ports have been placed. A gel mat on the table can increase the friction between the patient and the bed and minimize slippage. All pressure points should be padded and a face shield may be used to avoid inadvertent injury to the endotracheal tube and face due to robotic arm movement. Positioning injuries, neuropathy, and rhabdomyolysis are more common in prolonged procedures and we thus advocate that the patient is examined thoroughly at regular intervals throughout longer cases.

Veress access can be obtained transumbilically, as this is the area with the closest skin to peritoneum distance. Once insufflated, a long 12 mm camera port is preferred (Fig. 10.1) to maximize the utility of the camera during the surgery and

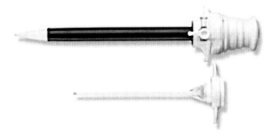

Fig. 10.1 Long 12 mm bladeless trocar used as camera port in obese patients

avoid port dislodgment. The camera port is placed approximately 16 cm cephalad from the pubic bone. We prefer using a visual obturator to introduce this initial port. It is critical to ensure that the holes on the insufflation port are intraperitoneal at all times during the procedure. This is because subcutaneous insufflation in addition to providing an inadequate working space will increase the skin to abdomen distance and may cause the ports to dislodge. Additionally, care should be taken to avoid angling ("skiving") the ports in obese patients as this will lead to decreased mobility of the robotic arms and assistant instruments. The lateral most ports on each side should be well away from the anterior superior iliac spine.

During the operation, obese patients can have extra adipose deposition in the posterior plane, making isolation of the seminal vesicles and vasa time-consuming. Opening the peritoneum widely here and judicious use of the assistant and fourth arm in this area is helpful. In cases with large amounts of fat and limited working space, the decision to drop the bladder and access the adnexal structures after incision of the bladder neck (anterior approach) may be time saving. Extensive periprostatic fat can complicate the incision of the endopelvic fascia and exposure of the dorsal vein. We meticulously release all this fat, especially at the apex, prior to incising the endopelvic fascia such that ideal visualization of these structures can be achieved (Fig. 10.2). Occasionally excessive bladder fat

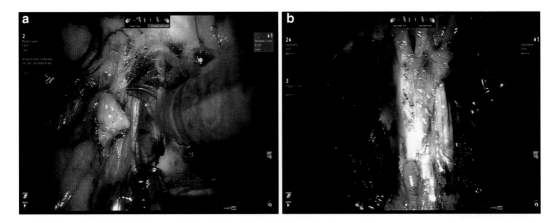

Fig. 10.2 (a) Meticulous removal of apical fat allows significantly improved visualization of the apex (b) in an obese patient with a large gland

or even mesenteric fat can push towards the prostate and obscure the surgical field. In this case, either the fourth arm or the assistant can aid with retraction. Additionally, while in non-obese patients a single camera angle (typically 0° lens) is adequate, the surgeon should not hesitate to change lens angles if need be to assist in visualization during certain parts of the procedure. For example a 30° down lens may be helpful during posterior bladder neck dissection. In our experience, the remainder of the procedure is relatively unaffected by the patients weight. As these patients often have narrow pelves, ample urethral length with a watertight tension-free anastomosis should be the goal. Should the shaft of the robotic instruments be clashing with the pelvis (particularly during the anastomosis), the bedside assistant can clutch the arm and move it into a more favorable position under direct vision of the surgical field while taking care to avoid any injury to adjacent organs.

Large Prostate

Patients with large prostates can cause a formidable challenge to the robotic surgeon due to decreased working space, impaired ability to retract the prostate to facilitate neurovascular bundle and pedicle exposure, and risk of violating the prostatic capsule during dissection. Existing literature regarding outcomes for large-gland RALP support its utilization and demonstrate feasibility. These studies have consistently documented higher operative times, slightly higher blood loss and lower positive margin rates in patients with glands >60 g compared with small or normal sized glands (Table 10.1) [12–15]. Long-term functional outcomes in this group have not been well characterized; however, there has been a suggestion of prolonged urinary incontinence in this group, most likely due to preexisting bladder dysfunction.

Table 10.1 Outcomes of RARP in patients with large prostates

Study	n	Prostate size (g)	OR time (min)	EBL (cc)	Positive margin (%)
Chan [12]	81	>75	234	152	9.9
Huang [13]	239	>63	164	214	10.3
Zorn [14]	31	>80	275	319	10.0
Link [15]	327	>70	192	250	21.2

Bladder Neck Identification and Transection

In patients with known large prostates, we prefer the posterior approach where the vasa and seminal vesicles are dissected and the prostate is freed off the rectum early in the case. The bladder neck dissection is notoriously difficult in these patients and having these structures pre-dissected simplifies this step.

The primary technical consideration in patients with large glands relates to the potential for significantly redundant bladder necks requiring reconstruction. In order to prevent this, we spend ample time making a precise determination of the prostatovesical junction prior to division. This can be facilitated by multiple maneuvers. The Foley catheter can be manipulated to see the site of balloon entrapment. Lateral displacement of the Foley catheter during this maneuver suggests a median lobe (see following section). Additionally, the bladder neck can be pinched by the robotic instruments on either side to trap the prostate. In this way the junction can be "palpated" when the prostate feels like it gives way into the bladder (Fig. 10.3). Lastly, the lateral contour of the prostate can be followed to the midline, where the transition from prostatic to perivesical fat signals the end of the bladder and start of the prostate.

Once the anterior bladder neck is incised, the catheter is visualized, pulled back and towards the anterior abdominal wall by the surgeon's

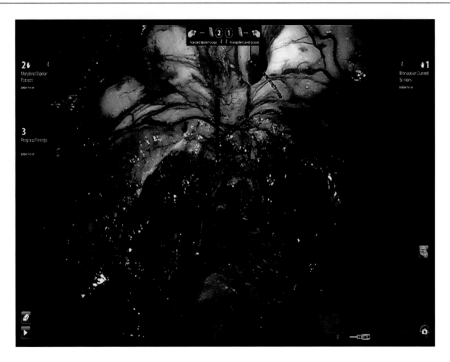

Fig. 10.3 Method of bladder neck identification using "palpation" of the prostatovesical junction

fourth arm or assistant. The posterior bladder neck is visualized and incised. In larger prostates changing to a 30° down lens can help better orient the surgeon during this step. Once the posterior mucosa has been incised through and through, it is grasped by the surgeon and retracted cephalad. The plane between the bladder and the prostate is entered. Care must be taken to avoid incising back towards the surgeon, which may result in "button-holing" of the bladder trigone close to the ureteral orifices. Expression of cloudy fluid usually suggests caudal deviation and entry into the prostate. Thin clear fibers signal entry into the correct plane, under which the seminal vesicles and vasa can be found. These are brought through the opening (if initially dissected at the start of the operation), retracted superiorly, and pedicle ligation and nerve dissection are performed in the standard manner.

Bladder Neck Reconstruction

An excessively large bladder neck can be tailored using a variety of techniques. If the ureteral orifices are far, we perform an anterior tennis racket repair. The bladder and urethra are brought together posteriorly per routine. As the anastomosis proceeds anteriorly, a separate suture is used to close the bladder anteriorly. Most of the time a single figure-of-eight stitch is all that is needed, but occasionally a longer suture line is required. The anastomosis is then completed.

If the ureteral orifices are close, we internalize them and tailor the bladder neck by the placement of a figure-of-eight closure stitch on each side of the bladder neck. At this point a routine anastomosis can be initiated and completed. The ureteral orifices are now internalized and thus not directly involved in the anastomosis.

Management of Median Lobe

Median lobes are more common in large prostates, and have an incidence of roughly 10–20 % based on intraoperative RALP documentation [16, 17]. Similar to large prostates, the main concern with this clinical scenario lies in the potential to lose the true anatomy of the bladder neck during posterior bladder neck division and potentially injure the ureteral orifices. Although preoperative

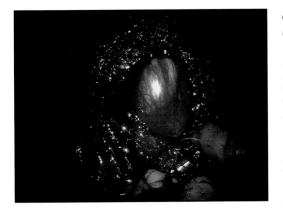

Fig. 10.4 Utilization of suture retraction of large median lobe to aid in bladder neck dissection

cystoscopy, cross-sectional imaging or transrectal ultrasound can all identify this variant, we do not believe this should alter the initial approach to the bladder neck and thus do not perform these procedures routinely preoperatively. A Foley balloon deviated off the midline or poor catheter drainage of the bladder can tip off the surgeon to a median lobe. Regardless, we utilize the same approach to the bladder neck as previously mentioned. If a median lobe is suspected, the bladder can be entered slightly more cranially to fully visualize the lobe. Once the catheter is identified and pulled up, a 2-0-polysorb suture is placed in a figure-of-eight fashion through the anterior part of the median lobe. If the median lobe is small it can be grasped with the fourth arm directly without an additional suture. The catheter is released and the fourth arm is used to hold this suture (or median lobe directly) and retract it towards the anterior abdominal wall (Fig. 10.4). This allows adequate inspection of the posterior bladder neck and identification of the plane between the adenoma and the trigone. Excessive bleeding during this step could indicate entry into the prostate as the plane between the adenoma and bladder is relatively avascular. Indigo carmine can be utilized if there is concern about the proximity of the ureteral orifices. This is usually not necessary, however, and once the median lobe is sufficiently elevated the posterior bladder neck dissection can proceed as previously described. Large bladder necks fre-

quently result and can be reconstructed as previously described.

The published results of RALP in patients with median lobes suggest that in experienced hands, the presence of a median lobe prolongs operative time but has no impact on perioperative or functional outcomes [16–18].

Previous Bladder Outlet Surgery

Fibrosis at the bladder neck following previous surgery for BPH (Greenlight, HoLEP, TURP) can complicate RARP and cause similar bladder neck concerns as the previous clinical scenarios. Additionally, a thickened bladder wall and scarred urethra may compromise the anastomosis and increase the risk of postoperative incontinence. Unlike the case of a large prostate or median lobe, existing data suggest uniformly worse outcomes in patients undergoing minimally invasive radical prostatectomy after TURP, including higher rates of incontinence and positive surgical margins [19–21]. Given the potential for severe periprostatic inflammation following a bladder outlet procedure (especially TURP), it is advised to wait for at least 3 months prior to performing radical prostatectomy. In our experience, the inflammatory process is particularly pronounced if the prostatic capsule had been violated during the outlet procedure. The prostatovesical junction is often quite scarred and careful attention to the ureteral orifices and the lateral contour of the prostate is necessary to avoid entering an unfavorable plane. Nerve-sparing, particularly at the apex can be difficult, and typical intraoperative cues regarding cancer extent can be lost.

Prior Hernia Repair

An increasing proportion of patients with prior hernia repairs are being encountered during RALP. The use of mesh during inguinal hernia repair was once thought to be a relative contraindication for radical prostatectomy due to obliteration of the space of Retzius. This is especially worrisome with laparoscopic inguinal hernia repair, as the mesh is placed directly into the preperitoneal space and tacked to the pelvic bones. This has not proven to be the case, however, as multiple series in both the open and minimally invasive literature suggest feasibility with no difference in safety, oncologic, or functional outcomes compared to patients without hernia repair [22–24]. Adequate pelvic lymphadenectomy in patients with mesh has been a recurrent concern in open and laparoscopic RP series; however, the robotic literature has not shown a difference in adequacy of lymph node yield [24]. Mesh repairs appear to elicit a greater inflammatory response and therefore have been associated with longer RALP operative times [23]. In most cases of repaired inguinal hernias, the edge of the mesh can be located lateral to the appropriate plane of dissection to drop the bladder off the anterior abdominal wall. Occasionally, bowel or bladder contents can become adherent to the fibrotic mesh and sharp dissection is needed to free these structures from the mesh. Rarely, the mesh itself needs to be incised to safely drop the bladder. If the surgeon is encountering difficulty with this step, the bladder can be filled to delineate its borders for safer dissection. If significant disruption to the hernia repair is needed to perform the prostatectomy, permanent sutures can be used to reinforce the hernia defect prior to completion of the operation. In cases of unrepaired inguinal hernias repairs, a tongue of bladder can rarely slip into the hernia sac; this must be treated with caution and the hernia sac extracted from the hernia defect as much as possible prior to ligation, otherwise an inadvertent cystotomy may result.

In cases of existing umbilical hernias, usually Veress access is obtained laterally on the abdominal wall to avoid possible injury of hernia sac contents. Once the abdomen is insufflated and visualized, the midline camera port can be slightly adjusted to avoid any mesh or hernia sac present. Reports of utilizing the hernia defect as the robotic camera port have also been described [25]. Following the conclusion of the procedure, the extraction site should be extended to include the midline defect, and the hernia sac should be excised and removed with the prostate. The fascial closure serves as the hernia repair and can be sufficient to prevent recurrence.

Prior Abdominal/GI Surgery

A thorough surgical history and inspection of a patient's abdomen preoperatively is important prior to RARP. Extensive abdominal surgery raises the risk of intraabdominal adhesions and altered anatomy and should be approached with extreme caution. A study of 4,000 robotic prostatectomy patients indicated a threefold increased rate of adhesiolysis performed in patients with prior abdominal or inguinal surgery compared to those without [26]. In this study prior colectomy carried the highest incidence of adhesiolysis requirement (72 %). Reports of an extraperitoneal approach to RARP have been advocated and may facilitate the procedure in patients with prior transperitoneal operations [27, 28]. Our approach is to obtain Veress access at a point safely away from abdominal scars. In the case of a previous lower midline incision, we place the Veress needle around Palmer's point in the left upper quadrant below the costal margin. Following adequate abdominal insufflation, the laparoscope is place through a 12 mm visual obturator port and the layers of the abdomen are carefully entered under vision. Upon abdominal entry, the degree and nature of abdominal adhesions can be ascertained. In many cases the traditional port placement can be minimally modified and the procedure can be started without significant adhesiolysis. In severe cases, however, another port can be placed and laparoscopic adhesiolysis can facilitate port placement. If placement of another port is not feasible, a "working" laparoscope or nephroscope with a built-in working channel can be utilized and the adhesions taken down through a single trocar [29].

Once the procedure is underway, any further adhesions in the pelvis can usually be taken down robotically. Especially in cases where extended lymphadenectomy (eLND) is planned, this adhesiolysis is important to fully delineate retroperitoneal anatomy. In experienced hands, the presence of prior abdominal surgery does not appear to affect the incidence of bowel injury, operative time, or overall outcomes [26]. It is important, however, to counsel the patient preoperatively regarding the risk of bowel injury and discuss the existence and safety of alternative extraperitoneal surgical techniques.

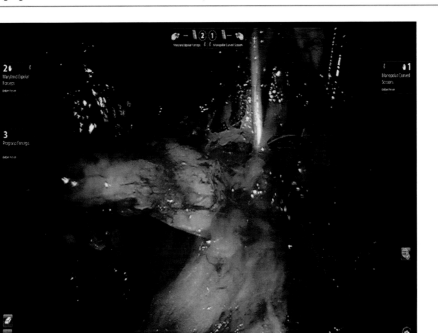

Fig. 10.5   Exposure of the obturator nerve while mobilizing a large nodal packet during ePLND

Extended Lymphadenectomy

Multiple studies have suggested a therapeutic (in addition to prognostic) ability of LND in prostate cancer [30, 31]. Furthermore, there appears to be a continued benefit in intermediate- or high risk men with an extended pelvic lymph node dissection (ePLND) in terms of overall and positive nodes retrieved. EPLND has been traditionally defined as bilateral excision of the external iliac, obturator, and hypogastric nodal groups. Available data in the robotic era suggest slight increases in operative time with ePLND, and however no increase in complications (lympoceles or others) [32]. Our preference is to perform ePLND on intermediate and high-risk patients. Following the posterior dissection of the adnexa and prior to releasing the bladder from the anterior abdominal wall, ePLND is performed. The pulsation of the external iliac artery is identified, and the posterior peritoneum is incised just medial to this. Blunt dissection is used to find the external iliac vein, and the lymphadenectomy is begun at the medial aspect of this

landmark, which serves as the lateral boundary of the dissection. The plane deep to this towards the back wall is found, and all fibrofatty tissue is released from the bifurcation of the iliac artery to the iliofemoral (Cloquet's node) junction distally. Once this is accomplished, attention is turned to the medial borders of the lymphadenectomy. The medial umbilical ligament is isolated and the fourth arm or the assistant retracts this structure medially. This maneuver prevents inadvertent ureteral dissection (the ureter will always be medial to the ligament) and allows identification of a loose areolar plane that serves as the medial border of dissection. The packet can now be taken en bloc starting distally. Care must be taken to identify and avoid the obturator nerve, which is seen once the obturator fossa is exposed as the packet is mobilized proximally (Fig. 10.5). Following excision the packet can be placed in an endocatch bag and retrieved immediately or placed in the abdomen and retrieved with the prostate at the conclusion of the procedure. It is important to note that we advocate the use of clips for lymphostasis, as the intraperitoneal technique does not eliminate the risk of lymphocele formation. In our experience, this dissection adds 20–30 min to overall operative time, and however clearly has increased overall nodal yield without any increase in complications or perioperative morbidity.

References

1. Jemal A, Siegel R, Ward E, et al. Cancer statistics, 2008. CA Cancer J Clin. 2008;58:71.
2. Intuitive Surgical, Inc. 10-K Annual report pursuant to section 13 and 15(d), filed on 2/1/11, filed period 12/31/10. http://phx.corporate-ir.net/phoenix.zhtml?c=122359&p=irol-sec&secCat011_rs=1&secCat01.1_re-10
3. Flegal KM, Carroll MD, Ogden CL, et al. Prevalence and trends in obesity among US adults, 1999–2000. JAMA. 2002;288:1723–7.
4. Calle EE, Rodriguez C, Walker-Thurmond K, et al. Overweight, obesity, and mortality from cancer in a prospectively studied cohort of U.S. adults. N Engl J Med. 2003;348:1625–38.
5. Amling CL, Riffenburgh RH, Sun L, et al. Pathologic variables and recurrence rates as related to obesity and race in men with prostate cancer undergoing radical prostatectomy. J Clin Oncol. 2004;22:439–45.
6. MacInnis RJ, English DR. Body size and composition and prostate cancer risk: systematic review and meta-regression analysis. Cancer Causes Control. 2006;17: 989–1003.
7. Capitanio U, Suardi N, Briganti A, et al. Influence of obesity on tumour volume in patients with prostate cancer. BJU Int. 2012;109:678–84.
8. Campeggi A, Xylinas E, Ploussard G, et al. Impact of body mass index on perioperative morbidity, oncological, and functional outcomes after extraperitoneal laparoscopic radical prostatectomy. Urology. 2012; 80:576–84.
9. Wiltz AL, Shikanov S, Eggener SE, et al. Robotic radical prostatectomy in overweight and obese patients: oncological and validated-functional outcomes. Urology. 2009;73(2):316–22.
10. Castle EP, Atug F, Woods M, et al. Impact of body mass index on outcomes after robot assisted radical prostatectomy. World J Urol. 2008;26(1):91–5.
11. Ahlering TE, Eichel L, Edwards R, et al. Impact of obesity on clinical outcomes in robotic prostatectomy. Urology. 2005;65(4):740–4.
12. Chan RC, Barocas DA, Chang SS, et al. Effect of a large prostate gland on open and robotically assisted laparoscopic radical prostatectomy. BJU Int. 2008; 101(9):1140–4.
13. Huang AC, Kowalczyk KJ, Hevelone ND, et al. The impact of prostate size, median lobe, and prior benign prostatic hyperplasia intervention on robot-assisted laparoscopic prostatectomy: technique and outcomes. Eur Urol. 2011;59(4):595–603.
14. Zorn KC, Orvieto MA, Mikhail AA, et al. Effect of prostate weight on operative and postoperative outcomes of robotic-assisted laparoscopic prostatectomy. Urology. 2007;69(2):300–5.
15. Link BA, Nelson R, Josephson DY, et al. The impact of prostate gland weight in robot assisted laparoscopic radical prostatectomy. J Urol. 2008;180(3):928–32.
16. Rehman J, Chughtai B, Guru K, et al. Management of an enlarged median lobe with ureteral orifices at the margin of the bladder neck during robotic-assisted laparoscopic prostatectomy. Can J Urol. 2009;16:4490–4.
17. Coelho RF, Chauhan S, Guglielmetti GB, et al. Does the presence of median lobe affect outcomes of robot-assisted laparoscopic radical prostatectomy? J Endourol. 2012;26(3):264–70.
18. Meeks JJ, Zhao L, Greco KA, et al. Impact of prostate median lobe anatomy on robotic-assisted laparoscopic prostatectomy. Urology. 2009;73(2):323–7.
19. Gupta NP, Singh P, Nayyar R, et al. Outcomes of robot-assisted radical prostatectomy in men with previous transurethral resection of the prostate. BJU Int. 2011;108(9):1501–5.
20. Jaffe J, Stakhovsky O, Cathelineau X, et al. Surgical outcomes for men undergoing laparoscopic radical prostatectomy after transurethral resection of the prostate. J Urol. 2007;178:483–7.
21. Katz R, Borkowski T, Hoznek A, et al. Laparoscopic radical prostatectomy in patients following transurethral resection of the prostate. Urol Int. 2006;77: 216–21.
22. Erdogru T, Teber D, Frede T, et al. The effect of previous transperitoneal laparoscopic inguinal herniorrhaphy on transperitoneal laparoscopic radical prostatectomy. J Urol. 2005;173(3):769–72.
23. Laungani RG, Kaul S, Muhletaler F, et al. Impact of previous inguinal hernia repair on transperitoneal robotic prostatectomy. Can J Urol. 2007;14(4):3635–9.
24. Hiafler M, Benjamin B, Ghinea R, et al. The impact of previous laparoscopic hernia repair on radical prostatectomy. J Endourol. 2012;26(11):1458–62.
25. Kim W, Abdelshehid C, Lee HJ, et al. Robotic-assisted laparoscopic prostatectomy in umbilical hernia patients: University of California, Irvine, technique for port placement and repair. Urology. 2012;79(6):1412–7.
26. Siddiqui SA, Krane LS, Bhandari A. The impact of previous inguinal or abdominal surgery on outcomes after robotic radical prostatectomy. Urology. 2010; 75(5):1079–82.
27. Atug F, Castle EP, Woods M, et al. Transperitoneal versus extraperitoneal robotic-assisted radical prostatectomy: is one better than the other? Urology. 2006;68(5):1077–81.

28. Horstmann M, Vollmer C, Schwab C, et al. Single-centre evaluation of the extraperitoneal and transperitoneal approach in robotic-assisted radical prostatectomy. Scand J Urol Nephrol. 2012;46(2): 117–23.

29. Boylu U, Oommen M, Raynor M, et al. Robot-assisted laparoscopic radical prostatectomy in patients with previous abdominal surgery: a novel laparoscopic adhesiolysis technique. J Endourol. 2010; 24(2):229–32.

30. Joslyn SA, Konety BR. Impact of extent of lymphadenectomy on survival after radical prostatectomy for prostate cancer. Urology. 2006;68:121–5.

31. Hyndman ME, Mullins JK, Pavlovich CP. Pelvic node dissection in prostate cancer: extended, limited, or not at all? Curr Opin Urol. 2010;20(3):211–7.

32. Yuh BE, Ruel NH, Mejia R, et al. Standardized comparison of robot-assisted limited and extended pelvic lymphadenectomy for prostate cancer. BJU Int. 2013;112(1):81–8.

Postoperative Management: Erectile Function

11

Robert L. Segal, Arthur L. Burnett, and Trinity J. Bivalacqua

Abbreviations

cGMP   Cyclic guanosine monophosphate
ED   Erectile dysfunction
EHS   Erection hardness score
EPO   Erythropoietin
ICI   Intracavernous injection
IIEF   International index of erectile function
IUA   Intraurethral alprostadil
MCID   Minimally clinical important difference
MUSE   Medicated urethral system for erection
NO   Nitric oxide
NVB   Neurovascular bundle
PDE   5-Phosphodiesterase-5
PFBT   Pelvic floor biofeedback training
QEQ   Quality of erection questionnaire
SHIM   Sexual health inventory for men
VED   Vacuum erection device

R.L. Segal, M.D., F.R.C.S. (C)
A.L. Burnett, M.D., M.B.A.
T.J. Bivalacqua, M.D., Ph.D. (✉)
Urology Department, Johns Hopkins Hospital,
600 N. Wolfe St., Marburg 409, Baltimore,
MD 21287, USA
e-mail: tbivala1@jhmi.edu

Introduction

The two most common long-term complications following radical prostatectomy are erectile dysfunction and urinary incontinence. The complication that is perhaps most feared, however, may be ED [1]. In fact, in one study, the impact of ED on quality of life was more severe than urinary incontinence [2]. While in most series the risk of persistent incontinence is low, the risk for ED is much higher, even in the ideal surgical candidate (most urologic oncologists choose young, healthy men who have the greatest ability to recover erections after bilateral nerve-sparing radical prostatectomy). Furthermore, even if recovery is achieved, it very often is a long, protracted course which can take years, whereas urinary continence is often recovered within weeks to months. As such, although incontinence may be encountered on a daily basis, because it is transient, ED may actually be more impactful overall. Moreover, global sexual function can be impacted postprostatectomy beyond solely the absence of rigid erections, which may affect the perception of how impotence (a catch-all term for sexual dysfunction, often used interchangeably with ED) has compromised quality of life. This includes reduced sexual drive/libido (especially in the context of adjuvant androgen deprivation therapy), dysorgasmia, anorgasmia, climacturia, loss of penile length, and penile curvature. Nevertheless, the purpose of this chapter is to review ED following radical prostatectomy. The prevalence, pathophysiology, assessment of and treatments for post-prostatectomy ED will be discussed. Additionally, the concept of and examples for penile rehabilitation, as well as future directions for necessary research, are covered.

Prevalence of Post-prostatectomy Erectile Dysfunction

The exact prevalence of ED post-radical prostatectomy is not truly known, and there is a wide reported range within the literature, from 20 to 90 % [1, 3, 4]. Even in more contemporary series, rates are still wide-ranging, ranging from 63 to 94 % [5]. The reasons for this disparity are numerous, and relate to patient-, disease-, and surgeon-related factors, as well as reporting biases.

It is well established that patient systemic comorbidity (obesity, hypertension, dyslipidemia, diabetes mellitus, atherosclerotic cardiovascular disease, smoking, and hypogonadism) contributes to organic ED [6, 7], and should not be ignored in patients undergoing radical prostatectomy. Furthermore, other patient factors, such as age, race, body mass index, and pretreatment erectile function are associated with postoperative erectile functional recovery [8, 9].

Features of prostate cancer, including preoperative serum prostate-specific antigen level, as well as pathological features such as clinical and pathological staging and Gleason score [8, 10], have been shown to influence erection recovery.

Surgeon-related factors ultimately have the greatest influence which would include degree and quality of nerve-sparing [11, 12]. Interestingly, while increasing surgical experience and progression along the learning curve for robotic-assisted radical prostatectomy has shown improvements in mean operative time, blood loss, positive surgical margin rates, and continence, this has not translated to recovery of erections [13]. It is still up for debate whether surgical approach (open, laparoscopic, robotic-assisted radical prostatectomy) impacts on erectile functional recovery [14–16]. The rate of erection recovery and thus ED rates is more a factor of surgeon expertise and nerve-sparing, and not the surgical approach.

Inconsistencies between studies and overall lack of uniformity of definitions preclude definitive understanding of the true impact of radical prostatectomy on ED and functional recovery. For example, in a recent meta-analysis, Tal et al. [17] reported that after evaluation of over 200 studies, there were 22 ways of defining favorable erectile functional recovery. Furthermore, variations in outcomes have been reported based on whether the study derived from single/multisurgeon or single/multicenter authors [18]. Another issue which is important to acknowledge is time to recovery. Intuitively, as time passes from surgery, erectile recovery will improve. Historically, most recovery was expected within 2 years of surgery [19]. Further study has demonstrated that recovery may extend beyond 2 years, and continue up to 4 years after prostatectomy [20]. Another concept that is perhaps not yet adequately addressed in the literature is "back-to-baseline," the ability for men to return to their preoperative erectile function after surgery, which is potentially considerably different than the return of erections capable of penetrative intercourse. Only 4–27 % of patients have been noted to achieve this outcome [18, 21]. Finally, selection bias, use of erectile aids such as phosphodiesterase-5 (PDE-5) inhibitors and use of validated questionnaires to define potency or the absence thereof, reported within the studies, can influence the appreciation of true post-prostatectomy ED.

When counseling patients prior to undergoing surgery, it is incumbent upon the surgeon to be honest and forthcoming about his/her own operative outcomes, such as experience and controllable factors such as quality of nerve-sparing, so that the patient has a realistic expectation of what his recovery potential may be postoperatively.

Pathophysiology of Post-prostatectomy ED

There are several underlying mechanisms of ED post-radical prostatectomy. Perhaps the most significant contributor is injury to the cavernous nerves, which may result from traction, thermal injury, or transection. These nerves evoke erection primarily via stimulation of nitric oxide (NO), which results in smooth muscle relaxation via intracellular calcium sequestration and potassium egress, as a result of cyclic guanosine monophosphate (cGMP) production from guanylate cyclase [22, 23]. Neural trauma may lead to a reduction in neuronal nitric oxide synthase [24], and corporal smooth muscle atrophy and fibrosis [25]. The delay in return of erectile function post-prostatectomy may reflect a healing neuropraxia.

Arteriogenic ED, resulting in insufficient penile arterial circulation, beyond systemic causes (smoking, dyslipidemia, hypertension), may result from transection of accessory or aberrant pudendal arteries, which can be the sole arterial supply to the corpora cavernosa unilaterally or bilaterally. This is not universal, however, as these are absent in up to 25 % of men [26]. Nevertheless, preservation of these vessels may lead to improved outcomes [27]. In assessing men up to 1 year after radical prostatectomy, one study revealed evidence for arterial insufficiency in 59 % of men [28].

Venogenic ED is based on corporal smooth muscle fibrosis, with evidence of increased expression of pro-fibrotic cytokines such as TGF-β which lead to heightened collagen expression [29]. This scarring results in veno-occlusive dysfunction, in that the tunica albuginea are incapable of expanding sufficiently to allow for compression of subtunical venules and blood retention within the penis. Clinically, even in the presence of good arterial penile inflow, this manifests as the patient being able to achieve, but not maintain, an erection satisfactory for penetrative intercourse. Mulhall et al. [28] demonstrated that the risk of this phenomenon increases over time, with a peak at 12 months post-prostatectomy, in up to 50 % of patients. Furthermore, a statistically significantly smaller proportion of patients with venogenic ED subsequently recover functional erections compared to patients with arteriogenic ED.

Finally, Peyronie's disease has been noted to be more common in men post-prostatectomy than in the general population [30]. Risk factors for Peyronie's development specifically in post-prostatectomy patients include younger age and Caucasian race. In patients with Peyronie's disease, the risk of ED is up to 50 % [31]. While a direct link between the surgery itself and the subsequent development of Peyronie's has not been found, it has been speculated that penile curvature results from attempts at intercourse with a relatively flaccid penis, with ensuing tunical injury and scarring [32]. This scarring results in veno-occlusive dysfunction.

Measurement of Erectile Function

Although the diagnosis of ED is clinical and can be derived from a thorough history and physical examination, the severity, degree of bother and response to therapy are not as easy to decipher. It is well established that the definition of potency may vary amongst patients [33], and surgeons' estimation of symptoms do not correlate with patient self-assessment, with a great tendency for underestimation [34, 35]. As such, it is critical for clinicians to rely upon patient self-reported outcomes for such assessments. Furthermore, the use of such standard questionnaires enables data comparisons between institutions, and facilitates communication between healthcare professionals. Caution must be taken to allow the patients to respond to quality of life questionnaires without the influence of outside parties, especially the surgeon, which will introduce bias.

There are several validated questionnaires available to aid in the assessment of ED. A relatively new tool employed for mostly research use is the Expanded Prostate Cancer Index Composite (EPIC), a 50-item instrument designed specifically to assess health-related quality of life in men with prostate cancer, derived from the University of California-Los Angeles Prostate Cancer Index (UCLA-PCI) [36, 37]. It can be used for men undergoing any prostate cancer treatment modality and covers several areas: urinary function, bowel habits, sexual function, hormonal function, and overall satisfaction. There are 13 questions relating to sexual function, including bother. The EPIC has been shortened to a 26-item questionnaire for use in the clinic [38]. ED Severity can be estimated using validated questionnaires-the Erectile Function domain of the International Index of Erectile Function (IIEF-EF) [39] is a six question survey derived from the overall 15-question IIEF which assesses erectile function over the previous 4 weeks, scored on a scale of 1–30. Severity is determined based on overall score: ≥ 26, no ED; 18–25, mild ED; 11–17, moderate ED; ≤ 10, severe ED. Similarly, the Sexual Health Inventory for Men (SHIM) [40] is a 5-question survey with a score range of 1–25, which assesses erectile function over the previous 6 months: ≥ 22, no ED; 17–21, mild ED; 12–16, mild–moderate ED; 8–11 moderate ED; ≤ 7, severe ED.

There are two questionnaires which directly address the issue of erectile rigidity. The Quality of Erection Questionnaire (QEQ) [41] is a six question survey that ranges from 0 to 100 with higher scores representing better rigidity, and should take approximately 3 min to complete. The Erection Hardness Score (EHS) [42] is a 4-question survey, with the scores defined as: (1) penis is larger but not hard, (2) penis is hard, but not hard enough for penetration, (3) penis is hard enough for penetration, but not fully hard, and (4) penis is completely hard and fully rigid. These scores have been shown to be well associated with the likelihood of successful sexual intercourse [43].

The aforementioned questionnaires may be employed at different time points (such as baseline prior to radical prostatectomy, prior to and after initiating therapy) to assess any differences in scores, which may reflect significant improvement in the overall condition. The concept of "minimally clinical important difference" (MCID) when employing validated questionnaires has been emphasized in sexual dysfunction research [44]. Specific calculations of the MCID have been calculated for the IIEF-EF [45] and QEQ [46]. For questionnaires wherein the MCID has not been specifically calculated, a reliable estimate is one-half of the standard deviation [47]. Alternatively, to assess patient satisfaction with an ED treatment, which incorporates the success of the treatment, one may use the Erectile Dysfunction Inventory of Treatment Satisfaction (EDITS), an 11-point questionnaire which specifically explores outcomes with medical ED treatments [48].

The ideal cutoff to determine erectile functional recovery after radical prostatectomy has yet to be unequivocally defined. Ficarra et al. [49] proposed that a cutoff of 17 on the IIEF-EF correlated with a higher health-related quality of life, whereas another study defined erectile recovery as IIEF-EF ≥ 22 [50]. Indeed, it has been shown that 28 % of men with IIEF-EF scores of 22–25 are able to definitely "have sex whenever [they] want" [51]. As will be evident upon review of the studies presented later in this chapter, there is indeed no standardized cutoff employed for the definition of potency post-prostatectomy, which may limit the generalizability of the outcomes of these studies, and underscores the need for more stringent criteria in this area.

Post-prostatectomy ED Treatment

There are several options for treatment of ED post-prostatectomy, including PDE-5 inhibitors, intracavernosal penile injection therapy, vacuum erection devices, intraurethral suppositories, and penile prostheses. There is abundant evidence for each supporting their use, and decisions regarding which option to try should be based on a thorough discussion between clinician and patient. In terms of issues to consider when discussing treatment for ED following radical prostatectomy are the potential benefits, risks, side effects, complications and cost of each option, but also the goals and expectations of the patient and their partner. Expectations are particularly critical to discuss, as post-prostatectomy ED, especially for men who prior to surgery had normal function, can be very difficult to adjust to. The prospect of natural recovery certainly offers hope and optimism, but the protracted course of recovery is still challenging. Patients must be counseled that while rigid erections for penetrative intercourse can almost certainly be restored depending on how far they are willing to go with these therapeutic options, each has their own drawbacks. The options will be discussed in detail below.

PDE-5 Inhibitors

The currently available PDE-5 inhibitors in the USA include sildenafil, vardenafil, and tadalafil. A new drug, avanafil, a more rapid-acting PDE-5 inhibitor, has been approved by the FDA and will soon be available in the USA [52]. They all function by inhibiting the enzyme phosphodiesterase subtype 5, which prevents the metabolism of cGMP and promotes cavernosal smooth muscle relaxation. They are considered first-line therapy for ED treatment, including those patients that suffer from ED post-radical prostatectomy [53–55]. This relates to their general tolerability (although possible side effects include headache, flushing, dizziness, gastrointestinal upset, cyanopsia for sildenafil, and low back pain for tadalafil) and facility in use. In the post-prostatectomy context, success is more likely if a nerve-sparing approach to surgery has been employed, although still possible even in a non-nerve-sparing situation [56]. Furthermore, reasonable expectations are that success with PDE-5 inhibitors will be greater if patients are able to generate spontaneous partial erections prior to attempts at using this pharmacotherapy; if men are unable to generate any spontaneous erectile tumescence, the likelihood of satisfactory erections for penetrative intercourse is low with PDE-5 inhibitor usage. Finally, although the optimal dosing strategy is debatable, the approach at our institution is to initiate the patient on the highest dose to maximize potential efficacy, and to titrate down based on effect or development of adverse effects.

There is ample evidence of successful use of PDE-5 inhibitors for ED treatment post-radical prostatectomy. The majority of reported data is based upon sildenafil use. While multiple studies have confirmed the potential utility of sildenafil in this circumstance [57–59], the data suggests that outcomes are best for bilateral nerve-sparing surgeries (compared to unilateral or non-nerve-sparing surgeries), and for younger men. These studies are limited by their single-institutional nature, small subject population, lack of validated erectile functional assessments and/or heterogenous follow-up. It can be variable at what

point following surgery the treatment may demonstrate efficacy. However, it has been shown that the benefit of sildenafil for ED treatment can be sustained: in a small, single-institutional study, after 3 years, 31/43 (73 %) patients were still satisfactorily using sildenafil. Only 5/43 (11.6 %) reported loss of efficacy of the medication [60].

Nehra and colleagues [61] studied 440 patients who had previously undergone nerve-sparing surgery (mean 1.7 years prior to enrollment) who were randomized to placebo, vardenafil 10 mg or vardenafil 20 mg to take in an on-demand fashion for 12 weeks after a 4 week treatment-free screening period. Patients in the vardenafil groups were noted to have significantly higher scores in IIEF intercourse satisfaction, orgasmic function and overall sexual satisfaction domains, as well as erection hardness scores, compared to placebo. Additionally, vardenafil 20 mg was also noted to lessen depressive symptoms.

The effect of tadalafil, the longer-acting PDE-5 inhibitor, on ED therapy post-prostatectomy has been confirmed [62]. In this placebo-controlled, double-blind randomized study, 303 men 12–48 months following bilateral nerve-sparing surgery were assessed, randomized to receive tadalafil 20 mg on demand ($n = 201$) or placebo ($n = 102$) for 12 weeks after a 4-week treatment-free run-in period. Patients in the tadalafil group had a statistically significantly higher IIEF-EF score and reported higher proportion of successful penetration and intercourse attempts.

A placebo-controlled, randomized trial assessing the efficacy of avanafil in the treatment of ED following bilateral nerve-sparing radical prostatectomy has been conducted, although not yet published [63]. Two hundred and ninety-eight men, mean age 58.4 years, mean 19.2 months after surgery with resultant ED, were randomized to receive either placebo, avanafil 100 or 200 mg for 12 weeks. Mean IIEF-EF score prior to initiating therapy was 9.2, and 72 % of men categorized their ED as "severe." Erectile function was followed at 4-week intervals, and after 12 weeks, both avanafil doses were significantly superior to placebo. Improvements in IIEF-EF scores of 3.6 (40 %) and 5.2 (55 %) points were noted for the avanafil 100 mg and 200 mg groups, respectively, compared to 0.1 (1 %) for placebo.

Overall, PDE-5 inhibitors can be efficacious in post-prostatectomy ED therapy. When presenting all treatment options, clinicians should present realistic expectations about the efficacy of these medications, and should consider their judicious use, perhaps more enthusiastically in younger men with bilateral nerve-sparing surgeries.

Intracavernosal Injection Therapy

Intracavernosal Injection (ICI) is a very effective treatment for ED. It generally involves instruction in the clinic as to the injection technique, and often includes the patient performing a test injection under supervision, to assess ability to actually perform the injection, to ensure no complications, and to gauge the proper injection drug cocktail and dosing. There are a variety of drug choices to be used, such as alprostadil (synthetic prostaglandin E1), papaverine, phentolamine, forskolin and atropine. These drugs may be used individually, or can be mixed together, and different concentrations of each drug may be employed. Overall, injections are well tolerated, although the patient should be counseled as to the possible adverse effects, including bleeding/hematoma, pain at the injection site, penile pain (predominantly from alprostadil injection), penile fibrosis/scarring (predominantly from papaverine), priapism, and lack of efficacy of the therapy. The patient must be detumesced prior to discharge from the clinic, to make certain that priapism will not result. The only absolute contraindication to considering ICI use is inability for either the patient or his partner to perform the injections, although caution should be taken in patients with a previous history of or tendency towards priapism, as well as those patients on anticoagulation or with bleeding tendencies.

ICI has been shown in studies to be an effective post-prostatectomy ED treatment. In an observational study, Ciaro et al. [64] retrospectively demonstrated that in 168 men with normal preoperative erectile function, among whom over 40 % had failed prior ED treatments, ICI with triple therapy (alprostadil, papaverine, and phentolamine) yielded successful intercourse with a rigid erection in 94.6 % of patients. In a study assessing long-term efficacy and compliance with ICI, Raina et al. [65] showed that one-third of men post-prostatectomy who presented with ED (102/306) chose ICI as first-line therapy. Of these, 48 % (49/102) continued long-term therapy (mean 3.7 years), with significant increases in SHIM scores compared to the immediate postoperative status. Furthermore, SHIM scores while using ICI were similar to preoperative scores. Finally, although pain with ICI is possible, it has been demonstrated that subjective pain scores decrease over time [66].

In an interesting study, a progressive protocol for ED treatment post-prostatectomy was assessed [67]. Most surgeries were non-nerve-sparing, and treatments were started 1.5–2.5 months after surgery. Patients were initiated on VED therapy, and were progressed to the next phase of ED treatment only if treatment failed. While 92 % of patients had "successful" treatment with VED, only 14 % were satisfied with the treatment. As such, they were progressed to sildenafil therapy, of whom only 20 % had a positive response. Those patients who did not have a response to sildenafil were given ICI with papaverine, phentolamine and prostaglandin E1, with 85 % having successful responses. For those who did not, the final progression was to ICI + VED. After 1 year of follow-up, 76/80 men were still successfully using therapy, with 9 % using VED, 14 % sildenafil, 71 % ICI and 5 % ICI + VED. Overall, these studies, although hampered by the use of non-validated erectile questionnaires, demonstrated that a thorough progressive approach to ED management post-prostatectomy can be successful, with ICI being the most effective nonsurgical therapy.

Vacuum Erection Device

The vacuum erection device (VED) is a popular choice for post-prostatectomy ED treatment by virtue of its noninvasive nature and the fact that no medication is required. The device is applied to the penis, and when activated, deoxygenated blood is drawn into the penis by vacuum effect, which results in engorgement and rigidity. Often times, a constriction ring is applied to the base of the penis to prevent blood egress. Drawbacks of the VED include atypical erection, which can feel cold and not as rigid as a natural erection, with possible erectile instability proximal to the constriction ring. Furthermore, the patient may experience penile numbness, as well as bruising and discomfort from the presence of the ring, which may bother the partner as well.

There are actually few studies specifically examining the role of VED in the treatment of post-prostatectomy ED, so data must be extrapolated from overall ED studies. Overall, there is a dropout rate of over 50 %, although patient satisfaction may be as high as 89 % [68].

Intraurethral Suppositories

Intraurethral Alprostadil (prostaglandin E1) suppositories (IUA) (otherwise known as MUSE-Medicated Urethral System for Erection) have been documented to be successful in treating organic ED [69]. The medication is absorbed from the urethra into the corpus spongiosum, and then into the corpora cavernosa, resulting in the erectile response. Typically patients are instructed as to the technique in clinic, and a test dose administered under clinical supervision to ensure correct suppository application, to verify proper dosing and to confirm absence of side effects, which principally include penile/urethral pain and hypotension.

IUA has been successful in treating post-prostatectomy ED. Costabile et al. [70] compared outcomes for men with organic ($n = 1127$) versus post-prostatectomy ($n = 384$) ED, and found the overall success rate for intercourse for IUA was 40 %. Post-prostatectomy ED patients had lower likelihood of treatment resulting in successful intercourse (57.1 % vs. 67.8 %, $p = 0.033$). The proportion of administrations of the medication which resulted in intercourse increased over time, from 63 % in the first month of therapy to 73 % by the third month.

In another study of 54 men with impaired erectile function prior to prostatectomy, 48 % of patients achieved successful intercourse with IUA, with a mean increase in their SHIM score of 10 points [71] over 2.3 years, to approximately 16. There was no difference in SHIM scores in men who had undergone non-nerve-sparing versus nerve-sparing surgery. Of those men who stopped IUA therapy, 57.1 % cited insufficient erections as the causative reason, with the remainder being switch to another therapy, return of spontaneous erections and side effects (14.7 % each).

Overall, IUA has utility in treating post-prostatectomy ED. Patients must be properly counseled as to the correct application of the therapy, and be provided with realistic expectations of the success of the treatment. Opponents of this therapy cite high dropout rates, side effects, and lack of efficacy as reasons not to advocate strongly for this treatment.

Combination Therapy

Multiple combinations of individual therapies have been utilized, with reported greater success than individual treatments alone. These include salvage IUA after failure of PDE5 inhibitor (sildenafil) [72], salvage PDE-5 inhibitor (sildenafil) after failure of VED alone [73], and salvage ICI (with prostaglandin E1) after suboptimal response to PDE5 inhibitor (sildenafil and/or vardenafil) [74] (see Table 11.1).

Penile Prostheses

Penile prostheses are typically employed as a definitive treatment for ED, including post-prostatectomy ED, should other treatments prove ineffective or unacceptable. In fact, since the introduction of PDE5 inhibitors, it has been demonstrated that the etiology of ED for men undergoing penile prosthesis implantation has changed, with vascular disease being the predominant etiology before sildenafil, and radical pelvic surgery (including radical prostatectomy) predominating

Table 11.1 Summary of combination therapy for post-prostatectomy ED

Failed agent	Salvage agent	Salvage regimen	Outcome	Reference
Sildenafil	MUSE	Sildenafil 100 mg 1 h prior to intercourse; 500 mcg MUSE immediately before intercourse	83 % patients reported improvements in EF (mean IIEF-5: 18.6 in salvage vs. 13.2 in sildenafil) and penile rigidity	[72]
VED	Sildenafil	Sildenafil 100 mg 1–2 h prior to VED use for intercourse	77 % patients reported improvements in penile rigidity and sexual satisfaction	[73]
Sildenafil or Vardenafil	ICI (alprostadil)	Alprostadil 15 or 20 mcg; timing of treatments not specified	68 % patients reported improvements in EF (mean SHIM: 23.4 salvage vs. 14.3 sildenafil alone; 24.1 vs. 14.9 vardenafil alone)	[74]

since [75]. Although multiple types of penile prostheses are available, including semirigid (non-inflatable) and two-piece inflatable prostheses, the gold standard prostheses are the three-piece inflatable models, currently the most commonly used penile prostheses [76, 77].

When counseling men and their partners about penile prostheses, reasonable expectations must be outlined. These are mechanisms by which to achieve rigid erections for intercourse; sensation, orgasm and actual penile length should not be affected, for better or worse. They must understand that once a penile prosthesis is in place, they cannot simply revert to another ED therapy should they not like it. Opportunities for independent review of information on the prostheses and for discussion with patients who have already undergone the procedure to ascertain their personal experiences should be provided.

The benefits of the prostheses are the assurance that a rigid erection will be achieved for penetrative intercourse, as well as the relative spontaneity with which an erection can be generated. The drawbacks include their irreversible nature and the need for surgery with all of the attendant risks. Specific risks for penile prostheses include device infection, erosion and malfunction requiring surgical revision or replacement. Especially for the inflatable penile prostheses, with recent advances in the devices including reinforced cylinders, kink-proof tubing, pre-connected pumps and antibiotic coating, these risks are lower than ever, and the devices consistently demonstrate good longevity [78–80].

For men who started a regimen of ED therapy post-prostatectomy, the overall treatment discontinuation rate at 18 months post-surgery was 73 % [81]. Reasons for discontinuation included treatment effect below expectation (with or without dose titration) and loss of interest in sex (either patient or partner). Other possible reasons, although not cited in this study, include cost and treatment side effects. It is also established that the use of penile prostheses can significantly improve quality of life [82]. They may, however, be underused: in one SEER-Medicare analysis, approximately 1 % of men post-prostatectomy ultimately underwent penile prosthesis insertion [83]. In another analysis, while it was found that 50 % of men post-prostatectomy elected to try ED therapy, only 1.9 % underwent implantation of penile prosthesis, the least commonly used therapy [84]. It was, however, reported to be the most helpful ED treatment.

Overall, satisfaction rates for penile prostheses are quite high (69–98 %) [85]. Uncommonly, patients may be dissatisfied as a result of the glans not being rigid to the same extent as the penile shaft, also known as "floppy glans syndrome." In this case, concomitant use of PDE5 inhibitors, IUA [86] or VED [87] may be attempted for supplemental glanular engorgement.

Given the upsurge of robotic-assisted approaches for prostate extirpation, there is scrutiny as to placement of abdomino-pelvic reservoirs for three-piece inflatable devices. For patients status post open radical prostatectomy, typically, reservoirs are easily placed through or adjacent to (traversing through the transversalis fascia) the external inguinal ring into the retropubic space of Retzius. With the robotic approach, this space may be obliterated, and assumed extraperitoneal reservoir placement may in fact be intraperitoneal [88]. This fact has led to the novel approach of ectopic reservoir placement in the abdominal wall [89]. Alternatively, a counter-incision may be employed for safe reservoir placement [90].

Other surgical considerations include the fact that radical prostatectomies are safely performed in men with preexisting inflatable penile prostheses (and their abdomino-pelvic reservoirs) [91–93]. Finally, Ramsawh and colleagues [94] examined the benefits of simultaneous placement of penile prosthesis at the time of radical prostatectomy. The patients who opted for this procedure reported greater overall quality of life, erectile function and more frequent sexual contact than those who underwent RP alone. This may be a reasonable option for patients in whom nerve-sparing is not possible, or who have severe ED refractory to medical options prior to surgery.

Penile Rehabilitation

Penile rehabilitation is defined as medical treatment at the time of or after prostatectomy to improve the restoration of natural penile mechanics which results in spontaneous erectile function [32]. This is different (perhaps subtly) than ED treatment post-prostatectomy, which is characterized by the administration of medication to achieve a more rigid erection which permits penetrative intercourse. In the former, the goal is to bring about recovery of the erectile mechanism so that, at least ideally, the patient is not dependent on any erectile aid, and can generate erections as he did prior to his surgery. The goal of the latter, however, is the attainment of a rigid erection. The importance of this distinction cannot be understated, and many patients and clinicians may not fully appreciate the difference.

The rationale for penile rehabilitation is that the ultimate erectile capacity of the penis is compromised as a result of the chronic absence of erections that the patient experiences postoperatively. Due to this inability to achieve erections, the normal cycling of arterial blood flow to the penis is disrupted and theoretically penile hypoxia results, which leads to intracorporal fibrosis [95]. In preclinical models of post-prostatectomy ED, improved oxygenation of cavernosal tissue, either via hyperbaric oxygen administration or PDE-5 inhibitors, yields improved erectile hemodynamics and prevention of smooth muscle loss and fibrosis [96–100].

Based on this knowledge, it is recommended that some form of treatment or penile rehabilitation be employed following radical prostatectomy, as this "…is undoubtedly better than leaving the erectile tissue to its unassisted, unfavorable fate" [101]. Furthermore, initiating therapy/rehabilitation early postoperatively may confer advantage to commencing in a more delayed fashion, although there is currently insufficient evidence to support specific time recommendations. Indeed, surveys of clinicians reveal that over 80 % recommend some sort of rehabilitation to their patients [102, 103]. Although all treatment options were employed, the most common initial therapy was PDE-5 inhibitors, and treatment was most commonly initiated at catheter removal, and lasted for 12–18 months. There were similar findings for members of the International Society of Sexual Medicine (ISSM) [102], wherein more members had formal sexual medicine training, although treatment duration tended to be for 12 months or less. Interestingly, 97 % of responders did not expect full rigidity with rehabilitation. As well, those clinicians who perform radical prostatectomy or who assessed more than 50 such patients annually were more likely to utilize penile rehabilitation. Finally, for those who do not employ rehabilitation, 50 % cited cost, 25 % the absence of evidence-based therapy, and 25 % the lack of familiarity with penile rehabilitation as their reasons.

The majority of data available for the utility of penile rehabilitation address the use of PDE-5 inhibitors. For many practitioners, they are considered first-line therapy for rehabilitative purposes as well, relating to their ease of use and safety. Bannowsky et al. [104] showed a benefit of nightly low-dose sildenafil (25 mg) in recovery of erectile function in patients following nerve-sparing radical prostatectomy in a small study. Forty-three patients, following catheter removal at 7–14 days following surgery, were studied, with 23 patients randomized to sildenafil 25 mg nightly starting the day following catheter removal, and a control group of 18 patients were followed without sildenafil administration. IIEF scores were then recorded at various timepoints after surgery. Over the course of the first postoperative year, there was a gradual increase in the IIEF scores for patients in both groups. In the nightly sildenafil group, however, there was a significantly higher IIEF score at 36 and 52 weeks post-op, compared to controls (9.6 vs. 6.4, 14.1 vs. 9.3, respectively). At 52 weeks, 47 % of men taking nightly sildenafil were able to achieve and maintain erections sufficient for intercourse, compared to 28 % in the control group ($p < 0.001$). Furthermore, when on-demand sildenafil 50–100 mg was used for patients in both groups, the overall potency of the nightly sildenafil group increased to 86 % compared to 66 % in the control group. The conclusion of the authors, that "…daily low-dose sildenafil leads to significant improvement in the recovery of erectile function," is limited by the small patient population and the absence of a true control group (i.e., patients administered a placebo). A higher dose of nightly sildenafil, 50 or 100 mg, and its impact on recovery of erectile function was assessed by Padma-Nathan et al. [105]. In a randomized, double-blind, placebo-controlled study of men having undergone nerve-sparing radical prostatectomy, patients were assigned to placebo, sildenafil 50 mg or sildenafil 100 mg nightly commencing 4 weeks postoperatively for 36 weeks. At 48 weeks, 4 % of the placebo group were deemed to have responded, whereas 26 % of those in the sildenafil 50 mg nightly group were responders, and 29 % of those in the sildenafil 100 mg group were responders (both $p < 0.05$). Based on these results, the authors concluded that nightly use of sildenafil markedly increased the return of normal spontaneous erections. These conclusions, however, are tempered by the substantial limitations of the study: the

small number of patients enrolled, the dropout rate, the significantly lower placebo response rate than that published in the literature, and the non-validated primary outcome of the study (responders were defined based on individual questions from the IIEF-EF, not the overall score).

Vardenafil had been studied for efficacy in improving recovery of erectile function [106]. Of particular importance in this study was that patients underwent unilateral nerve-sparing surgery, and that there was no significant difference between 5 and 10 mg vardenafil dosing in erectile recovery according to the IIEF-5 (equivalent to the SHIM questionnaire). The utility of nightly versus on-demand therapy with vardenafil on erectile function recovery following bilateral nerve-sparing radical prostatectomy was assessed [107]. The design consisted of a 9-month double-blind treatment period, a 2-month single-blind washout period and an optional 2-month open-label period, to start within 2 weeks of surgery. The primary outcome measure was the percentage of subjects with an IIEF-EF score of >22 after the washout period. The intention-to-treat population consisted of 628 men randomized to treatment. Whereas at the end of the treatment period there was noted to be a significantly higher proportion of patients with IIEF-EF > 22 in the on-demand group, there were no significant differences between on-demand and nightly dosing at the end of the washout period. The authors concluded that these results support a paradigm shift toward on-demand dosing in a rehabilitative context in men post-prostatectomy. While certainly interesting, the trial is limited by the potential inexact definition of potency according to the IIEF-EF, as well as the failure to report the number of tablets consumed in the on-demand group. As such, it is unclear (though unlikely) whether patients in the on-demand group used similar doses to those in the nightly dosing group.

There are no clinical studies specifically addressing the role of tadalafil for penile rehabilitation for recovery of erectile function post-prostatectomy.

Montorsi [108] was the first to conceive of a penile rehabilitative concept, utilizing ICI with alprostadil. In that study, after bilateral nerve-sparing radical retropubic prostatectomy, 30 men were randomized into two groups: 15 men underwent alprostadil injection three times per week for 12 weeks, and 15 men observation with no erectogenic treatment. After 6 months, in the control group, only 3/15 (20 %) patients had normal erectile function, compared to the experimental group (8/12–67 %, $p < 0.01$). Despite there being several notable limitations to this study, including small sample size, preoperative parameters of erectile function and patient comorbidities not discussed and despite the claim of "spontaneous recovery of erections" erectogenic aids still being required, this served as the basis for further studies assessing penile rehabilitation, employing different ED treatments and protocols. Another study of penile rehabilitation involving ICI assessed the combination of intracavernous alprostadil or triple therapy with sildenafil started at the time of hospital discharge following bilateral nerve-sparing radical prostatectomy [109]. Injections were started within 3 weeks of catheter removal. This early combination therapy was shown to facilitate early sexual intercourse, improve patient satisfaction and possibly promote earlier return of spontaneous erections in 22 men. Sildenafil was taken daily and the ICI was done 2–3 times per week until natural erections occurred. The combination also allowed for a lower dose of ICI, which minimized penile discomfort. This study is limited by the small patient number as well as the absence of a control group.

The data supporting the use of the VED in the context of penile rehabilitation exceeds that available for primary ED treatment. In a pilot study of early (starting 1 month postoperatively, daily 10-min device application) VED use, Kohler et al. [110] demonstrated not only better erectile function at 3 and 6 months postoperatively according to the IIEF in the early VED use (compared to a control group), but also maintained stretch penile length, which was significantly shorter in the control group. In another prospective study [111], daily VED use (no constriction ring unless attempting intercourse) was compared to no erectogenic treatment in 109 men starting 1 month following surgery for a total of 9 months. A modest benefit was noted in the VED group for vaginal penetration without erectile aid. While these studies suggest a role for VED in penile rehabilitation, opponents would argue that by virtue of the fact that no more than 60 % of blood drawn to the penis using a VED is arterial [112], the potential benefit of VED in this context is limited compared to treatments which target and are meant to enhance penile arterial blood flow, such as PDE5 inhibitors, ICI or IUA.

IUA has been demonstrated to be of benefit in the rehabilitative setting. In a prospective study of 91 men after bilateral nerve-sparing radical prostatectomy with a median follow-up of 6 months, 56 men treated with 125 or 250 μg of intraurethral prostaglandin E1 three times per week starting 12–15 days after catheter removal reported higher SHIM scores, and had a higher proportion of men recovering spontaneous erections compared to the control group who had no rehabilitative treatment [113]. Notable is the 32 % dropout rate for patients in the IUA group. Drawbacks of this study include lack of intent-to-treat analysis and randomization, and self-selection of intervention, as well as the absence of statistical analysis between groups. In another study [114], a prospective randomized trial comparing nightly intraurethral alprostadil (IUA) versus sildenafil for post-prostatectomy penile rehabilitation was conducted. Two hundred and twelve patients were randomized to receive nightly intraurethral alprostadil IUA (initially 125 μg, with titration up to 250 μg at 1 month post-op) or sildenafil, and were followed up regularly over the first 12 postoperative months. By the end of the study period, there were no differences noted in the IIEF-EF scores or intercourse success rates between the 2 groups. The dropout rate for patients in the IUA group was higher than in the sildenafil group (30 % vs. 19 %), and the drug compliance rate (measured by the dispensed-to-returned medication ratio) was lower (79 % vs. 98 %). The rationale for the use of a subtherapeutic dose (125 μg) of IUA initially was that higher doses may have led to an unacceptably high dropout rate due to local adverse effects. Practically speaking, given the absence of a clear benefit with IUA versus sildenafil, it seems

Table 11.2 Summary of penile rehabilitative strategies

Treatment	Dose	Regimen	Duration	Success	Level of evidence	Reference
Sildenafil	25 mg	Nightly, starting the day of catheter removal	52 weeks	Improvement in IIEF-5	2b	[104]
Sildenafil	50–100 mg	Nightly, starting 4 weeks after surgery	36 weeks	Improvement in spontaneous EF and satisfaction	2b	[105]
Vardenafil	10 mg nightly; 5/20 mg on demand	Nightly versus on-demand	9 months	No difference in IIEF-EF between nightly versus on-demand	1b	[107]
Alprostadil ICI	Optimized per patient (2.5–14 mcg, mean 8 mcg)	Three times weekly, starting 1 month after surgery	12 weeks	Recovery of spontaneous erections	2b	[108]
Alprostadil/trimix ICI + sildenafil	Alprostadil 1–4 mcg; trimix 20 U; sildenafil 50 mg at the time of hospital discharge	Injections 2–3 times weekly; sildenafil daily	6 months	50 % patients recovered partial spontaneous erections	4	[109]
VED	Not specified	Daily starting 2 weeks after surgery	9 months	Improvement in IIEF-5 in the early daily VED use	2b	[111]
MUSE	125 mcg, with possible titration to 250 mcg	Three times weekly starting 3 weeks after surgery	9 months	Improvement in SHIM	4	[113]
MUSE (vs. Sildenafil)	125 mcg (vs. 50 mg sildenafil)	Nightly starting within 1 month of surgery	9 months	No difference in recovery between MUSE and sildenafil groups	4	[114]

unlikely that clinicians and patients would elect to pursue nightly IUA for rehabilitation when a seemingly more convenient oral therapy yields similar outcomes. Nevertheless, for patients interested in some form of penile rehabilitation, should PDE5 inhibitors be contraindicated due to risk, adverse effect or cost, IUA may be considered (Table 11.2).

The success of a penile rehabilitative program is not solely defined by the ability for the participants to generate their own erections. Compliance is an important issue to consider: no matter what the potential is for achieving success, should the regimen be too intensive, costly or with too many adverse effects, patients will not adhere to the protocol, may not recover erections, and frustra-

tion and mistrust may develop. This unfortunate prospect has been proven: Polito et al. [115] showed that 36.5 % of 430 consecutive radical prostatectomy patients ultimately declined participation in a rehabilitation protocol involving ICI with alprostadil, and of those that participated, 18.6 % eventually withdrew from the program, for a total of 55.1 % of their overall patient cohort not participating in their program. Reasons for declining participation in the program included patient's lack of sexual interest (51.6 %), lack of interest by the partner (30.2 %), and presence of urinary incontinence (26.7 %), and reasons for withdrawal after initiation of the program included disappointment with treatment efficacy (64.7 %), injection pain (45 %), and difficulties with or fear of performing the injection by themselves or by the partner (35.2 %). Cost of the drug was not cited to be a cause for dropout. Men who declined or withdrew participation were significantly older, had inferior preoperative erectile function and sustained more adjuvant therapy (androgen deprivation and/or radiation therapy) than those who carried out the program. Although the exact rehabilitative regimen with regard to the frequency of injections was not specified, and that these results may not be generalizable to other rehabilitative regimens (especially with other ED treatment modalities), the important takeaway point of this study is that compliance with penile rehabilitation is an important issue to consider.

Another issue to resolve is which patients should be considered for rehabilitation, that is, who is most likely to benefit from a rehabilitative protocol. Briganti et al. [116] attempted to help define this concept, by retrospectively analyzing 435 patients who had undergone bilateral nerve-sparing radical prostatectomy, who were stratified into three groups according to their risk of post-prostatectomy ED. Low-risk patients were those who were below 65 years of age, had a preoperative IIEF-EF score ≥ 26 and a Charlson Comorbidity Index (CCI) of ≤ 1; intermediate-risk patients were 66–69 years of age, preoperative IIEF-EF score 11–25 and CCI ≤ 1; high-risk patients were ≥ 70 years of age, IIEF-EF ≤ 10 and CCI ≥ 2. In the low- and high-risk groups, there was comparable efficacy of a rehabilitative protocol consisting of daily PDE-5 inhibitor use, whereas in the intermediate patient group, daily PDE-5 inhibitor use was associated with significantly greater erectile recovery at 3 years. A similar study by Müller et al. [117] found that on multivariate analysis, factors which predicted lack of success for a rehabilitation protocol (in this study consisting of thrice weekly sildenafil to achieve a penetration-rigidity erection for at least 18 months post-prostatectomy, with ICI to be used if oral therapy failed) included age >60 years, non-bilateral nerve-sparing surgery, presence of two or more vascular comorbidities (hypertension, dyslipidemia, coronary artery disease, diabetes mellitus), initiating the rehabilitation program >6

months after surgery, lack of response to sildenafil by 12 months post-surgery and the need for ICI trimix dosing of >50 units. Based on these two studies, it appears as though several factors, including patient demographic factors (age), preoperative erectile functional status, comorbid status, type of surgery (nerve-sparing), timing of rehabilitation initiation, and response to ED therapy should assist in determining the capacity to respond to a rehabilitation protocol.

Another issue that must be considered is whether penile rehabilitation is cost-effective. Although the cost of the use of these therapies has not been studied specifically in the context of rehabilitation, their cost in treating ED has been examined, with undecided results, with up to tenfold differences noted depending on the analysis [118, 119]. The reasons why an exact cost estimate cannot be ascribed to ED therapy are multiple, and include older studies with dated cost estimates, the upsurge in ED treatment use over time, the inability to capture the opportunity cost of how ED affects other aspects of life (such as other health problems [i.e., depression, relationship discord] and time missed from work) and the limitations of the various methods of answering the question (retrospective claims analyses, decision analytic models). Furthermore, most patients must cover most, or at times, all of the costs associated with ED treatment out of pocket: for example, in the USA, approximately 60 % of sildenafil prescriptions are paid out of pocket [120]. As such, many of the expenses associated with ED therapies are not even accounted for in these studies. Therefore, while an exact monetary figure cannot be estimated for the different therapies either for primary ED treatment or penile rehabilitation, the socioeconomic impact on the patient, as well as society, is not negligible, and should at least be considered, when prescribing these therapies.

Overall, when counseling patients and their partner about the prospect of penile rehabilitation post-radical prostatectomy, many factors should be considered: patient-related (preexisting comorbidities, motivation, recovery from surgery), partner-related (presence or absence of a regular sexual partner, motivation, partner comorbidities which may preclude regular sexual attempts, motivation), and disease-related (pathological stage and need for adjuvant therapy). As in other aspects of managing post-prostatectomy ED, managing patient and partner expectations is critical, and provision of reliable and honest data is important for patients to make their best informed decision about participation in a penile rehabilitation protocol.

Future Directions

There is much regarding ED treatment and how erectile function can be optimally recovered after radical prostatectomy that still remains elusive and must be clarified. There are a variety of avenues still to be explored, and for which exciting new research is being conducted, including surgical, pharmacological, and several novel approaches.

Surgery

Refinements in surgical technique to continue to improve upon Walsh's seminal work [121] in nerve-sparing prostatectomy are currently being explored, for both open and robotic laparoscopic-assisted radical prostatectomy. These include visual magnification, high anterior release of the levator fascia, intrafascial neurovascular bundle (NVB) preservation, early NVB dissection, "Veil of Aphrodite" prostatic fascia preservation, digital haptic feedback during NVB sparing, avoidance of NVB counter-traction during dissection, and cautery-free NVB dissection [122–127]. Other surgical modifications include the investigation of the possible benefits of nerve interposition grafting in situations where one or both cavernous nerves must be sacrificed for oncological control. Sural, ilioinguinal, and genitofemoral nerve grafting has been studied, with limited benefit having been demonstrated thus far [128–131]. Further research into cavernous nerve regeneration using acellular nerve grafts has had promising results in rats [132]. Finally, another innovative surgical concept is cavernous nerve stimulation. This can serve the dual purpose of

facilitation of cavernous nerve localization at the time of surgery, as well as the ultimate purpose of retention of the implanted electrodes for chronic cavernous nerve stimulation for the preservation of erectile tissue health. This has been studied in pilot projects, with successful demonstration of penile tumescence as well as enhanced penile blood flow with nerve stimulation at the time of surgery [133–135].

Medications

Erythropoietin (EPO), a cytokine that stimulates erythropoiesis under hypoxic conditions, has also demonstrated utility in hastening functional nerve recovery in animal models of nerve damage [136–138]. Indeed, in humans, a recent trial demonstrated the efficacy of recombinant human EPO in recovery following acute ischemic cerebrovascular accident [139]. EPO as a neuromodulatory agent for treating neurogenic ED has also been assessed in preclinical studies, with the expression of the EPO receptor proven in the human urogenital tract [140]. Furthermore, in a rat model, EPO administration promoted the recovery of erectile function following cavernous nerve injury. On electron microscopy, axonal regeneration was promoted [141]. There has been a single human study retrospectively assessing EPO in erectile recovery following radical prostatectomy [142]. Fifteen patients undergoing nerve-sparing radical retropubic prostatectomy elected to receive a 40,000 IU subcutaneous injection of EPO on their preoperative day, and were compared to a control group consisting of 21 patients who did not undergo injection. IIEF questionnaire data were compiled at 3, 6, and 12 months postoperatively, with patients in the treatment group demonstrating significantly higher IIEF-5 scores than those in the control group. As well, although the rate of patients who were sexually active was not significantly different, a significantly higher proportion of patients in the EPO group reported clinically meaningful erections allowing for completion of sexual intercourse than in the control group. The authors concluded that men who received a single dose of EPO preoperatively recovered functionally relevant erections more significantly than those who did not, and that this therapy holds promise for treatment of ED post-prostatectomy. A randomized, prospective, double-blind clinical trial assessing three perioperative doses of subcutaneous EPO versus placebo is being conducted by the same group, with results still pending.

Irbesartan, an antihypertensive medication within the angiotensin-receptor blocker (ARB) class, may facilitate accelerated erectile functional recovery post-prostatectomy. Segal et al. [143] assessed this in a retrospective cohort analysis, based on preclinical data showing that low- and high-dose losartan, another ARB, preserved erectile function after bilateral cavernous nerve crush injury in rats [144]. In the clinical study, 17 men were treated with 300 mg irbesartan starting on postoperative day 1, and their IIEF-5 outcomes at various timepoints compared with men who elected not to be treated. While by 24 months there was no difference between IIEF-5 scores between groups, at 12 months, the scores were significantly higher in the irbesartan group, suggesting that early recovery (<12 months) may be improved by the administration of this drug. The limitations of this study include small patient number, the absence of a true control group, and the open-label and retrospective nature of the study. Nevertheless, this "proof-of-principle" study justifies further research, in the form of a randomized, double-blind clinical trial.

It has been postulated that the regular use of "statins," HMG-CoA reductase inhibitors, can impact on the early return of potency after radical prostatectomy, based on their protective effect on vascular endothelium. A study from Korea [145] tried to prove this, showing that men who took atorvastatin 10 mg daily for 3 months starting on postoperative day 1 showed statistically significantly higher IIEF-5 scores 6 months after surgery. There are multiple methodological flaws with this study, including small study population, absence of a placebo group, and arbitrary potency definition, and conclusive statements about the true utility of statins in this context are still elusive.

Although human studies have not yet been published, immunosuppressant medications have shown promise in animal models in terms of erectile recovery after cavernous nerve injury [146–148]. Specifically, immunophilin ligands, such as FK-506 and rapamycin, possibly by virtue of effects on neuronal nitric oxide, antioxidative, and antiapoptotic mechanisms, may be an avenue of further study going forward.

Other Strategies

Pelvic floor biofeedback training (PFBT), classically applied to treat incontinence, has been studied to assess possible benefits for erectile recovery. This was initially noted in a case series which showed improvement in IIEF scores (of at least three points, in line with MCID findings) in 3 men after a 4-month PFBT regimen, initiated 12–18 months after radical prostatectomy [149]. This finding was corroborated in a rehabilitative fashion in a prospective, randomized trial [150], wherein weekly PFBT starting at postoperative day 15 (after catheter removal) for 12 weeks resulted in a significantly higher proportion of men recovering potency (defined as IIEF-5 ≥ 20) in the treatment versus control groups (47.1 % vs. 12.5 %, $p=0.032$) at 1 year postoperatively. Furthermore, recovery of potency was correlated with recovery of continence. This trial was limited by small patient population (a total of 33 patients finished the protocol), high dropout rate and the arbitrary definition of potency.

Improvement in lifestyle, such as exercise/improved fitness, weight loss and behavior modification to live an overall healthier life have been shown to be protect against development of ED, and may be helpful in maintaining erectile function in type 2 diabetic men [151, 152]. Adopting these lifestyle modifications intuitively benefits patients who are recovering from surgery, but these have not been assessed for how they may impact quality of life recovery after radical prostatectomy. A planned trial in Germany aims to do just that, enrolling patients 8–12 weeks after radical prostatectomy in a rehabilitative sports program and assessing resultant aerobic fitness and quality of life outcomes, including urinary incontinence and erectile dysfunction [153].

Although no formal clinical studies have been completed thus far, there is interest in penile vibratory stimulation for the treatment of ED, including post-prostatectomy ED, and even for penile rehabilitation. This takes advantage of genital afferent nerve stimulation which may lead to reflexogenic erections by activation of several reflexes, including the pudendo-cavernosal and bulbocavernosus reflexes [154]. In theory, the ability to stimulate erections independent of the function of the cavernous nerve would be advantageous post-prostatectomy. An FDA-cleared device for the treatment of ED, the handheld Viberect®, is available for purchase by patients. Rigorous studies are needed to prove the utility of this device and treatment modality.

With regard to penile rehabilitation, while the myriad of studies previously discussed allude to the beneficial effect of some sort of rehabilitative regimen, more research in the field is still needed. Up until now, there has not been any randomized trial comparing different rehab protocols, in an effort to prove which is most efficacious. It is not known which ED treatment modality (if any) is best, and for each modality, what the optimal timing, dose, frequency and duration of therapy is, respectively, to achieve maximal erectile recovery. Furthermore, as implied by the Montorsi study [107], perhaps on-demand therapy, if the patient is motivated and engages in attempted sexual intercourse frequently enough (ample frequency itself not being adequately defined as of yet), is sufficient to rehabilitate post-prostatectomy erectile function. If so, this may be of interest to patients, as it enables them to not have to rely on a daily dose of medication, and limits the cost and possible adverse effects of the therapy. Indeed, patient (as well as partner) motivation has been noted to be a key factor in determining the type of rehabilitation protocol in which to enlist the couple [155].

In all likelihood, there is no one rehabilitation protocol that will be definitely shown to be superior to all others; more likely, therapy will have to be tailored to patients, based on their goals, expectations, motivation, socioeconomic and relationship status, medical comorbidities and need for any adjuvant cancer treatment, which in turn can also effect erectile and sexual function. Of equal importance to note is that the key will likely be a rehabilitation protocol which involves not a single drug, but multiple treatments, which may include a cocktail of medications, the application of devices and lifestyle modifications in both the perioperative and postoperative periods to maximally enhance erectile recovery. The physiology of human erection is complex, and integrates neural, vascular, endocrine, and psychological components to achieve the end result. All of these may be exploited using available and yet-to-be-defined therapies to achieve erectile recovery post-prostatectomy.

Conclusion

Erectile dysfunction is a common adverse effect from radical prostatectomy, whose impact can be severe for both patient and partner. Fortunately, based on an improved understanding of the erectile mechanism, there are a variety of available treatment options which can restore functionality. Furthermore, with the concept of penile rehabilitation, there are methods which may help restore function independent of the need for erectile aids. When counseling patients about treatment options, realistic expectations should be fostered, and treatment for patients should be selected based on the best chance for their success and realizing patients' goals. More research is needed to better define the concepts of erectile functional recovery and penile rehabilitation.

References

1. Litwin MS, Flanders SC, Pasta DJ, Stoddard ML, Lubeck DP, Henning JM. Sexual function and bother after radical prostatectomy or radiation for prostate cancer: multivariate quality of-life analysis from CaPSURE. Cancer of the prostate strategic urologic research endeavor. Urology. 1999;54:503–8.
2. Arai Y, Okubo K, Aoki Y, Maekawa S, Okada T, Maeda H, et al. Patient-reported quality of life after radical prostatectomy for prostate cancer. Int J Urol. 1999;6:78–86.

3. Catalona WJ, Basler JW. Return of erections and urinary continence following nerve sparing radical retropubic prostatectomy. J Urol. 1993;150:905–7.

4. Jonler M, Messing EM, Rhodes PR, Bruskewitz RC. Sequelae of radical prostatectomy. Br J Urol. 1994;74:352–8.

5. Ficarra V, Novara G, Ahlering TE, Costello A, Eastham JA, Graefen M, et al. Systematic review and meta-analysis of studies reporting potency rates after robot-assisted radical prostatectomy. Eur Urol. 2012;62:418–30.

6. Feldman HA, Goldstein I, Hatzichristou DG, Krane RJ, McKinlay JB. Impotence and its medical and psychosocial correlates: results of the Massachusetts Male Aging Study. J Urol. 1994;151:54–61.

7. Teloken PE, Nelson CJ, Karellas M, Stasi J, Eastham J, Scardino PT, et al. Defining the impact of vascular risk factors on erectile function recovery after radical prostatectomy. BJU Int. 2013;111(4):653–7. doi:10.1111/j.1464-410X.2012.11321.x.

8. Alemozaffar M, Regan MM, Cooperberg MR, Wei JT, Michalski JM, Sandler HM, et al. Prediction of erectile function following treatment for prostate cancer. JAMA. 2011;306:1205–14.

9. Ko WJ, Truesdale MD, Hruby GW, Landman J, Badani KK. Impacting factors for recovery of erectile function within 1 year following robotic-assisted laparoscopic radical prostatectomy. J Sex Med. 2011;8:1805–12.

10. Pierorazio PM, Spencer BA, McCann TR, McKiernan JM, Benson MC. Preoperative risk stratification predicts likelihood of concurrent PSA-free survival, continence, and potency (the trifecta analysis) after radical retropubic prostatectomy. Urology. 2007;70:717–22.

11. Moskovic DJ, Alphs H, Nelson CJ, Rabbani F, Eastham J, Touijer K, et al. Subjective characterization of nerve sparing predicts recovery of erectile function after radical prostatectomy: defining the utility of a nerve sparing grading system. J Sex Med. 2011;8:255–60.

12. Levinson AW, Pavlovich CP, Ward NT, Link RE, Mettee LZ, Su L. Association of surgeon subjective characterization of nerve sparing quality with potency following laparoscopic radical prostatectomy. J Urol. 2008;179:1510–4.

13. Zorn KC, Wille MA, Thong AE, Katz MH, Shikanov SA, Razmaria A, et al. Continued improvement of perioperative, pathological and continence outcomes during 700 robot-assisted radical prostatectomies. Can J Urol. 2009;16:4742–9.

14. Hu JC, Gu X, Lipsitz LR, Barry MJ, D'Amico AV, Weinberg AC, et al. Comparative effectiveness of minimally invasive vs open radical prostatectomy. JAMA. 2009;302:1557–64.

15. Ficarra V, Novara G, Artibani W, Cestari A, Galfano A, Graefen M, et al. Retropubic, laparoscopic, and robot-assisted radical prostatectomy: a systematic review and cumulative analysis of comparative studies. Eur Urol. 2009;55:1037–63.

16. Boorjian SA, Eastham JA, Graefen M, Guillonneau B, Karnes RJ, Moul JW, et al. A critical analysis of the long-term impact of radical prostatectomy on cancer control and function outcomes. Eur Urol. 2012;61:664–75.

17. Tal R, Alphs HH, Krebs P, Nelson CJ, Mulhall JP. Erectile function recovery rate after radical prostatectomy: a meta-analysis. J Sex Med. 2009;6:2538–46.

18. Mulhall JP. Defining and reporting erectile function outcomes after radical prostatectomy: challenges and misconceptions. J Urol. 2009;181:462–71.

19. Burnett AL. Erectile dysfunction following radical prostatectomy. JAMA. 2005;293:2648–53.

20. Glickman L, Godoy G, Lepor H. Changes in continence and erectile function between 2 and 4 years after radical prostatectomy. J Urol. 2009;181:731–5.

21. Levinson AW, Lavery HJ, Ward NT, Su LM, Pavlovich CP. Is a return to baseline sexual function possible? An analysis of sexual function outcomes following laparoscopic radical prostatectomy. World J Urol. 2011;29:29–34.

22. Burnett AL, Lowenstein CJ, Bredt DS, Chang TS, Snyder SH. Nitric oxide: a physiologic mediator of penile erection. Science. 1992;257:401–3.

23. Lue TF. Erectile dysfunction. N Engl J Med. 2000;342:1802–13.

24. Gratzke C, Strong TD, Gebska MA, Champion HC, Stief CG, Burnett AL, et al. Activated RhoA/Rho kinase impairs erectile function after cavernous nerve injury in rats. J Urol. 2010;184:2197–204.

25. User HM, Hairston JH, Zelner DJ, McKenna KE, McVary KT. Penile weight and cell subtype specific changes in a post-radical prostatectomy model of erectile dysfunction. J Urol. 2003;169:1175–9.

26. Walz J, Burnett AL, Costello AJ, Eastham JA, Graefen M, Guillonneau B, et al. A critical analysis of the current knowledge of surgical anatomy related to optimization of cancer control and preservation of continence and erection in candidates for radical prostatectomy. Eur Urol. 2010;57:179–92.

27. Rogers CG, Trock BP, Walsh PC. Preservation of accessory pudendal arteries during radical retropubic prostatectomy: Surgical technique and results. Urology. 2004;64:148–51.

28. Mulhall JP, Slovick R, Hotaling J, Aviv N, Valenzuela R, Waters WB, et al. Erectile dysfunction after radical prostatectomy: hemodynamic profiles and their correlation with the recovery of erectile function. J Urol. 2002;167:1371–5.

29. Leungwattanakij S, Bivalacqua TJ, Usta MF, Yang DY, Hyun JS, Champion HC, et al. Cavernous neurotomy causes hypoxia and fibrosis in rat corpus cavernosum. J Androl. 2003;24:239–45.

30. Tal R, Heck M, Teloken P, Siegrist T, Nelson CJ, Mulhall JP. Peyronie's disease following radical prostatectomy: incidence and predictors. J Sex Med. 2010;7:1254–61.

31. Bella AJ, Perelman MA, Brant WO, Lue TF. Peyronie's disease. J Sex Med. 2007;4:1527–38.

32. Segal R, Burnett AL. Erectile preservation after radical prostatectomy. Ther Adv Urol. 2011;3:35–46.

33. Krupski TL, Saigal CS, Litwin MS. Variation in continence and potency by definition. J Urol. 2003;170:1291–4.

34. Litwin MS, Lubeck DP, Henning JM, Carroll PR. Differences in urologist and patient assessments of health related quality of life in men with prostate cancer: results of the CaPSURE database. J Urol. 1998;159:1988–92.

35. Lee SR, Kim HW, Lee JW, Jeong WJ, Rha KH, Kim JH. Discrepancies in perception of urinary incontinence between patient and physician after robotic radical prostatectomy. Yonsei Med J. 2010;51(6): 883–7.

36. Wei JT, Dunn RL, Litwin MS, Sandler HM, Sanda MG. Development and validation of the expanded prostate cancer index composite (EPIC) for comprehensive assessment of health-related quality of life in men with prostate cancer. Urology. 2000;56: 899–905.

37. Litwin MS, Hays RD, Fink A, Ganz PA, Leake B, Brook RH. The UCLA Prostate Cancer Index: development, reliability, and validity of a health-related quality of life measure. Med Care. 1998;36: 1002–12.

38. Szymanski KM, Wei JT, Dunn RL, Sanda MG. Development and validation of an abbreviated version of the expanded prostate cancer index composite instrument for measuring health-related quality of life among prostate cancer survivors. Urology. 2010;76:1245–50.

39. Rosen RC, Riley R, Wagner G, Osterloh IH, Kirkpatrick J, Mishra A. International index of erectile function (IIEF): a multidimensional scale for assessment of erectile dysfunction. Urology. 1997;49:822–30.

40. Cappelleri JC, Rosen RC. The Sexual Health Inventory for Men (SHIM): a 5-year review of research and clinical experience. Int J Impot Res. 2005;17:307–19.

41. Porst H, Gilbert C, Collins S, Huang X, Symonds T, Stecher V, et al. Development and validation of the quality of erection questionnaire. J Sex Med. 2007;4:372–81.

42. Mulhall JP, Goldstein I, Bushmakin AG, Cappelleri JC, Hvidsten K. Validation of the erection hardness score. J Sex Med. 2007;4:1626–34.

43. Goldstein I, Mulhall JP, Bushmakin AG, Cappelleri JC, Hvidsten K, Symonds T. The erection hardness score and its relationship to successful sexual intercourse. J Sex Med. 2008;5:2374–80.

44. Albersen M, Lue TF. Sexual dysfunction: MCID provides new perspective on erectile function research. Nat Rev Urol. 2011;8:591–2.

45. Rosen RC, Allen KR, Ni X, Araujo AB. Minimal clinically important differences in the erectile function domain of the International Index of Erectile Function scale. Eur Urol. 2011;60:1010–6.

46. Hvidsten K, Carlsson M, Stecher VJ, Symonds T, Levinson I. Clinically meaningful improvement on the quality of erection questionnaire in men with erectile dysfunction. Int J Impot Res. 2010;22: 45–50.

47. Norman GR, Sloan JA, Wyrwich KW. Interpretation of changes in health-related quality of life: the remarkable universality of half a standard deviation. Med Care. 2003;41:582–92.

48. Althof AE, Corty EW, Levine SB, Levine F, Burnett AL, McVary K, et al. EDITS: development of questionnaires for evaluating satisfaction with treatments for erectile dysfunction. Urology. 1999;53:793–9.

49. Ficarra V, Novara G, Galfano A, Stringari C, Baldassarre R, Cavalleri S, et al. Twelve-month self-reported quality of life after retropubic radical prostatectomy: a prospective study with Rand 36-Item Health Survey (Short Form-36). BJU Int. 2006;97:274–8.

50. Briganti A, Di Trapani E, Abdollah F, Gallina A, Suardi N, Capitanio U, et al. Choosing the best candidates for penile rehabilitation after bilateral nerve-sparing radical prostatectomy. J Sex Med. 2012;9: 608–17.

51. Teloken P, Valenzuela R, Parker M, Mulhall J. The correlation between erectile function and patient satisfaction. J Sex Med. 2007;4:472–6.

52. Segal R, Burnett AL. Avanafil for the treatment of erectile dysfunction. Drugs Today (Barc). 2012;48: 7–15.

53. Montague DK, Jarow JP, Broderick GA, Dmochowski RR, Heaton JP, Lue TF, et al. Chapter 1: The management of erectile dysfunction: an AUA update. J Urol. 2005;174:230–9.

54. Hatzimouratidis K, Amar E, Eardley I, Giuliano F, Hatzichristou D, Montorsi F, et al. Guidelines on male sexual dysfunction: erectile dysfunction and premature ejaculation. Eur Urol. 2010;57:804–14.

55. Carson CC, Lue TF. Phosphodiesterase type 5 inhibitors for erectile dysfunction. BJU Int. 2005;96: 257–80.

56. García-Cardoso J, Vela R, Mahillo E, Mateos-Cáceres PJ, Modrego J, Macaya C, et al. Increased cyclic guanosine monophosphate production and endothelial nitric oxide synthase level in mononuclear cells from sildenafil citrate-treated patients with erectile dysfunction. Int J Impot Res. 2010;22:68–76.

57. Zippe CD, Jhaveri FM, Klein EA, Kedia S, Pasqualotto FF, Kedia A, et al. Role of viagra after radical prostatectomy. Urology. 2000;55:241–5.

58. Zagaja GP, Mhoon DA, Aikens JE, Brendler CB. Sildenafil in the treatment of erectile dysfunction after radical prostatectomy. Urology. 2000;56: 631–4.

59. Feng MI, Huang S, Kaptein J, Kaswick J, Aboseif S. Effect of sildenafil citrate on post-radical prostatectomy erectile dysfunction. J Urol. 2000; 164:1935–8.

60. Raina R, Lakin MM, Agarwal A, Sharma R, Goyal KK, Montague DK, et al. Long-term effect of sildenafil citrate on erectile dysfunction after radical prostatectomy: 3-year follow-up. Urology. 2003; 62:110–5.

61. Nehra A, Grantmyre J, Nadel A, Thibonnier M, Brock G. Vardenafil improved patient satisfaction with erectile hardness, orgasmic function and sexual experience in men with erectile dysfunction following nerve sparing radical prostatectomy. J Urol. 2005;173:2067–71.

62. Montorsi F, Padma Nathan H, McCullough A, Brock GB, Broderick G, Ahuja S, et al. Tadalafil in the treatment of erectile dysfunction following bilateral nerve sparing radical retropubic prostatectomy: a randomized, double-blind, placebo controlled trial. J Urol. 2004;172:1036–41.

63. Mulhall JP, Burnett AL, Wang R, McVary KT, Moul JW, Bowden CH, et al. A phase 3, placebo-controlled study of the safety and efficacy of avanafil for the treatment of erectile dysfunction following nerve-sparing radical prostatectomy. J Urol. 2013;189(6):2229–36. doi:10.1016/j.juro.2012.11.177. http://dx.doi.org/.

64. Ciaro J, de Aboim J, Maringolo M, Andredo E, Agular W, Noguera M, et al. Intracavernous injection in the treatment of erectile dysfunction after radical prostatectomy: an observational study. Sao Paulo Med J. 2001;119:135–7.

65. Raina R, Lakin MM, Thukral M, Agarwal A, Ausmundson S, Montague DK, et al. Long-term efficacy and compliance of intracorporeal (IC) injection for erectile dysfunction following radical prostatectomy: SHIM (IIEF-5) analysis. Int J Impot Res. 2003;15:318–22.

66. Yiou R, Cunin P, de la Taille A, Salomon L, Binhas M, Lingombet O, et al. Sexual rehabilitation and penile pain associated with intracavernous alprostadil after radical prostatectomy. J Sex Med. 2011;8:575–82.

67. Baniel J, Israilov S, Segenreich E, Livne PM. Comparative evaluation of treatments for erectile dysfunction in patients with prostate cancer after radical retropubic prostatectomy. BJU Int. 2001;88: 58–62.

68. Hellstrom WJG, Montague DK, Moncada I, Carson C, Minhas S, Faria G, et al. Implants, mechanical devices, and vascular surgery for erectile dysfunction. J Sex Med. 2010;7:501–23.

69. Padma-Nathan H, Hellstrom WJ, Kaiser FE, Labasky RF, Lue TF, Nolten W, The Medicated Urethral System for Erection (MUSE) Study Group, et al. Treatment of men with erectile dysfunction with transurethral alprostadil. NEJM. 1997;336:1–7.

70. Costabile RA, Spevak M, Fishman IJ, Govier FE, Hellstrom WJG, Shabsigh R, et al. Efficacy and safety of transurethral alprostadil in patients with erectile dysfunction following radical prostatectomy. J Urol. 1998;160:1325–8.

71. Raina R, Agarwal A, Zaramo CE, Ausmundson S, Mansour D, Zippe CD. Long-term efficacy and compliance of MUSE for erectile dysfunction following radical prostatectomy: SHIM (IIEF-5) analysis. Int J Impot Res. 2005;17:86–90.

72. Raina R, Nandipati KC, Agarwal A, Mansour D, Kaelber DC, Zippe CD. Combination therapy: medicated urethral system for erection enhances sexual satisfaction in sildenafil citrate failure following nerve-sparing radical prostatectomy. J Androl. 2005;26:757–60.

73. Raina R, Agarwal A, Allamaneni SSR, Lakin MM, Zippe CD. Sildenafil citrate and vacuum constriction device combination enhances sexual satisfaction in erectile dysfunction after radical prostatectomy. Urology. 2005;65:360–4.

74. Mydlo JH, Viterbo R, Crispen P. Use of combined intracorporal injection and a phosphodiesterase-5 inhibitor therapy for men with a suboptimal response to sildenafil and/or vardenafil monotherapy after radical retropubic prostatectomy. BJU Int. 2005;95:843–6.

75. Cortés-Gonzalez JR, Glina S. Have phosphodiesterase-5 inhibitors changed the indications for penile implants? BJU Int. 2009;103:1518–21.

76. Lotan Y, Roehrborn CG, McConnell JD, Hendin BN. Factors influencing the outcomes of penile prosthesis surgery at a teaching institution. Urology. 2003;62:918–21.

77. Chung E, Van CT, Wilson I, Cartmill RA. Penile prosthesis implantation for the treatment of male erectile dysfunction: clinical outcomes and lessons learnt after 955 procedures. World J Urol. 2013;31(3):591–5. doi:10.1007/s00345-012-0859-4.

78. Wilson SK, Delk JR, Salem EA, Cleves MA. Long-term survival of inflatable penile prostheses: single surgical group experience with 2384 first-time implants spanning two decades. J Sex Med. 2007;4:1074–9.

79. Carson III CC, Mulcahy JJ, Harsch MR. Long-term infection outcomes after original antibiotic impregnated inflatable penile prosthesis implants: up to 7.7 years of follow-up. J Urol. 2011;185:614–8.

80. Mulcahy JJ, Carson III CC. Long-term infection rates in diabetic patients implanted with antibiotic-impregnated versus nonimpregnated inflatable penile prostheses: 7-year outcomes. Eur Urol. 2011;60:167–72.

81. Salonia A, Gallina A, Zanni G, Briganti A, Deho F, Sacca A, et al. Acceptance of and discontinuation rate from erectile dysfunction oral treatment in patients following bilateral nerve-sparing radical prostatectomy. Eur Urol. 2008;53:564–70.

82. Hassan A, El-Hadidy M, El-Deeck BS, Mostafa T. Couple satisfaction to different therapeutic modalities for organic erectile dysfunction. J Sex Med. 2008;5:2381–91.

83. Tal R, Jacks LM, Elkin E, Mulhall JP. Penile implant utilization following treatment for prostate cancer: analysis of the SEER-Medicare database. J Sex Med. 2011;8:1797–804.

84. Stephenson RA, Mori M, Hsieh Y, Beer TM, Stanford JL, Gilliland FD, et al. Treatment of erectile

dysfunction following therapy for clinically localized prostate cancer: patient reported use and outcomes from the surveillance, epidemiology, and end results prostate cancer outcomes study. J Urol. 2005;174:646–50.

85. Bernal RM, Henry GD. Contemporary patient satisfaction rates for three-piece inflatable penile prostheses. Adv Urol. 2012;2012:707321. Epub 2012 Jul 26

86. Benevides MD, Carson CC. Intraurethral application of alprostadil in patients with failed inflatable penile prosthesis. J Urol. 2000;163:785–7.

87. Soderdahl DW, Petroski RA, Mode D, Schwartz BF, Thrasher JB. The use of an external vacuum device to augment a penile prosthesis. Tech Urol. 1997; 3:100–2.

88. Sadeghi-Nejad H, Munarriz R, Shah N. Intra-abdominal reservoir placement during penile prosthesis surgery in post-robotically assisted laparoscopic radical prostatectomy patients: a case report and practical considerations. J Sex Med. 2011;8:1547–50.

89. Perito PE. Ectopic reservoir placement–no longer in the space of Retzius. J Sex Med. 2011;8:2395–8.

90. Hartman RJ, Helfand BT, McVary KT. Outcomes of lateral retroperitoneal reservoir placement of three-piece penile prosthesis in patients following radical prostatectomy. Int J Impot Res. 2010;22:279083.

91. Tiguert R, Hurely PM, Gheiler EL, Tefilli MV, Gudziak MR, Dhabuwala CB. Treatment outcome after radical prostatectomy is not adversely affected by a pre-existing penile prosthesis. Urology. 1998;52:1030–3.

92. Deho F, Salonia A, Briganti A, Zanni G, Gallina A, Rokkas K, et al. Anatomical radical retropubic prostatectomy in patients with a preexisting three-piece inflatable prosthesis: a series of case reports. J Sex Med. 2009;6:578–83.

93. Erdeljian P, Brock G, Pautler SE. Robot-assisted laparoscopic prostatectomy in patients preexisting three-piece inflatable penile prosthesis. J Sex Med. 2011;8:306–9.

94. Ramsawh HJ, Morgentaler A, Covino N, Barlow DH, DeWolf WC. Quality of life following simultaneous placement of penile prosthesis with radical prostatectomy. J Urol. 2005;174:1395–8.

95. Iacono F, Gianella R, Somma P, Manno G, Fusco F, Mirone V. Histological alterations in cavernous tissue after radical prostatectomy. J Urol. 2005;173: 1673–6.

96. Muller A, Tal R, Donohue JF, Akin-Olugbade Y, Kobylarz K, Paduch D, et al. The effect of hyperbaric oxygen therapy on erectile function recovery in a rat cavernous nerve injury model. J Sex Med. 2008;5:562–70.

97. Ferrini MG, Davila HH, Kovanecz I, Sanchez SP, Gonzalez-Cadavid NF, Rajfer J. Vardenafil prevents fibrosis and loss of corporeal smooth muscle that occurs after bilateral cavernosal nerve resection in the rat. Urology. 2006;68:429–35.

98. Kovanecz I, Rambhatla A, Ferrini M, Vernet D, Sanchez S, Rajfer J, et al. Long-term continuous sildenafil treatment ameliorates corporal veno-occlusive dysfunction (CVOD) induced by cavernosal nerve resection in rats. Int J Impot Res. 2008;20:202–12.

99. Kovanecz I, Rambhatla A, Ferrini MG, Vernet D, Sanchez S, Rajfer J, et al. Chronic daily tadalafil prevents the corporal fibrosis and veno-occlusive dysfunction that occurs after cavernosal nerve resection. BJU Int. 2008;101:203–10.

100. Vignozzi L, Filippi S, Morelli A, Ambrosini S, Luconi M, Vannelli GB, et al. Effect of chronic tadalafil administration on penile hypoxia induced by cavernous neurotomy in the rat. J Sex Med. 2006;3:419–31.

101. Salonia A, Burnett AL, Graefen M, Hatzimouratidis K, Montorsi F, Mulhall JP, et al. Prevention and management of postprostatectomy sexual dysfunctions part 2: recovery and preservation of erectile function, sexual desire, and orgasmic function. Eur Urol. 2012;62:273–86.

102. Teloken P, Mesquita G, Montorsi F, Mulhall J. Post-radical prostatectomy pharmacological penile rehabilitation: practice patterns among the international society for sexual medicine practitioners. J Sex Med. 2009;6:2032–8.

103. Tal R, Teloken P, Mulhall JP. Erectile function rehabilitation after radical prostatectomy: practice patterns among AUA members. J Sex Med. 2011; 8:2370–6.

104. Bannowsky A, Schulze H, van der Horst C, Hautmann S, Junemann KP. Recovery of erectile function after nerve-sparing radical prostatectomy: improvement with nightly low-dose sildenafil. BJU Int. 2008;101:1279–83.

105. Padma-Nathan H, McCullough AR, Levine LA, Lipshultz LI, Siegel R, Montorsi F, et al. Randomized, double-blind, placebo-controlled study of postoperative nightly sildenafil citrate for the prevention of erectile dysfunction after bilateral nerve-sparing radical prostatectomy. Int J Impot Res. 2008; 20:479–86.

106. Bannowsky A, van Ahlen H, Loch T. Increasing the dose of vardenafil on a daily basis does not improve erectile function after unilateral nerve-sparing radical prostatectomy. J Sex Med. 2012;9:1448–53.

107. Montorsi F, Brock G, Lee J, Shapiro J, Van Poppel H, Graefen M, et al. Effect of nightly versus on-demand vardenafil on recovery of erectile function in men following bilateral nerve-sparing radical prostatectomy. Eur Urol. 2008;54:924–31.

108. Montorsi F, Guazzoni G, Strambi LF, Da Pozzo LF, Nava L, Barbieri L, et al. Recovery of spontaneous erectile function after nerve-sparing radical retropubic prostatectomy with and without early intracavernous injections of alprostadil: results of a prospective, randomized trial. J Urol. 1997;158: 1408–10.

109. Nandipati K, Raina R, Agarwal A, Zippe CD. Early combination therapy: intracavernosal injections and sildenafil following radical prostatectomy increases sexual activity and the return of natural erections. Int J Impot Res. 2006;18:446–51.

110. Kohler TS, Pedro R, Hendlin K, Utz W, Ugarte R, Reddy P, et al. A pilot study on the early use of the vacuum erection device after radical retropubic prostatectomy. BJU Int. 2007;100:858–62.

111. Raina R, Agarwal A, Ausmundson S, Lakin M, Nandipati KC, Montague DK, et al. Early use of vacuum constriction device following radical prostatectomy facilitates early sexual activity and potentially earlier return of erectile function. Int J Impot Res. 2006;18:77–81.

112. Bosshardt RJ, Farwerk R, Sikora R, Sohn M, Jakse G. Objective measurement of the effectiveness, therapeutic success and dynamic mechanisms of the vacuum device. Br J Urol. 1995;75:786–91.

113. Raina R, Pahlajani G, Agarwal A, Zippe CD. The early use of transurethral alprostadil after radical prostatectomy potentially facilitates an earlier return of erectile function and successful sexual activity. BJU Int. 2007;100:1317–21.

114. McCullough AR, Hellstrom WG, Wang R, Lepor H, Wagner KR, Engel JD. Recovery of erectile function after nerve-sparing radical prostatectomy and penile rehabilitation with nightly intraurethral alprostadil versus sildenafil citrate. J Urol. 2010;183:2451–6.

115. Polito M, d'Anzeo G, Conti A, Muzzonigro G. Erectile rehabilitation with intracavernous alprostadil after radical prostatectomy: refusal and dropout rates. BJU Int. 2012;110(11 Pt C):E954–7. doi:10.1111/j.1464-410X.2012.11484.x.

116. Briganti A, Di Trapani E, Abdollah F, Gallina A, Suardi N, Capitanio U, et al. Choosing the best candidates for penile rehabilitation after bilateral nerve-sparing radical prostatectomy. J Sex Med. 2012;9:608–17.

117. Müller A, Parker M, Waters BW, Flanigan RC, Mulhall JP. Penile rehabilitation following radical prostatectomy: predicting success. J Sex Med. 2009;6:2806–12.

118. Sun P, Deftel A, Swindle R, Ye W, Pohl G. The costs of caring for erectile dysfunction in a managed care setting: evidence from a large national claims database. J Urol. 2005;174:1948–52.

119. Tan HL. Economic cost of male erectile dysfunction using a decision analytic model: for a hypothetical managed-care plan of 100,000 members. Pharmacoeconomics. 2000;17:77–107.

120. Anastasiadis AG, Ghafar MA, Burchardt M, Shabsigh R. Economic aspects of medical erectile dysfunction therapies. Expert Opin Pharmacother. 2002;3:257–63.

121. Walsh PC, Donker PJ. Impotence following radical prostatectomy: insight into etiology and prevention. J Urol. 1982;128:492–7.

122. Hubanks JM, Umbreit EC, Karnes RJ, Myers RP. Open radical retropubic prostatectomy using high anterior release of the levator fascia and constant haptic feedback in bilateral neurovascular bundle preservation plus early postoperative phosphodiesterase type 5 inhibition: a contemporary series. Eur Urol. 2012;61:878–84.

123. Khoder WY, Schlenker B, Waidelich R, Buchner A, Kellhammer N, Stief CG, et al. Open complete intrafascial nerve-sparing retropubic radical prostatectomy: technique and initial experience. Urology. 2012;79:717–21.

124. Masterson TA, Serio AM, Mulhall JP, Vickers AJ, Eastham JA. Modified technique for neurovascular bundle preservation during radical prostatectomy: association between technique and recovery of erectile function. BJU Int. 2008;101:1217–22.

125. Kowalczyk KJ, Huang AC, Hevelone ND, Lipsitz SR, Yu HY, Ulmer WD, et al. Stepwise approach for nerve sparing without countertraction during robot-assisted radical prostatectomy: technique and outcomes. Eur Urol. 2011;60:536–47.

126. Ahlering TE, Skarecky D, Borin J. Impact of cautery versus cautery free preservation of neurovascular bundles on early return of potency. J Endourol. 2006;20:586–9.

127. Kaul S, Bhandari A, Hemal A, Savera A, Shrivastava A, Menon M. Robotic radical prostatectomy with preservation of the prostatic fascia: a feasibility study. Urology. 2005;66:1261–5.

128. Joffe R, Klotz LH. Results of unilateral genitofemoral nerve grafts with contralateral nerve sparing during radical prostatectomy. Urology. 2007;69:1161–4.

129. Zorn KC, Bernstein AJ, Gofrit ON, Shikanov SA, Mikhail AA, Song DH, et al. Long-term functional and oncological outcomes of patients undergoing sural nerve interposition grafting during robot-assisted laparoscopic radical prostatectomy. J Endourol. 2008;22:1005–12.

130. Davis JW, Chang DW, Chevray P, Wang R, Shen Y, Wen S, et al. Randomized phase II trial evaluation of erectile function after attempted unilateral cavernous nerve-sparing retropubic radical prostatectomy with versus without unilateral sural nerve grafting for clinically localized prostate cancer. Eur Urol. 2009;55:1135–43.

131. Secin FP, Koppie TM, Scardino PT, Eastham JA, Patel M, Bianco FJ, et al. Bilateral cavernous nerve interposition grafting during radical retropubic prostatectomy: Memorial Sloan-Kettering Cancer Center experience. J Urol. 2007;177:664–8.

132. Connolly SS, Yoo JJ, Abouheba M, Soker S, McDougal WS, Atala A. Cavernous nerve regeneration using acellular nerve grafts. World J Urol. 2008;26:333–9.

133. Burnett AL, Teloken PE, Briganti A, Whitehurst T, Montorsi F. Intraoperative assessment of an implantable electrode array for cavernous nerve stimulation. J Sex Med. 2008;5:1949–54.

134. Klotz L, Herschorn S. Early experience with intraoperative cavernous nerve stimulation with penile

tumescence monitoring to improve nerve sparing during radical prostatectomy. Urology. 1998;52: 537–42.

135. Axelson HW, Johansson E, Bill-Axelson A. Intraoperative cavernous nerve stimulation and laser-doppler flowmetry during radical prostatectomy. J Sex Med. 2012. doi: 10.1111/j.1743-6109.2012.02892.x.

136. Celik M, Gökmen N, Erbayraktar S, Akhisaroglu M, Konakc S, Ulukus C, et al. Erythropoietin prevents motor neuron apoptosis and neurologic disability in experimental spinal cord ischemic injury. Proc Natl Acad Sci U S A. 2002;99:2258–63.

137. Erbayraktar S, Grasso G, Sfacteria A, Xie QW, Coleman T, Kreilgaard M, et al. Erythropoietin is a nonerythropoietic cytokine with broad neuroprotective activity in vivo. Proc Natl Acad Sci U S A. 2003;100:6741–6.

138. Brines ML, Ghezzi P, Keenan S, Agnello D, de Lanerolle NC, Cerami C, et al. Erythropoietin crosses the blood–brain barrier to protect against experimental brain injury. Proc Natl Acad Sci U S A. 2000;97:10526–31.

139. Ehrenreich H, Hasselblatt M, Dembowski C, Cepek L, Lewczuk P, Stiefel M, et al. Erythropoietin therapy for acute stroke is both safe and beneficial. Mol Med. 2002;8:495–505.

140. Liu T, Allaf ME, Lagoda G, Burnett AL. Erythropoietin receptor expression in the human urogential tract: immunolocalization in the prostate, neurovascular bundle and penis. BJU Int. 2007; 100:1103–6.

141. Allaf ME, Hoke A, Burnett AL. Erythropoietin promotes the recovery of erectile function following cavernous nerve injury. J Urol. 2005;174:2060–4.

142. Burnett AL, Allaf ME, Bivalacqua TJ. Erythropoietin promotes erection recovery after nerve-sparing radical retropubic prostatectomy: a retrospective analysis. J Sex Med. 2008;5:2392–8.

143. Segal RL, Bivalacqua TJ, Burnett AL. Irbesartan promotes erection recovery after nerve-sparing radical retropubic prostatectomy: a retrospective longterm analysis. BJU Int. 2012;110(11):1782–6. doi:10.1111/j.1464-410X.2012.11098.x.

144. Canguven O, Lagoda G, Sezen SF, Burnett AL. Losartan preserves erectile function after bilateral cavernous nerve injury via antifibrotic mechanisms in male rats. J Urol. 2009;181:2816–22.

145. Hong SK, Han BK, Jeong SJ, Byun SS, Lee SE. Effect of statin therapy on early return of potency after nerve sparing radical retropubic prostatectomy. J Urol. 2007;178:613–6.

146. Lagoda G, Sezen SF, Burnett AL. FK506 and rapamycin neuroprotect erection and involve different immunophilins in a rat model of cavernous nerve injury. J Sex Med. 2009;6:1914–23.

147. Lagoda G, Xie Y, Sezen SF, Hurt KJ, Liu L, Musicki B, et al. FK506 neuroprotection after cavernous nerve injury is mediated by thioredoxin and glutathione redox systems. J Sex Med. 2011;8(12):3325–34. doi:10.1111/j.1743-6109.2011.02500.x.

148. Mulhall JP, Müller A, Donohue JF, Golijanin D, Tal R, Akin-Olugbade Y, et al. FK506 and erectile function preservation in the cavernous nerve injury model: optimal dosing and timing. J Sex Med. 2008;5:1334–44.

149. Sighinolfi MC, Rivalta M, Mofferdin A, Micali S, De Stefani S, Bianchi G. Potential effectiveness of pelvic floor rehabilitation treatment for postradical prostatectomy incontinence, climacturia, and erectile dysfunction: a case series. J Sex Med. 2009;6:3496–9.

150. Prota C, Gomes CM, Ribeiro LH, de Bessa J, Jr NE, Dall'Oglio M, et al. Early postoperative pelvic-floor biofeedback improves erectile function in men undergoing radical prostatectomy: a prospective, randomized, controlled trial. Int J Impot Res. 2012;24:174–8.

151. Rosen RC, Wing RR, Schneider S, Wadden TA, Foster GD, West DS, et al. Erectile dysfunction in type 2 diabetic men: relationship to exercise fitness and cardiovascular risk factors in the Look AHEAD trial. J Sex Med. 2009;6:1414–22.

152. Wing RR, Rosen RC, Fava JL, Bahnson J, Brancati F, Gendrano III IN, et al. Effects of weight loss intervention on erectile function in older men with type 2 diabetes in the Look AHEAD trial. J Sex Med. 2010;7:156–65.

153. Zopf EM, Braun M, Machtens S, Zumbé J, Bloch W, Baumann FT. Implementation and scientific evaluation of rehabilitative sports groups for prostate cancer patients: study protocol of the ProRehab Study. BMC Cancer. 2012;12:312–8.

154. Tajkarimi K, Burnett AL. The role of genital nerve afferents in the physiology of the sexual response and pelvic floor function. J Sex Med. 2011;8: 1299–312.

155. Jamal JE, Engel JD. Management of postprostatectomy erectile dysfunction. Can J Urol. 2011;18:5726–30.

Postoperative Management and Preoperative Considerations: Urinary Incontinence and Anastomotic Stricture

Jaspreet S. Sandhu

Introduction

Urinary adverse events after radical prostatectomy, particularly urinary incontinence and formation of an anastomotic stricture, are bothersome and can lead to significant decrease in quality of life [1–5]. In addition to having knowledge of standard treatment options for these maladies, it is important to understand the risk factors for development of persistent urinary incontinence and anastomotic stricture. The natural history of recovery of urinary function is extremely important in determining when intervention is needed. In this chapter, we review preoperative evaluation, risk factors, and management of voiding dysfunction—urinary incontinence and anastomotic strictures—after radical prostatectomy.

Preoperative Evaluation

Preoperative urinary function has an important influence on subsequent voiding dysfunction after radical prostatectomy (RP). A pretreatment assessment of baseline urinary function using a validated instrument is, therefore, important to

identify men at risk of urinary dysfunction after RP. The International Prostate Symptom Score (IPSS) along with a measure of any degree of urinary incontinence is one set of measures that can be used to measure preoperative function and to follow patients postoperatively to document recovery of urinary function. Alternatives to the IPSS specific for measuring quality of life (QoL) after prostate cancer treatment, such as Prostate Cancer Index (PCI) or Expanded Prostate Cancer Index Composite (EPIC) assess both urinary symptoms and urinary incontinence. The presence of urinary incontinence preoperatively is uncommon and should prompt further evaluation. The presence of neurologic disease, history of prostate or urethral surgery, or the use medicine for lower urinary tract symptoms (e.g., Alpha blockers) is important to note. Measurement of post-void residual urine, uroflowmetry, or formal urodynamics may be needed for patients with preoperative urinary dysfunction, particularly for patients with preoperative urinary incontinence. If the urinary incontinence is due to prostate obstruction, it is reasonable to expect continence to improve after RP because of relief of obstruction.

Setting realistic expectations with respect to the recovery of urinary continence after RP should be a standard component of preoperative counseling. Understanding the risk factors for voiding dysfunction after RP, particularly those related to the formation of anastomotic stricture and persistent urinary incontinence is critical. Furthermore, knowledge of the natural history of

J.S. Sandhu, M.D. (✉)
Department of Surgery, Urology Service, Memorial Sloan-Kettering Cancer Center, 1275 York Avenue, New York, NY 10065, USA
e-mail: sandhuj@mskcc.org

J.A. Eastham and E.M. Schaeffer (eds.), *Radical Prostatectomy: Surgical Perspectives*,
DOI 10.1007/978-1-4614-8693-0_12, © Springer Science+Business Media New York 2014

recovery of urinary function is important in deciding if and when patients need further specialized postoperative management [5].

Pelvic floor muscle exercises (PFME) should be taught, if feasible, in the preoperative setting. Patients should be encouraged to perform PFME in the preoperative and immediate postoperative setting to help hasten recovery of continence.

Natural History of Post-prostatectomy Voiding Function

The recovery of urinary function after RP has been the subject of much study. RP, regardless of approach, leads to changes in urinary function, including urinary incontinence, that usually resolve by the end of the first postoperative year. The rate of urinary incontinence after RP depends on the definition of urinary incontinence and the methodology used to collect the data [6, 7]. Walsh et al. [1] assessed the continence rate at 10 years in their first 593 patients undergoing anatomical nerve-sparing RP. They reported that 6 % wore 1 or more pads per day and 2 men required placement of an artificial urinary sphincter (AUS). No patient was reported as totally incontinent. Eastham et al. [8] reported a continence rate of 91 % at 2 years post RP with continence defined as those patients who did not use pads or who used a pad occasionally although they were consistently dry with moderate exercise.

Patient-reported QoL studies, as measured by PCI or EPIC, show significant worsening of urinary function immediately after RP followed by slow recovery over the ensuing year. Sanda et al. [9] prospectively evaluated 1,201 patients, 603 of whom underwent RP, for changes in self-reported QoL using the EPIC instrument. They noted a significant decline in urinary incontinence score at 3 months post-RP, with recovery and stabilization at 12 months. The incontinence score improved slowly up to 2 years, but remained below the baseline score. The urinary irritation or obstruction scores, on the other hand, declined at 3 months, but surpassed the baseline scores at 6 months.

Urinary Incontinence

Urinary incontinence is one of the most bothersome complications of RP. Persistent urinary incontinence is associated with significant patient dissatisfaction [3, 5, 9]. Most authorities consider persistent urinary incontinence as incontinence that is present 1 year after RP. Figure 12.1 illustrates the general management of urinary function before and after RP.

Risk Factors

Risk factors for urinary incontinence after RP are varied and for the sake of simplicity can be broken up into demographic, disease-specific, or technique-specific/intra-operative [10, 11]. Further, they can be classified as those known preoperatively and possibly correctable, and those known immediately postoperatively. Table 12.1 summarizes these risk factors.

Demographic Risk Factors

Multiple risk factors have been associated with delayed return of continence after RP including patient age, body mass index (BMI) or obesity, prostate size, membranous urethral length, presence of comorbidities, history of transurethral resection of the prostate, previous history of incontinence, or a history of lower urinary tract obstructive symptoms.

Age is one of the strongest predictors of decreased return of continence at 1 year. Licht [12], in a prospective analysis of 206 patients, showed that age greater than 65 was an independent predictor of incomplete return of urinary function after RP. Eastham et al. [8] evaluated 581 consecutive patients over a 2 year period, to determine which factors predicted an earlier return of continence. The strongest risk factor in a multivariate analysis was age. Karakiewicz [13] made a similar observation in a population based study. Age is associated with worsening continence in the general male population. Anger et al. [14] found an overall prevalence of incontinence of 17 % in men over 60 years in a

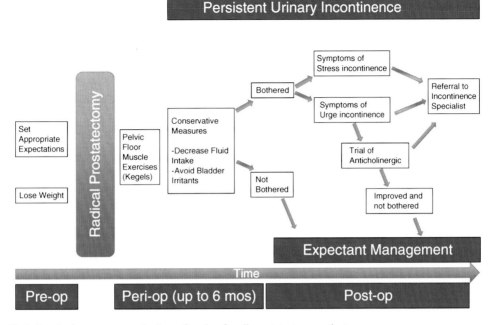

Fig. 12.1 Standard management of urinary function for all prostatectomy patients

Table 12.1 Risk factors for post-prostatectomy urinary incontinence

Demographic factors
Age
BMI/physical activity
Prostate volume
Previous TURP
Medical comorbidities
Previous LUTS
Membranous urethral length
Disease specific factors
Nerve-sparing surgery
Previous RT
Grade, stage, PSA
Technique related factors
Surgeon experience
Surgical approach (Open versus MIS)
Anastomotic technique/stricture
Urethral fixation
Puboprostatic sparing
Bladder neck preservation
Reconstruction of periurethral tissue
Intraoperative slings

population-based study. The prevalence of incontinence in the general population increased from 11 % in men 60–64 years of age to 31 % in men over the age of 85. It is no surprise, therefore, that age is consistently one of the strongest factors associated with recovery of continence after RP.

BMI or obesity has been implicated in delayed recovery of continence after RP. Mulholland et al. [15] studied the effect of BMI on urinary incontinence after RP by sending questionnaires related to voiding function to 268 consecutive patients over a 2-year period. Based on the 182 responses, no association with urinary function and body mass index was identified. However, this study had limited number of subjects and relied on correlation between degree of leakage and BMI. Anast et al. [16], on the other hand, found that BMI was indeed associated with worse urinary function, but not overall health related QoL. Their study, on a subset of 672 patients from the CapSURE registry, found that higher BMI was associated with higher rates of urinary incontinence on univariate analysis and a similar trend was observed on multivariate analysis. More recent studies have shown that obesity is indeed associated with delayed return of urinary incontinence. Wolin et al. [17] evaluated the role of physical activity and obesity in a cohort of 589 patients. They found that at 58 weeks, patients that were obese and inactive were more likely to be incontinent (59 %) than men who were non-obese and inactive (25 %) or men who were obese and active (24 %). Men who were non-obese and active had the best outcomes as related to urinary continence (16 %). Similarly, Ahlering et al. [18] noted, in a study of 100 patients undergoing robotic radical prostatectomy, that obese patients had delayed return of urinary continence.

Medical comorbidities, particularly diabetes mellitus (DM), have been associated with delayed recovery of continence after RP. Karakeiwitz et al. [19] found a strong relationship between lifetime prevalence of comorbidities and worse urinary function in a survey-based study. Teber [20] evaluated the role of DM in patients undergoing laparoscopic RP and noted that diabetic patients had later recovery of continence. In addition, a longer duration of DM was associated with later return of continence.

A history of previous TURP [8, 21–24], presence of preoperative LUTS [5, 25], and increasing prostate volume [8, 23, 26, 27] have all been suggested as risk factors, but their relation to continence recovery after RP remains controversial. Membranous urethral length has also been implicated in return of continence post RP. Membranous urethral length can be measure by performing urethral pressure profiles during urodynamics testing or via preoperative prostate imaging such as MRI. Hammerer and Huland [28] performed urodynamic evaluations in 82 men pre- and post-RP. Continent men had longer preoperative membranous urethral length than incontinent men. Similarly, Coakley et al. [29] measured membranous urethral length on preoperative endorectal-coil prostate MRI obtained in 211 consecutive patients. They noted men with shorter membranous urethral length had delayed recovery of continence than those with longer urethral length. Von Bodman et al. [30] confirmed this finding in a study which evaluated multiple soft-tissue parameters on preoperative MRI with respect to the ability to predict urinary incontinence. These authors found urethral volume and distance between the urethral edge and the levator muscles also predictive; however,

the addition of these other soft tissue parameters to urethral length did not meaningfully add to the predictive accuracy of a model with urethral length alone.

Disease Specific Risk Factors

Multiple disease specific factors may be related to subsequent postoperative urinary incontinence. Nerve sparing has been implicated in early recovery of continence [5, 8, 31]. Burkhard et al. [31] evaluated 536 consecutive patients and found that attempted nerve sparing was associated with improved urinary continence. These authors found a graded level of continence; the highest in the group that underwent attempted bilateral nerve sparing and the least in the group with no nerve sparing.

Previous radiation treatment is clearly implicated in worse urinary continence after RP. Stephenson et al. [32] evaluated 100 consecutive patients that underwent RP after radiotherapy for prostate cancer and found that the rate of urinary continence was 39 % at 5-year follow-up; much lower than the rate of continence in patients that underwent RP without prior radiotherapy by the same group. Subsequently, Masterson et al. [33] showed that patients that receive pelvic radiotherapy for non-prostate malignancies have similar urinary outcomes as those that receive prostate radiotherapy. Ward et al. [34] evaluated functional outcomes after salvage RP and noted that urinary continence ranged from 43 % to 56 %, with improvement in more contemporary cases. This "learning curve" is likely related to technical factors and will be discussed in the following section. Grade, stage and preoperative PSA have generally not been implicated with recovery of urinary incontinence after RP [5, 8, 35].

Technique Related Risk Factors

Surgeon experience and hospital volume have been associated with improved urinary outcomes. Begg et al. [36] evaluated 11,522 men that underwent RP from 1992 and 1996 and attempted to determine the effect of surgeon and hospital volume on urinary complications, including urinary incontinence. They found that hospital volume was not related to symptoms or procedures for urinary incontinence, but surgeon volume was, when controlled for case mix. Similarly, Hu et al. [37] have shown more recently that higher volume surgeons have lower rates of post RP urinary incontinence. These authors also showed that MIS surgery may be related to decreased urinary continence, although this must be considered in the setting of a new technique and may just be a manifestation of surgeons learning this technique.

Changes in surgical technique have been associated with earlier return of continence after RP. Eastham et al. [8] showed that after changing anastomotic technique, rates of urinary continence at 1 year improved from 72 % to 92 %. The technical modification used by the authors included fixing the urethral anastomosis to the periosteum of the pubic symphysis, simulating the puboprostatic ligaments. Others have shown that sparing the puboprostatic ligaments is related to improved continence. Poore et al. [38] compared 18 men who underwent puboprostatic ligament sparing RP versus 25 men who underwent standard open RP and noted that patients who underwent puboprostatic sparing had earlier return of continence (6.5 weeks vs. 12 weeks).

Bladder neck preservation is a surgical modification that has been associated with earlier return of continence by some. Multiple authors [39–41] have noted an earlier return to continence compared to other non-bladder neck sparing techniques. More recent studies, however, have shown higher rates of positive margins in groups that underwent bladder neck preservation [42] decreasing enthusiasm for this modification.

Mucosal eversion and reconstruction of the bladder neck are now considered standard parts of open RP. Furthermore, modifications in reconstruction of tissue around the urethrovesical junction have recently been proposed to improve continence. Rocco et al. [43] proposed a modification that included reconstruction of Denonvilliers' fascia prior to performing the urethrovesical anastomosis and noted a significant improvement in time to continence in 250 patients who underwent the technique compared to 50 who did not. This group also compared this technique in 31 patients undergoing MIS RP with 31 patients undergoing MIS RP without posterior

reconstruction and noted a similar hastening of continence in the group that underwent reconstruction [44]. Tewari et al. [45] compared 182 patients who underwent reconstruction of anterior and posterior periurethral tissue to 304 who underwent reconstruction of only anterior tissue to 214 who underwent no reconstruction and noted significantly shorter time to continence in the total reconstruction group.

Intrafascial dissection has been proposed as surgical modifications performed during MIS RP that lead to earlier return of continence. Neill et al. [46] compared continence rates in 240 patients who underwent laparoscopic RP with an intrafascial dissection to 270 patients who underwent standard dissection and noted earlier return of continence without any change in cancer control or potency in patients who underwent intrafascial dissection.

The use of slings at the time of RP has been attempted as a way to improve return of continence. Jorion [47] placed a strip of rectus fascia under the urethrovesical anastomosis in 30 consecutive men. He then compared return of continence to the previous 30 patients who did not undergo a sling and noted an earlier return of continence in the sling group. Jones [48] evaluated using an absorbable sling in a similar anatomic position and noted earlier return of continence, but did note a higher rate of anastomotic strictures.

Management of Post-prostatectomy Urinary Incontinence

A thorough evaluation is important when evaluating patients presenting for treatment of post-RP urinary incontinence. Figure 12.2 illustrates the management algorithm for patients with persistent post-RP incontinence. A simple history can help delineate the difference between urge urinary incontinence (UUI) and stress urinary incontinence (SUI)—an important distinction because of vastly different forms of treatment [49, 50]. UUI should be suspected in patients with significant urinary frequency, urinary

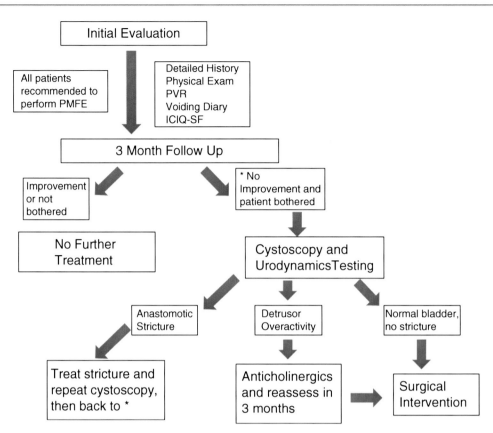

Fig. 12.2 Management of patients presenting for persistent post-prostatectomy incontinence

urgency, or nocturia often associated with night-time urinary incontinence. This form of incontinence often responds to medical management, whereas SUI rarely does. Regardless, both UUI and SUI are initially treated with conservative management. If conservative management fails, then additional testing in the form of urodynamics and/or cystoscopy or a trial of pharmacotherapy may be indicated.

Conservative Management

Conservative management is important in managing urinary incontinence after RP. In general, this includes limiting fluid intake, particularly at night, avoidance of known bladder irritants, such as caffeine and alcohol, and PFME. Bladder training and timed voiding have not been shown to be useful in men [51, 52].

Pelvic Floor Muscle Exercises/Behavior Modifications

Pelvic floor muscle exercises, also called "Kegel exercises," for the physician who popularized them, consist of intermittent voluntary contractions of the urethral sphincter muscle. If patients are unable to generate a urethral sphincter muscle contraction, aides including biofeedback might be helpful. PFME have been studied in the setting of post-prostatectomy incontinence and appear to be beneficial at hastening return of continence. A randomized control trial to evaluate the effect of PFME in men who had undergone RP used urinary continence at 3 months after surgery as the primary endpoint [53]. In this study, 88 % of the men in the treatment group achieved complete continence, measured by 24-h pad weight, significantly greater than 56 % of the men who achieved continence at 3 months in the placebo group. At 1 year, the difference between the two groups was only 14 %. Subsequently Filocamo et al. [54] randomized 300 consecutive patients who had undergone RP for clinically confined prostate cancer and showed an earlier return to continence with 74 % of the men performing PFME being dry, measured by pad usage, compared to 30 % in the untreated group at 3 months. While this difference was statistically significant, the difference at 1 year (98.7 % vs. 88 %) was not. Most men regain continence after RP; it appears that PFME can reduce time to continence, at least in the first postoperative year. Goode et al. [55] studied the effect of PFME on patients presenting with persistent post-prostatectomy urinary incontinence, defined as incontinence present after the first postoperative year. These authors randomized 208 men to one of three arm—one underwent 8 weeks of behavior therapy (PFME and bladder control strategies), the second included behavior therapy plus (addition of biofeedback and pelvic floor muscle stimulation), and a control arm (no treatment). They noted a 55 % decline in mean incontinence episodes at 8 weeks in the behavior therapy arm compared to 24 % in the control arm, a statistically significant improvement. Furthermore, they noted no significant improvement over behavior therapy with the addition of biofeedback and pelvic floor muscle stimulation. As such, a trial of pelvic floor exercises appears prudent for all men presenting for management of urinary incontinence after RP.

Biofeedback

Biofeedback has been evaluated to determine if it improves recovery of continence over PFME alone. Burgio et al. [56], studied the use of preoperative biofeedback assisted behavioral training to decrease post-RP incontinence. Participants were taught pelvic floor muscle control and received instructions in daily PFME. Patients were taught to contract the sphincter muscles during 2 to 10-s periods separated by 2–10 s of relaxation depending on initial ability. The main outcome measurements were duration of incontinence as derived from bladder diaries, severity of incontinence, distress from incontinence, and pad use. The Hopkins Symptom Checklist was used to measure psycho-

logical distress and the Medical Outcomes Study Short Form Health Survey (SF-36) was used to assess impact on QoL. They concluded that preoperative behavioral training could hasten the recovery of urine control and decrease the severity of incontinence following RP. A similar study done by Wille et al. [57], questioned the benefit of early biofeedback after RP, the outcomes measured included a 20-min pad test (an objective measure) and a urine symptom questionnaire.

Goode et al. [55] found that the addition of biofeedback to behavior therapy did not improve continence compared to behavior therapy alone, suggesting that if patients can perform PFME regularly, biofeedback has no role as adjunct therapy.

Management of UUI

Urge urinary incontinence is present in the minority of men who present for evaluation of post-RP incontinence [58, 59]. It is characterized by urinary frequency, urgency, and nocturia. Nighttime urinary incontinence is the hallmark of patients with urge urinary incontinence post-RP. The treatment of UUI in the post-RP setting has not been studied extensively, but just as in overactive bladder, anticholinergic medications have a primary role. If these medications are not efficacious or have intolerable side effects, second line treatment such as injection of botulinum toxin in the bladder or possibly sacral neuromodulation may have a role. It should be stressed, however, that data regarding these modalities and pharmacology for post-RP UUI is lacking.

Surgical Management of SUI

Surgical treatments, endoscopic or open, are usually not entertained for men with stress urinary incontinence until conservative treatments have failed. Given the natural history of urinary function recovery after RP, it is prudent to wait at least a year after surgery before undergoing evaluation and treatment for urinary incontinence. Surgical management remains the mainstay for the correction of post-RP SUI. Common surgical procedures currently used are endoscopic bulking

Table 12.2 Select reports of incontinence procedures with number of patients, success rate, efficacy measures used, and whether or not complications presented

Series	# patients	Success rate	Pads/day	Questionnaires used	Complications reported
Urethral bulking agents					
Cummings et al. [60]	19	21 %	Yes		No
Smith et al. [61]	62	38.70 %	Yes		No
Westney et al. [62]	322	17 %	Yes	Satisfaction score	No
Male sling					
Kaufman [64]	42	63 %	Yes		No
Schaeffer et al. [65]	64	56 %	Yes		Yes
Clemens et al. [66]	66	53 %	Yes	Custom, satisfaction score	Yes
Comiter [68]	21	76 %	Yes	UCLA/PCI	Yes
Ullrich and Commiter [69]	22	73 %	Yes	UCLA/PCI	Yes
Rajpurkar et al. [70]	46	37 %	Yes	UCLA/PCI, satisfaction score	Yes
Fischer et al. [71]	62	58 %	No	UCLA/PCI, ICIQ-SF, IIQ-7, PGI-I, UDI-6	Yes
Artificial urinary sphincter					
Scott et al. [74]	34	79 %	Yes/no leakage		No
Leibovich and Barrett [80]	417	88 %	Yes		Yes
Haab et al. [114]	68	79 %	Yes	Voiding and QOL	No
Elliot and Barrett [81]	323	NR	No		Yes
Venn et al. [82]	100	84 %	Yes		Yes
Montague et al. [78]	113	32 %	Yes	Satisfaction score	No
Gousse et al. [79]	71	58 %	Yes	Satisfaction score	Yes
Raj et al. [83]	554	Variable	xx		xx
Lai et al. [84]	218	Variable	xx		xx

agents, the artificial urinary sphincter, and a variety of male slings. Table 12.2 lists selected reports with the various modalities as well as the success rate.

Endoscopic Management/Urethral Bulking Agents

Urethral bulking agents have been used in female SUI and have also been applied to male SUI, particularly in the setting of post-RP SUI. Glutaraldehyde cross-linked collagen has been approved by the Food and Drug Administration for the treatment of intrinsic sphincter deficiency since 1993. In males with post-RP SUI, the technique consists of endoscopic injection of collagen in the submucosa overlying or just distal to the

urethral sphincter at four sites circumferentially until the urethra coapts. Collagen injection can be repeated after 4 weeks.

Cummings et al. [60] reviewed their initial series of glutaraldehyde cross-linked collagen used as an injectable bulking agent for the therapy of post-radical prostatectomy stress incontinence. Preoperative severity of incontinence was measured as mild (1–2 pads/day), moderate (3–4 pads/day) or severe (more than 4 pads/day or total incontinence). These authors reported that 58 % of patients had a "good" or "improved" result at a mean follow-up of 10.3 months. Smith et al. [61] reviewed their series of men with post-RP SUI who underwent injection of glutaraldehyde cross-linked collagen and stratified the patients as being "totally dry" or "socially continent" if they used no more than 1 pad daily. Their analysis of men who underwent collagen injection revealed that 8.1 % of the men were dry and 38.7 % of the men achieved social continence after a median of 4 injections. In a more recent review, Westney et al. [62] calculated pad usage before and after therapy. Treatment effect was stratified into quartiles of improvement of 0 % to 25 %, 26 % to 50 %, 51 % to 75 %, and 76 % to 100 %. 17 % of patients gained complete continence. Published success rates with urethral bulking agents is difficult to compare because of varying number of injections and multiple outcome measures used in studies, but ranges from 17 % to 38 % [60–62].

It should be noted that most authorities do not consider urethral bulking agents as a durable treatment for male SUI, particularly post-RP. In fact, the most recent International Consultation on Incontinence [63], a consensus meeting of incontinence experts, regarded urethral bulking agents as showing only modest success rates with low cure rates for male SUI.

Male Slings

Urethral compression procedures were introduced in 1972 when Kaufman published a series of manuscripts evaluating three different types of urethral compression techniques designed to improve continence after RP. The procedures consisted of using the penile crura with or without a buttress to compress the bulbar urethra. In his early description of this procedure he reported his success rates as excellent if there was no leakage, marked improvement in those with some leakage but no appliance and poor if a clamp was necessary. His final procedure, a silicone gel compressive implant placed just under the bulbar urethra, had a success rate, defined as dry without protection, of 63 % in 21 men with short-term follow-up [64]. These procedures, along with the success of the pubovaginal sling for female SUI, led to multiple types of male urethral slings. A male sling based on the needle suspension procedures for incontinence in females was subsequently introduced. This sling consists of three synthetic bolsters placed under the bulbar

urethra and suspended above the rectus fascia in the lower abdomen via sutures through the retropubic space. Schaeffer et al. [65] reviewed their results of this bulbourethral sling for PPI. Pad usage was measured daily and the patients were stratified into dry, improved (>50 % reduction in pad usage), and wet. The success rate, defined as being completely dry, in 64 men was 56 %. Clemens et al. [66] reviewed a series of patients undergoing the same procedure and introduced a satisfaction rate ("Would you undergo the procedure all over again?") as an outcome measure and reported a satisfaction rate of 90.2 %.

A bone-anchored variant of the male sling was reported in 2001 [67]. Initial success with this technique, defined as being dry or needing a pad for security without any episode of incontinence, was reported to be 87.5 % in 14 men followed for a mean of 12 months. Comiter [68] prospectively evaluated 21 men who underwent the bone-anchored sling surgery. Patients were stratified per their pad usage as well as their score on the UCLA/RAND Incontinence score. In this study, 76 % of men followed for a mean of 12 months demonstrated success, defined as the need for no pads.

Ullrich and Comiter [69] evaluated 22 patients with preoperative and postoperative pad usage and preoperative and postoperative urodynamic parameters, as well as UCLA/PCI questionnaire. Pad usage decrease from 4.6 to 0.74 and they found no significant change in maximum flow rate or detrusor pressure at maximum flow rate. In terms of satisfaction, they found that 73 % of patients report no or a very small problem after male sling surgery. Rajpurkar et al. [70] utilized a similar classification to assess cure in their series of 46 patients. They classified patients as "cured" if they were dry, "improved" if they were using 1–2 pads/day and "failed" if they utilized >2 pads/day. In addition to using the UCLA/PCI questionnaire, they reported patient satisfaction rates of 70 %.

More recently, Fischer et al. [71] evaluated the male perineal sling in 62 men and attempted to determine preoperative parameters that could predict success. Patients completed multiple validated questionnaires including the I-PSS (International

Prostate Symptom Score), UCLA/RAND Prostate Cancer Index urinary function score, ICIQ-SF (International Consultation on Incontinence short form), IIQ-7 (Incontinence Impact Questionnaire short form), PGI-I (Patient Global Impression of Improvement), and the UDI-6 (Urogenital Distress Index short form). Success was defined by the PGI-I, patient perception of their lower urinary tract condition, as very much or much improved. Failure was defined as a little better, no change, a little worse, or much worse. As defined by the PGI-I, these authors reported a success rate of 58 %. The successes and failures as defined by the PGI-I were then compared to their pad weights and the results of the postoperative questionnaires. They found that the patients' perception of success correlated with the 24 h pad weight as well as all the questionnaires. This study suggests that a global question is a reasonable way to measure outcomes.

A transobturator version of the male sling is now being used extensively in the USA and Europe [72]. This sling is made of polypropylene and is placed through a perineal incision and tensioned via trocars passed through a transobturator route. Initial results with this sling are comparable to initial results with the bone anchored sling. Published success rates with male slings range from 38 % to 76 % depending on outcome measures used [66–72].

Complications of the male sling procedure include infection (6 % rate in a recent series 47) and temporary urinary retention. Less common complications include persistent urinary retention (3 % rate [71]) or erosion (2 % rate [71]) of the sling into the urinary tract. Infection or erosion require removal of the sling, a procedure during which there is often quite a bit of fibrosis and the key is to find the sling and dissect in close proximity to the sling material. Urinary retention may be dealt with by incising the sling.

A modification of the transobturator sling is the "quadratic sling," which is a polypropylene mesh that has four arms—two that are tunneled through the transobturator route and two that are tunneled through a pre-pubic route. While efficacy with this sling variant has not been reported, Comiter et al. [73] reported that among 22 patients who underwent this sling, retrograde leak point pressure, a presumed measure of efficacy, increased after tensioning the transobturator arms and further increased after tensioning the pre-pubic arms.

There are also multiple variants of urethral compression devices on the international market that have not been approved for use in the USA [50].

Artificial Urinary Sphincter

The gold standard for post-RP SUI remains the AUS [74–76]. The first report of this device was published in the 1974. At that time, the device consisted of a urethral cuff placed at the bladder neck that was connected to an abdominal reservoir via two pumps—one to inflate the cuff, one to deflate. The technique has been modified over time. The current AUS consists of a urethral cuff, available in multiple sizes, a pressure regulating balloon (available in three different pressures), and a single control pump that is responsible for deflating the cuff and has an auto-refill mechanism.

In the original report by Scott et al. [74], describing placement of an AUS, the authors described long-term success as "no urinary leakage" with 100 % of patients reporting initial success. Leach et al. [77], subsequently used a "pad score," pre and postoperatively: 0—no protection required, 1—less than 2 pads daily, 2—2 to 4 pads daily, and 3—greater than 4 pads daily. The authors reported a decrease in pad score from 2.69 to 1.05 in 39 men who underwent an AUS placement. Montague et al. [78] and Gousse et al. [79] added a patient satisfaction score to their outcome measures, and both noted high rates of patient satisfaction. In addition to objective success, the reliability of the device has to be taken into consideration. Overall complication rates and AUS durability have been reported in multiple contemporary large series [80– 84]. Published success rates, generally reported as "socially continent rates," considered up to one pad per day, range from 58 % to 88 % [74, 78–84]. Multiple device modifications have been made in the original device—the most important one may have been the introduction of a narrow backing to the cuff that resulted in significantly better outcomes [85].

The operative technique for the AUS consists of placing a urethral cuff, measured to size, around the bulbar urethra through a perineal incision. A second incision in the lower abdomen allows exposure to the rectus fascia, below which the pressure-regulating balloon is placed. A control pump is then tunneled to the scrotum through the abdominal incision. The tubing from the urethral cuff is tunneled into the abdominal incision and all tubes are connected in a water-tight manner. See Fig. 12.3 for an illustration of AUS surgical technique. Changes in surgical technique have been introduced over the years, including the transverse scrotal approach [86], the transcorporal approach [87], and tandem cuff placement [88]. The transverse scrotal approach is an attempt to simplify the operation, by allowing the entire operation to be done through a high penoscrotal incision. However, there are concerns about its efficacy as compared to the standard perineal approach [89]. The tandem cuff is used typically in patients that have recurrent incontinence after a single cuff procedure has been performed or occasionally as a primary procedure in patients with severe urinary incontinence [88]. The transcorporal approach is used primarily in patients who have had erosion in the past and are not concerned about erectile function. It should be noted that results of the AUS in men after salvage RP for failed RT are similar to those after RP alone [87, 90]. The AUS has also been used in patients with recurrent incontinence after the placement of a male sling with reasonable results [91]. In this case the sling can be left in place or removed if feasible.

Common complications of an AUS include infection, erosion, and device malfunction. In a recent large series [84], the infection rate was 5.5 % at a median of 3.7 months from surgery and erosion rate was 6.0 % at 19.8 months from surgery. Device malfunction occurred in 6 % of patients at 68.1 months from surgery. With the advent of an antibiotic coated version of the urethral cuff introduced in 2007, infection rates may decrease. A common cause for erosion is urethral instrumentation, including urethral catheterization; therefore it is prudent to counsel patients regarding this etiology and if possible, have them

wear identification notifying medical professionals that they have an AUS implanted [76, 92]. If an infection of the AUS develops, the entire device should be removed and most surgeons wait 3–6 months prior to re-implanting another AUS. In the setting of erosion, the entire device usually needs to be removed; in addition, a urethral catheter needs to be left indwelling for about 3 weeks to allow the urethra to heal. Mechanical failure or recurrent incontinence due to urethral atrophy usually leads to entire device or specific malfunctioning component replacement.

While the reoperation rate is high with the AUS [83, 84, 93], there are known methods of decreasing this rate. Sandhu et al. [93] have shown that there is a clear association with surgeon experience with the procedure and subsequent re-operative rates. Other than improved surgical training, reoperations can be minimized by following strict operating room and postoperative protocols. Protocols should be instituted that decrease the risk of inadvertent urethral catheterization in patients that have an AUS in place such as requiring patients to wear a bracelet with an inscription stating that they have a sphincter in place, for example those provided by the MedicAlert Foundation (http://www.medicalert.org) [76, 92].

Anastomotic Stricture

Alterations in urinary function include the development of anastomotic strictures, also known as bladder neck contractures, which can lead to significant morbidity [94] (UDA). The economic impact of symptomatic urethral and anastomotic strictures in the USA has been documented and is high (over $6,000 per individual affected). A recent analysis of the CaPSURE database which evaluated RP outcomes in a community setting reported an anastomotic stricture rate of 8.4 % [95]. Similar findings were reported in a SEER-Medicare study with anastomotic stricture rates ranging from 5.8 % to 14.0 % depending on technique [37]. There is a wide variation in published rates of anastomotic stricture development post-RP and estimates vary from as low as 2.7 %

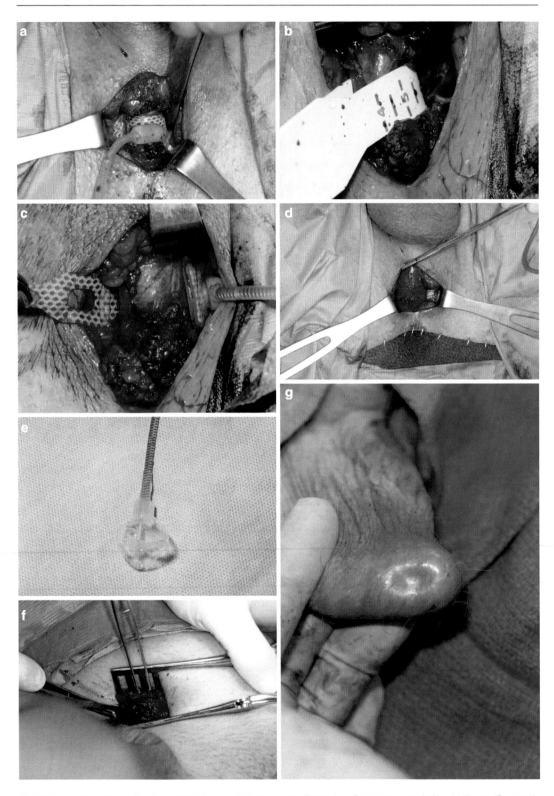

Fig. 12.3 (a) Dissection of bulbar urethra form underlying corporal bodies; (b) Measuring size of urethral cuff (sizes range from 3.5 cm to 6.5 cm, sized at time of surgery); (c) placement of urethral cuff; (d) Urethral cuff in place; (e) Example of pressure regulating balloon; (f) ectopic location of pressure regulating balloon—under the lateral border of rectus muscle; (g) control pump in situ (placed through tunnel from abdominal incision)

to as high as 25.7 % [96, 97]. This wide variation is likely a result of differences in patient population, individual surgical practice patterns, postoperative follow-up, and data collection.

Risk Factors

Similar to urinary incontinence, individual surgeon experience and technique have been shown influence the development of anastomotic strictures [36, 96]. Begg et al. [36] evaluated 11,522 men in the SEER-Medicare linked database and noted a lower rate of late urinary complications, the majority of which were anastomotic or urethral strictures, for higher volume surgeons. Hu et al. [37] later evaluated a SEER-Medicare linked database to evaluate the difference between minimally invasive and open RP and noted a lower rate of anastomotic strictures in the minimally invasive group (5.8 % vs. 14.0 %, $p<0.001$). Sandhu et al. [98] similarly showed that individual surgeon and surgical approach are predictors of the development of symptomatic anastomotic strictures. Furthermore, in their series of 4,592 patients, age, BMI, Charlson score, EBL, postoperative anastomotic urine leak, and postoperative hematoma were also all independent predictors of the development of a symptomatic anastomotic stricture. Surgical approach was the strongest predictor of development of an anastomotic stricture in their model with a roughly tenfold higher rate in patients that underwent open RP as opposed to minimally invasive RP.

CaPSURE investigators showed that in a community-wide cohort of 6,597 men, age and BMI are associated with development of urethral stricture after treatment for prostate cancer [95]. While these investigators evaluated patients treated with RP or RT and did not differentiate between anastomotic and other urethral strictures, they did show a much higher rate of strictures in men treated with RP than other modalities and therefore the analysis is likely driven by anastomotic stricture after RP.

In a retrospective review of 467 patients, Borboroglu et al. [99] found a significantly higher incidence of anastomotic strictures in current cigarette smokers (26 %) and in patients with CAD (26 %), HTN (19 %), and diabetes mellitus (21 %). An association with longer operative time and higher EBL was also identified. Multivariate analysis identified smoking as the strongest predictor. Surya et al. [100] identified prior TURP as another factor predictive of anastomotic stricture following RP.

Anastomotic disruption likely also contributes to the development of anastomotic strictures. In a series of 1,370 RPs, Hedican and Walsh [101] showed that three patients managed expectantly for postoperative hemorrhage requiring transfusion developed anastomotic strictures and long-term incontinence. In contrast, only one of four patients managed with surgical exploration developed mild incontinence suggesting that anastomotic distraction by pelvic hematoma may contribute to the development of anastomotic strictures.

An association between anastomotic urine leak and subsequent development of anastomotic strictures has also been studied. Surya et al. [100] retrospectively evaluated 156 patients who had undergone RP and identified 18 patients with anastomotic strictures (11.5 %). Significant predictors included anastomotic urine leak, excessive blood loss, and prior TURP. In contrast, Levy et al. [102] found that the identification of contrast extravasation on voiding cystourethrogram at 3 weeks postoperatively did not correlate with the subsequent development of anastomotic stricture provided that the Foley catheter was left in place until there was documented resolution. Sandhu et al. [98] found that a postoperative hematoma and a prolonged urine leak are both independently associated with formation of symptomatic anastomotic strictures.

Knowledge of known risk factors of anastomotic strictures can be useful in evaluating and counseling patients with voiding dysfunction post-RP. The threshold for cystoscopic evaluation of patients with obstructive voiding symptoms and known risk factors should be very low. Table 12.3 lists known risk factors for anastomotic strictures.

Table 12.3 Risk factors for anastomotic stricture

Age
BMI
History of previous TURP
Previous RT
Disease characteristics
Surgeon volume
Surgical technique/approach (open versus MIS)
Anastomotic technique
Anastomotic urinary leak
Pelvic hematoma
Cigarette smoking
Medical comorbidities (particularly cardiovascular, renal, or hematologic)

Diagnosis

When urinary function deviates from the known pattern of recovery, particularly if patients develop obstructive urinary symptoms (weak stream or difficulty emptying their bladder), an anastomotic stricture should be suspected. New onset irritative symptoms such as urinary urgency or nocturia can sometimes be symptoms of anastomotic stricture.

While uroflowmetry and ultrasound measurement of post-void residual urine may have a role in screening patients for anastomotic stricture, the definitive diagnosis in the current era is established via flexible cystoscopy. The inability to traverse the urethrovesical anastomosis with a 14–16F flexible cystoscope confirms the diagnosis. The widespread availability and ease of flexible cystoscopy has allowed it to replace retrograde urethrogram as the test of choice for anastomotic strictures.

Management

Management of anastomotic strictures usually follows a graded pattern with initial office dilation using either serial dilation or a urethral balloon dilator, followed by internal urethrotomy, and if needed, a transurethral resection of bladder neck contracture [103]. Figure 12.4 illustrates the management algorithm for anastomotic strictures.

Some authorities tailor their surgical approach based on the appearance of the stricture, as opposed to the graded approach favored by most. Regardless of approach, it is important to inform patients with anastomotic strictures about the risk of urinary incontinence—either new onset or worsening—after treatment of the stricture.

Urethral dilation is the initial treatment for anastomotic strictures and is often the only treatment needed. Multiple forms of urethral dilation can be used. A set of progressively increasing caliber stiff dilators can be introduced over a wire until an 18 or 20F opening is easily traversed. A urethral balloon dilator is another option—in this case a 6F balloon dilating catheter is introduced over a wire into the bladder and then the balloon is filled with 8–10 ml of fluid and left dilated for 2 min. In both of these options, a 16 or 18F urethral catheter should be left in place for a few days.

If initial dilation fails, internal urethrotomy is an option. This can be performed using a cold knife [104], an electrosurgical knife with cutting current [103], or a laser [105]. The adjunct use of intralesional mitomycin C has also been instituted by some [106] as have steroid injections [105]. The placement of an endoluminal metallic urethral stent for recalcitrant anastomotic strictures was greeted with enthusiasm [107, 108], but has subsequently fallen out of favor and the metallic stent is no longer available for general use. In each case of endoscopic intervention, care must be taken to avoid deep incisions posteriorly because of the risk of a recto-urethral fistula [109, 110] or anteriorly because of risk of pubovesical communication [111]. Most authorities perform deep incisions anterolaterally or laterally to the point that a 24F rigid cystoscope can be introduced without difficulty. An 18 or 20F urethral catheter is left in place for 7–10 days to allow the incision to heal in a fixed position.

The final endoscopic management option for anastomotic stricture is a formal transurethral resection of bladder neck contracture (TURBNC). As with an internal urethrotomy, care should be exercised while resecting posteriorly or anteriorly. A TURBNC is performed by first introducing a

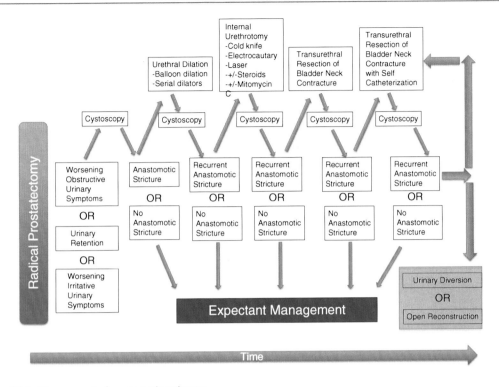

Fig. 12.4 Management of anastomotic strictures

resectoscope with a visual obturator and then if need performing an internal urethrotomy. An electrosurgical loop is used to reset scar tissue in an eccentric manner to open the urethrovesical anastomosis. After evacuating bladder neck chips, an 18 or 20F catheter is left in place for 7–10 days. In cases where multiple TURBNCs have been performed, a schedule of self-catheterization can be introduced—typically with an 18F catheter which is left in place for a few minutes and then removed. The duration of self-catheterization is variable. See Fig. 12.5 for an illustration of endoscopic incision of AS and TURBNC.

Finally, an open reconstruction or urinary diversion is an option for intractable anastomotic strictures. An open reconstruction should follow principles of posterior urethroplasty with the understanding that failure rates are high and essentially all patients that undergo successful reconstruction will be incontinent and will likely need an AUS [112].

As stated above, rates of urinary incontinence after treating anastomotic stricture are high. This has several implications—among them, urethral bulking agents are likely ineffective due to fibrosis at the anastomotic region, and care should be exercised in situations where an AUS is placed and anastomotic stricture reforms [113].

Conclusion

Urinary incontinence and anastomotic strictures are not uncommon after RP. Management of these maladies is reasonably straightforward and as shown in this chapter should be performed in a careful and systematic manner. Despite multiple treatment modalities, most patients can be managed safely and effectively.

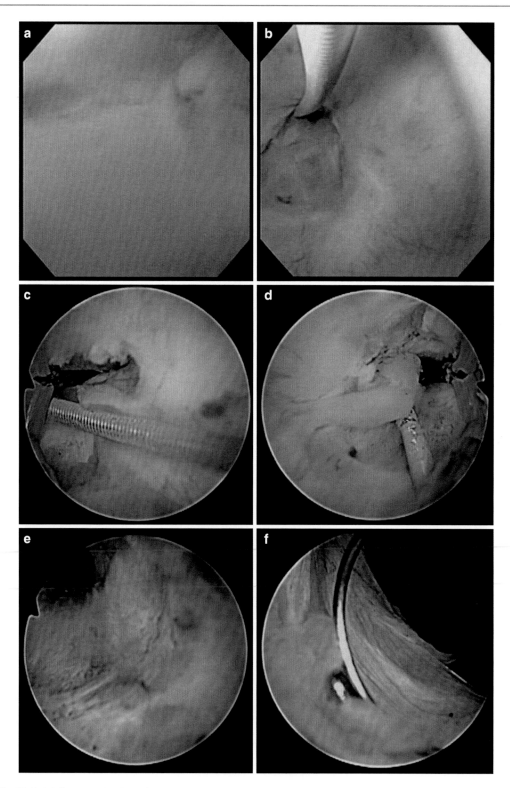

Fig. 12.5 (a) Cystoscopic view of anastomotic stricture; (b) passage of wire through stricture; (c) Incision with electrosurgical knife using cutting current; (d) Completion of incision with electrosurgical knife using cutting current; (e) Resection using cutting current; (f) Identification of foreign body (titanium clip); (g) Removal of foreign body; (h) Final view prior to placing 20 French catheter

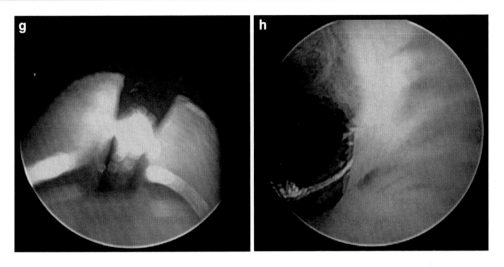

Fig. 12.5 (continued)

References

1. Walsh PC, Partin AW, Epstein JI. Cancer control and quality of life following anatomical radical retropubic prostatectomy: results at 10 years. J Urol. 1994; 152:1831–6.

2. Catalona WJ, Basler JW. Return of erections and urinary continence following nerve sparing radical retropubic prostatectomy. J Urol. 1993;150:905–7.

3. Potosky AL, Davis WW, Hoffman RM, Stanford JL, Stephenson RA, Penson DF, et al. Five-year outcomes after prostatectomy or radiotherapy for prostate cancer: the prostate cancer outcomes study. J Natl Cancer Inst. 2004;96:1358–67.

4. Stothers L, Thom DH, Calhoun EA. Urinary incontinence in men. In: Litwin MS, Saigal CS, editors. Urologic diseases in America. US Department of Health and Human Services, Public Health Service, National Institutes of Health, National Institute of Diabetes and Digestive and Kidney Diseases. Washington DC: US Government Publishing Office; 2007; NIH Publication No. 07-5512. p. 193–222.

5. Wei JT, Dunn RL, Marcovich R, Montie JE, Sanda MG. Prospective assessment of patient reported urinary continence after radical prostatectomy. J Urol. 2000;164:744–8.

6. Krupski TL, Saigal CS, Litwin MS. Variation in continence and potency by definition. J Urol. 2003; 170:1291–4.

7. Litwin MS, Lubeck DP, Henning JM, Carroll PR. Differences in urologist and patient assessments of health related quality of life in men with prostate cancer: results of the CaPSURE database. J Urol. 1998;159:1988–92.

8. Eastham JA, Kattan MW, Rogers E, et al. Risk factors for urinary incontinence after radical prostatectomy. J Urol. 1996;156:1707–13.

9. Sanda MG, Dunn RL, Michalski J, et al. Quality of life and satisfaction with outcome among prostate-cancer survivors. N Engl J Med. 2008;358:1250–61.

10. Sandhu JS, Eastham JA. Factors predicting early return of continence after radical prostatectomy. Curr Urol Rep. 2010;11:191–7.

11. Llughlin KR, Prasad MM. Post-prostatectomy urinary incontinence: a confluence of 3 factors. J Urol. 2010;183:871–7.

12. Licht MR, Klein EA, Tuason L, Levin H. Impact of bladder neck preservation during radical prostatectomy on continence and cancer control. Urology. 1994;44:883–7.

13. Karakiewicz PI, Tanquay S, Kattan MW, Elhilali MM, Aprikian AG. Erectile and urinary dysfunction after radical prostatectomy for prostate cancer in Quebec: a population-based study of 2415 men. Eur Urol. 2004;46:188–94.

14. Anger JT, Saigal CS, Stothers L, et al. The prevalence of urinary incontinence among community dwelling men: results from the National Health and Nutrition Examination survey. J Urol. 2006;176:2103–8.

15. Mulholland TL, Huynh PN, Huang RR, et al. Urinary incontinence after radical prostatectomy is not related to patient body mass index. Prostate Cancer Prostatic Dis. 2006;9:153–9.

16. Anast JW, Sadetshy N, Pasta DJ, et al. The impact of obesity on health related quality of life before and after radical prostatectomy (data from CaPSURE). J Urol. 2005;173:1132–8.

17. Wolin KY, Luly J, Sutcliffe S, Andriole GL, Kibel AS. Risk of urinary incontinence following prostatectomy: the role of physical activity and obesity. J Urol. 2010;183:629–33.

18. Ahlering TE, Eichel L, Edwards R, Skarecky DW. Impact of obesity on clinical outcomes in robotic prostatectomy. Urology. 2005;65:740–4.

19. Karakiewicz PI, Bhojani N, Neugut A, et al. The effect of comorbidity and socioeconomic status on

sexual and urinary function and on general health-related quality of life in men treated with radical prostatectomy for localized prostate cancer. J Sex Med. 2008;5:919–27.

20. Teber D, Sofikerim M, Ates M, et al. Is type 2 diabetes mellitus a predictive factor for incontinence after laparoscopic radical prostatectomy? A matched pair and multivariate analysis. J Urol. 2010;183:1087–91.

21. Colombo R, Naspro R, Salonia A, et al. Radical prostatectomy after previous prostate surgery: clinical and functional outcomes. J Urol. 2006;176: 2459–63.

22. Palisaar JR, Wenske S, Sommerer F, Hinkel A, Noldus J. Open radical retropubic prostatectomy gives favourable surgical and functional outcomes after transurethral resection of the prostate. BJU Int. 2009;104:611–5.

23. Elder JS, Gibbons RP, Correa Jr RJ, Brannen GE. Morbidity of radical perineal prostatectomy following transurethral resection of the prostate. J Urol. 1984;132:55–7.

24. Gupta NP, Singh P, Nayyar R. Outcomes of robot-assisted radical prostatectomy in men with previous transurethral resection of prostate. BJU Int. 2011;108:1501–5.

25. Lepor H, Kaci L. The impact of open radical retropubic prostatectomy on continence and lower urinary tract symptoms: a prospective assessment using validated self-administered outcome instruments. J Urol. 2004;171:1216–9.

26. Konety BR, Sadetsky N, Carroll PR, et al. Recovery of urinary continence following radical prostatectomy: the impact of prostate volume—analysis of data from the CaPSURE database. J Urol. 2007; 177:1423–5.

27. Pettus JA, Masterson T, Sokol A, et al. Prostate size is associated with surgical difficulty but not functional outcome at 1 year after radical prostatectomy. J Urol. 2009;182:949–55.

28. Hammerer P, Huland H. Urodynamic evaluation of changes in urinary control after radical retropubic prostatectomy. J Urol. 1997;157:233–6.

29. Coakley FV, Eberhardt S, Kattan MW, et al. Urinary continence after radical retropubic prostatectomy: relationship with membranous urethral length on preoperative endorectal magnetic resonance imaging. J Urol. 2002;168:1032–5.

30. von Bodman C, Matsushita K, Savage C, et al. Recovery of urinary function after radical prostatectomy: predictors of urinary function on preoperative magnetic resonance imaging. J Urol. 2012;187: 945–50.

31. Burkhard FC, Kessler TM, Fleischmann A, et al. Nerve sparing open radical retropubic prostatectomy—does it have an impact on urinary continence? J Urol. 2006;176:189–95.

32. Stephenson AJ, Scardino PT, Bianco Jr FJ, et al. Morbidity and functional outcomes of salvage radical prostatectomy for locally recurrent prostate cancer after radiation therapy. J Urol. 2004;172:2239–43.

33. Masterson TA, Wedmid A, Sandhu JS, Eastham JA. Outcomes after radical prostatectomy in men receiving previous pelvic radiation for non-prostate malignancies. BJU Int. 2009;104:482–5.

34. Ward JF, Sebo TJ, Blute ML, Zincke H. Salvage surgery for radiorecurrent prostate cancer: contemporary outcomes. J Urol. 2005;173:1156–60.

35. Cambio AJ, Evans CP. Minimising postoperative incontinence following radical prostatectomy: considerations and evidence. Eur Urol. 2006;50: 903–13.

36. Begg CB, Riedel ER, Bach PB, et al. Variations in morbidity after radical prostatectomy. N Engl J Med. 2002;346:1138–44.

37. Hu JC, Gu X, Lipsitz SR, et al. Comparative effectiveness of minimally invasive vs open radical prostatectomy. JAMA. 2009;302:1557–64.

38. Poore RE, McCullough DL, Jarow JP. Puboprostatic ligament sparing improves urinary continence after radical retropubic prostatectomy. Urology. 1998;51: 67–72.

39. Braslis KG, Petsch M, Lim A, Civantos F, Soloway MS. Bladder neck preservation following radical prostatectomy: continence and margins. Eur Urol. 1995;28:202–8.

40. Lowe BA. Comparison of bladder neck preservation to bladder neck resection in maintaining postrostatectomy urinary continence. Urology. 1996;48: 889–93.

41. Deliveliotis C, Protogerou V, Alargof E, Varkarakis J. Radical prostatectomy: bladder neck preservation and puboprostatic ligament sparing–effects on continence and positive margins. Urology. 2002;60:855–8.

42. Srougi M, Nesrallah LJ, Kauffmann JR, Nesrallah A, Leite KR. Urinary continence and pathological outcome after bladder neck preservation during radical retropubic prostatectomy: a randomized prospective trial. J Urol. 2001;165:815–8.

43. Rocco F, Carmignani L, Acquati P, et al. Early continence recovery after open radical prostatectomy with restoration of the posterior aspect of the rhabdosphincter. Eur Urol. 2007;52:376–83.

44. Rocco B, Gregori A, Stener S, et al. Posterior reconstruction of the rhabdosphincter allows a rapid recovery of continence after transperitoneal videolaparoscopic radical prostatectomy. Eur Urol. 2007;51:996–1003.

45. Tewari A, Jhaveri J, Rao S, et al. Total reconstruction of the vesico-urethral junction. BJU Int. 2008;101:871–7.

46. Neill MG, Louie-Johnsun M, Chabert C, Eden C. Does intrafascial dissection during nerve-sparing laparoscopic radical prostatectomy compromise cancer control? BJU Int. 2009;104:1730–3.

47. Jorion JL. Rectus fascial sling suspension of the vesicourethral anastomosis after radical prostatectomy. J Urol. 1997;157:926–8.

48. Jones JS, Vasavada SP, Abdelmalak JB, et al. Sling may hasten return of continence after radical prostatectomy. Urology. 2005;65:1163–7.

49. Sandhu JS. Treatment options for male stress urinary incontience. Nat Rev Urol. 2010;7:222–8.

50. Bauer RM, Gozzi C, Hubner W, et al. Contemporary management of postprostatectomy incontinence. Eur Urol. 2011;59:985–96.

51. Eustice S, Roe B, Paterson J. Prompted voiding for the management of urinary incontinence in adults. Cochrane Database Syst Rev. 2000; 2:CD0002113.

52. Wallace SA, Roe B, Williams K, et al. Bladder training for urinary incontinence in adults. Cochrane Database Syst Rev. 2004; 1:CD001308.

53. Van Kampen M, De Weerdt W, Van Poppel H, De Ridder D, Feys H, Baert L, et al. Effect of pelvic-floor re-education on duration and degree of incontinence after radical prostatectomy: a randomised controlled trial. Lancet. 2000;355:98.

54. Filocamo MT, Li Marzi V, Del Popolo G, et al. Effectiveness of early pelvic floor rehabilitation treatment for post-prostatectomy incontinence. Eur Urol. 2005;48:734.

55. Goode PS, Burgio KL, Johnson II TM, et al. Behavioral therapy with or without biofeedback and pelvic floor electrical stimulation for persistent post-prostatectomy incontinence. JAMA. 2011;305:151–9.

56. Burgio KL, Goode PS, Urban DA, et al. Preoperative biofeedback assisted behavioral training to decrease post-prostatectomy incontinence: a randomized, controlled trial. J Urol. 2006;175:196.

57. Wille S, Sobottka A, Heidenreich A, et al. Pelvic floor exercises, electrical stimulation and biofeedback after radical prostatectomy: results of a prospective randomized trial. J Urol. 2003;170:490.

58. Groutz A, Blaivas JG, Chaikin DC, et al. The pathophysiology of post-radical prostatectomy incontinence: a clinical and video urodynamic study. J Urol. 2000;163:1767–70.

59. Kielb SJ, Clemens JQ. Comprehensive urodynamic evaluation of 146 men with incontinence after radical prostatectomy. Urology. 2005;66:392–6.

60. Cummings JM, Boullier JA, Parra RO. Transurethral collagen injections in the therapy of post-radical prostatectomy stress incontinence. J Urol. 1996;155:1011.

61. Smith DN, Appell RA, Rackley RR, et al. Collagen injection therapy for post-prostatectomy incontinence. J Urol. 1998;160:364.

62. Westney OL, Bevan-Thomas R, Palmer JL, et al. Transurethral collagen injections for male intrinsic sphincter deficiency: the University of Texas-Houston experience. J Urol. 2005;174:994.

63. Herschorn S, Bruschini H, Comiter C, et al. Surgical treatment of stress incontinence in men. Neurourol Urodyn. 2010;29:179–90.

64. Kaufman JJ. Surgical treatment of post-prostatectomy incontinence: use of the penile crura to compress the urethra. J Urol. 1972;107:293.

65. Schaeffer AJ, Clemens JQ, Ferrari M, et al. The male bulbourethral sling procedure for post-radical prostatectomy incontinence. J Urol. 1998;159:1510.

66. Clemens JQ, Bushman W, Schaeffer AJ. Questionnaire based results of the bulbourethral sling procedure. J Urol. 1999;162:1972.

67. Madjar S, Jacoby K, Giberti C, et al. Bone anchored sling for the treatment of post-prostatectomy incontinence. J Urol. 2001;165:72.

68. Comiter CV. The male sling for stress urinary incontinence: a prospective study. J Urol. 2002;167:597.

69. Ullrich NF, Comiter CV. The male sling for stress urinary incontinence: urodynamic and subjective assessment. J Urol. 2004;172:204.

70. Rajpurkar AD, Onur R, Singla A. Patient satisfaction and clinical efficacy of the new perineal bone-anchored male sling. Eur Urol. 2005;47:237.

71. Fischer MC, Huckabay C, Nitti VW. The male perineal sling: assessment and prediction of outcome. J Urol. 2007;177:1414.

72. Rehder P, Gozzi C. Transobturator sling suspension for male urinary incontinence including post-radical prostatectomy. Eur Urol. 2007;52:860–6.

73. Comiter CV, Nitti V, Elliot C, Rhee E. A new quadratic sling for male stress incontinence: retrograde leak point pressure as a measure of urethral resistance. J Urol. 2012;187:563–8.

74. Scott FB, Bradley WE, Timm GW. Treatment of urinary incontinence by an implantable prosthetic urinary sphincter. J Urol. 1974;112:75.

75. Van der Aa F, Drake MJ, Kasyan GR, et al. The artificial urinary sphincter after a quarter of a century: a critical systematic review of its use in male non-neurogenic incontinence. Eur Urol. 2013;63:681–9.

76. Sandhu JS. Artificial urinary sphincter: the workhorse for treatment of male stress urinary incontinence. Eur Urol. 2013;63:690–1.

77. Leach GE, Trockman B, Wong A, et al. Post-prostatectomy incontinence: urodynamic findings and treatment outcomes. J Urol. 1996;155:1256.

78. Montague DK, Angermeier KW, Paolone DR. Long-term continence and patient satisfaction after artificial sphincter implantation for urinary incontinence after prostatectomy. J Urol. 2001;166:547.

79. Gousse AE, Madjar S, Lambert MM, et al. Artificial urinary sphincter for post-radical prostatectomy urinary incontinence: long-term subjective results. J Urol. 2001;166:1755.

80. Leibovich BC, Barrett DM. Use of the artificial urinary sphincter in men and women. World J Urol. 1997;15:316.

81. Elliott DS, Barrett DM. Mayo Clinic long-term analysis of the functional durability of the AMS 800 artificial urinary sphincter: a review of 323 cases. J Urol. 1998;159:1206.

82. Venn SN, Greenwell TJ, Mundy AR. The long-term outcome of artificial urinary sphincters. J Urol. 2000;164:702.

83. Raj GV, Peterson AC, Toh KL, et al. Outcomes following revisions and secondary implantation of the artificial urinary sphincter. J Urol. 2005;173:1242.

84. Lai HH, Hsu EI, Teh BS, et al. 13 years of experience with artificial urinary sphincter implantation at Baylor College of Medicine. J Urol. 2007;177:1021.

85. Leo ME, Barrett DM. Success of the narrow-backed cuff design of the AMS800 artificial urinary

sphincter: analysis of 144 patients. J Urol. 1993; 150:1412–4.

86. Sotelo TM, Westney OL. Outcomes related to placing an artificial urinary sphincter using a single-incision, transverse-scrotal technique in high-risk patients. BJU Int. 2008;101:1124–7.

87. Guralnick ML, Miller E, Toh KL, Webster GD. Transcorporal artificial urinary sphincter cuff placement in cases requiring revision for erosion and urethral atrophy. J Urol. 2002;167:2075–8.

88. DiMarco DS, Elliott DS. Tandem cuff artificial urinary sphincter as a salvage procedure following failed primary sphincter placement for the treatment of post-prostatectomy incontinence. J Urol. 2003;170: 1252–4.

89. Henry GD, Graham SM, Cleves MA, et al. Perineal approach for artificial urinary sphincter implantation appears to control male stress incontinence better than the transscrotal approach. J Urol. 2008;179: 1475–9.

90. Gomha MA, Boone TB. Artificial urinary sphincter for post-prostatectomy incontinence in men who had prior radiotherapy: a risk and outcome analysis. J Urol. 2002;167:591–6.

91. Fisher MB, Aggarwal N, Vuruskan H, Singla AK. Efficacy of artificial urinary sphincter after failed bone-anchored male sling for postprostatectomy incontinence. Urology. 2007;70:942–4.

92. Anusionwu II. EJ Wright: Indications for revision of artificial urinary sphincter and modifiable risk factors for device related morbidity. Neurourol Urodyn. 2013;32:63–5.

93. Sandhu JS, Mashino AC, Vickers AJ. The surgical learning curve for artificial urinary sphincter procedures compared to typical surgeon experience. Eur Urol. 2011;60:1285–90.

94. Santucci RA, Joyce GF, Wise M. Male urethral stricture disease. J Urol. 2007;177:1667.

95. Elliott SP, Meng MV, Elkin EP, et al. Incidence of urethral stricture after primary treatment for prostate cancer: data From CaPSURE. J Urol. 2007;178:529.

96. Hu JC, Gold KF, Pashos CL, et al. Role of surgeon volume in radical prostatectomy outcomes. J Clin Oncol. 2003;21:401.

97. Kao TC, Cruess DF, Garner D, et al. Multicenter patient self-reporting questionnaire on impotence, incontinence and stricture after radical prostatectomy. J Urol. 2000;163:858.

98. Sandhu JS, Gotto GT, Yunis LH, et al. Age, obesity, medical co-morbidities, and surgical technique are predictive of symptomatic anastomotic strictures following contemporary radical prostatectomy. J Urol. 2011;185:2148–52.

99. Borboroglu PG, Sands JP, Roberts JL, et al. Risk factors for vesicourethral anastomotic stricture after radical prostatectomy. Urology. 2000;56:96.

100. Surya BV, Provet J, Johanson KE, et al. Anastomotic strictures following radical prostatectomy: risk factors and management. J Urol. 1990;143:755.

101. Hedican SP, Walsh PC. Postoperative bleeding following radical retropubic prostatectomy. J Urol. 1994;152:1181.

102. Levy JB, Ramchandani P, Berlin JW, et al. Vesicourethral healing following radical prostatectomy: is it related to surgical approach? Urology. 1994;44:888.

103. Gousse AE, Tunuquntla HS, Leboeuf L. Two-stage management of severe postprostatectomy bladder neck contracture associated with stress incontinence. Urology. 2005;65:316–9.

104. Yurkanin JP, Dalkin BL, Cui H. Evaluation of cold knife urethrotomy for the treatment of anastomotic stricture after radical prostatectomy. J Urol. 2001; 165:1545–8.

105. Eltahawy E, Gur U, Virasoro R, et al. Management of recurrent anastomotic stenosis following radical prostectomy using holmium laser and steroid injection. BJU Int. 2008;102:796–8.

106. Vanni AJ, Zinman LN, Buckley JC. Radial urethrotomy and intralesional mitomycin C for the management of recurrent bladder neck contractures. J Urol. 2011;186:156–60.

107. Elliott DS, Boone TB. Combined stent and artificial urinary sphincter for management of severe recurrent bladder neck contracture and stress incontinence after prostatectomy: a long-term evaluation. J Urol. 2001;165:413–5.

108. Anger JT, Raj GV, Delvecchio FC, Webster GD. Anastomotic contracture and incontinence after radical prostatectomy: a graded approach. J Urol. 2005; 173:1143–6.

109. Lane BR, Stein DE, Remzi FH, et al. Management of radiotherapy induced rectourethral fistula. J Urol. 2006;175:1382–7.

110. Linder BJ, Umbreit EC, Larson D, et al. Effect of prior radiotherapy and ablative therapy on surgical outcomes for the treatment of rectourethral fistulas. J Urol. 2013; epub ahead of print.

111. Matsushita K, Ginsburg L, Mian BM, et al. Pubovesical fistula: a rare complication after treatment of prostate cancer. Urology. 2012;80:446–51.

112. Elliott SP, McAninch JW, Chi T, et al. Management of severe urethral complications of prostate cancer therapy. J Urol. 2006;176:2508–13.

113. Weissbart SJ, Chughtai B, Elterman D, Sandhu JS. Management of anastomotic stricture after artificial urinary sphincter placement in patients who underwent salvage prostatectomy. Urology. 2013;82(2):476–9.

114. Haab F, Trockman BA, Zimmern PE, Leach GE. J Urol. 1997 Aug;158(2):435–9.

Index